Natural Language Processing in Healthcare Informatics: Challenges and Future Directions

Edited by

A. Shankar
Department of ECE
Manakula Vinayagar Institute of Technology
Puducherry, India
Current Affiliation
Department of ECE
Hindusthan College of Engineering & Technology
Coimbatore, India

Saranya Jayapalan
Department of Bioinformatics
Pondicherry University
Puducherry, India
Current Affiliation
SS TechLogix, C42
Centre of Excellence in Biotechnology
Tamil Nadu Agricultural University Campus
Coimbatore - 641003, India

&

Basant. K. Tiwary
Department of Bioinformatics
Pondicherry University
Puducherry, India

Natural Language Processing in Healthcare Informatics: Challenges and Future Directions

Editors: A. Shankar, Saranya Jayapalan & Basant. K. Tiwary

ISBN (Online): 979-8-89881-492-2

ISBN (Print): 979-8-89881-493-9

ISBN (Paperback): 979-8-89881-494-6

First published in 2026.

Bentham Science Publishers Pte. Ltd.
No. 9 Raffles Place
Office No. 26-01
Singapore 048619
Singapore
Email: subscriptions@benthamscience.net

BENTHAM SCIENCE

CONTENTS

FOREWORD

In today's rapidly evolving healthcare technology landscape, the intersection of Artificial Intelligence (AI) and Natural Language Processing (NLP) stands as a beacon of innovation and transformation. As an NLP researcher, I found this book as a comprehensive guide to navigating the complexities and opportunities presented by connecting the power of AI-driven NLP in healthcare informatics. From its foundational principles to cutting-edge applications, this book offers invaluable insights into how NLP techniques can be leveraged to unlock the potential of unstructured clinical text data, driving improvements in patient care, clinical decision-making, and biomedical research. The authors have meticulously explored both the theoretical foundations and the practical implications of these technologies, providing valuable insights for researchers, clinicians, and anyone interested in the future of healthcare. This collection is a vital resource for navigating the complex and rapidly evolving world of AI and NLP in healthcare.

As we embark on this journey through the pages of this book, we are reminded of the immense potential of AI and NLP to revolutionize the healthcare industry. Through insightful discussions, case studies, and future projections, this book serves as a resource for healthcare professionals, researchers, and stakeholders to embrace and harness the transformative power of AI-driven NLP.

This collection of chapters delves into the cutting-edge developments, challenges, and future directions of this dynamic field. From drug discovery to mental health care, and from rare disease prediction to public health surveillance, the authors explore various applications poised to revolutionize how we understand, diagnose, and treat illnesses.

I commend the editors for their dedication and expertise in compiling this comprehensive resource. I am confident that it will inspire and empower readers to embark on their own journey toward leveraging AI and NLP for the betterment of healthcare worldwide.

N. Jeyakumar
Department of Bioinformatics
Bharathiar University
Coimbatore–641 046
Tamilnadu, India

PREFACE

Integrating healthcare and Artificial Intelligence (AI), particularly Natural Language Processing (NLP), holds great potential to significantly transform clinical practice, data-driven research, disease diagnosis, and drug discovery workflows. Healthcare is inherently information-rich, yet much of this information resides in unstructured formats: clinical notes, Electronic Health Records (EHRs), research publications, and patient feedback. Bridging the gap between this unstructured data and actionable knowledge is achieved through NLP. By enabling computers to understand, interpret, and generate human language, NLP empowers us to unlock patterns, trends, and crucial information that would otherwise remain hidden. In this book, we explore the fascinating realm of AI and NLP within the healthcare context. Our aim is to provide readers with a broad understanding of the principles, methodologies, and applications of AI-enhanced NLP in healthcare. From core concepts to advanced techniques and real-world case studies, this book is designed to equip healthcare professionals and researchers with the knowledge and insights needed to leverage NLP technologies for improving patient outcomes, clinical decision-making, and biomedical research.

As we begin our exploration of AI and NLP in healthcare, it is imperative to acknowledge the promise these technologies hold in revolutionizing the delivery of patient care and advancing medical research. Through synthesizing theoretical knowledge and practical visions, this book is intended for a diverse audience, including researchers, clinicians, data scientists, healthcare professionals, and students. Each chapter, spanning from initial conceptualization to practical implementation, provides readers with a deep dive into NLP's methodologies, challenges, data handling, its role in disease prediction, chatbots, and future trends within NLP-associated healthcare informatics. This book, "Natural Language Processing in Healthcare Informatics: Challenges and Future Directions," investigates this interdisciplinary discipline, exploring the intricate ways NLP is applied to extract meaningful insights from the vast sea of healthcare data.

We hope it is a valuable resource for understanding the NLP’s ability to reshape and inspire further innovation in this critical field. The editors thank all contributing authors and supporting institutions that enabled the completion of this volume.

A. Shankar
Department of ECE
Manakula Vinayagar Institute of Technology
Puducherry, India
Current Affiliation
Department of ECE
Hindusthan College of Engineering & Technology
Coimbatore, India

Saranya Jayapalan
Department of Bioinformatics
Pondicherry University
Puducherry, India

Current Affiliation
SS TechLogix, C42
Centre of Excellence in Biotechnology
Tamil Nadu Agricultural University Campus
Coimbatore - 641003, India

&

Basant K. Tiwary
Department of Bioinformatics
Pondicherry University
Puducherry, India

List of Contributors

A. Britto Manoj	Advanced Computer Science and Engineering, Vignan's Foundation for Science, Technology, and Research, Vadlamudi (Post), Guntur (Dist.), India
A. Shankar	Department of ECE, Manakula Vinayagar Institute of Technology, Puducherry, India
Arockiyajainmary Michealsamy	Independent Researcher, Chennai, Tamilnadu, India
Avantika Sharma	School of Life and Basic Sciences, Jaipur National University, Jaipur, Rajasthan, India
Balu Bhasuran	eHEALTH Lab, College of Communication and Information, Florida State University, TallahasseeFL, 32306-2100, USA
Basant K. Tiwary	Department of Bioinformatics, Pondicherry University, Puducherry, India
Bharath Addepalli	Department of Computing Technologies, SRM Institute of Science and Technology, Kattankulathur, India
Divyanshi Salundiya	School of Life and Basic Sciences, Jaipur National University, Jaipur, Rajasthan, India
Forhan Bin Emdad	eHEALTH Lab, College of Communication and Information, Florida State University, TallahasseeFL, 32306-2100, USA
G. Sekar	Department of Electronics and Communication Engineering, VSB College of Engineering Technical Campus, Coimbatore, India
Guneswar Sethi	Center for Companion Animal New Drug Development, Korea Institute of Toxicology, 30 Baehak 1-gil, Jeongeup, Jeollabuk-do - 56212, Republic of Korea
Gurusamy Murugesan	Department of Computer Science and Engineering, Koneru Lakshmaiah Education Foundation, Vaddeswaram, Guntur, Andhra Pradesh-522302, India
Jeong Ho Hwang	Center for Companion Animal New Drug Development, Korea Institute of Toxicology, 30 Baehak 1-gil, Jeongeup, Jeollabuk-do - 56212, Republic of Korea
Jeyaraman Jeyakanthan	Structural Biology and Biocomputing Lab, Department of Bioinformatics, Alagappa University, Karaikudi-630003, Tamil Nadu, India Department of Bioinformatics (4th Floor), Science Block, Alagappa University, Karaikudi – 630003, Tamil Nadu, India
Jishnu K. S.	Department of Computing Technologies, School of Computing, CET, SRM Institute of Science and Technology, Kattankulathur Campus, Chennai, Tamil Nadu, India
Juhi Sharma	School of Life and Basic Sciences, Jaipur National University, Jaipur, Rajasthan, India
K. P. Naveen	Pondicherry Institute of Medical Sciences, Puducherry, India

K. Suresh Joseph	Department of Computer Science, Pondicherry University, Puducherry, India
Karthika Alagesan	Department of Bioinformatics (4th Floor), Science Block, Alagappa University, Karaikudi – 630003, Tamil Nadu, India
Kratika Pathak	School of Life and Basic Sciences, Jaipur National University, Jaipur, Rajasthan, India
L. Sankar Ganesh	School of Computer Science and Engineering, Vellore Institute of Technology, Vellore, India
Maharaja Muthuvairam Subbulakshmi	Structural Biology and Biocomputing Lab, Department of Bioinformatics, Alagappa University, Karaikudi-630003, Tamil Nadu, India
Manikandan Jayaraman	Structural Biology and Biocomputing Lab, Department of Bioinformatics, Alagappa University, Karaikudi-630003, Tamil Nadu, India
M. K. Bhanuja	Department of Computer Science, Pondicherry University, Puducherry, India
Mohammad Ishtiaque Rahman	Department of Information Systems, University of Maryland - Baltimore County, USA
N. Priyadharshini	Department of Computer Technology and Data Science, Sri Krishna Arts and Science College, Coimbatore, India
P. Mohan Kumar	School of Computer Science and Engineering, Vellore Institute of Technology, Vellore, India
P. M. Benson Mansingh	Advanced Computer Science and Engineering, Vignan's Foundation for Science, Technology, and Research, Vadlamudi (Post), Guntur (Dist.), India
Pradeep Kumar Sriram	Structural Biology and Biocomputing Lab, Department of Bioinformatics, Alagappa University, Karaikudi-630003, Tamil Nadu, India
R. Brindha	Department of Computing Technologies, School of Computing, CET, SRM Institute of Science and Technology, Kattankulathur Campus, Chennai, Tamil Nadu, India
R. K. Pongiannan	Department of Computing Technologies, School of Computing, CET, SRM Institute of Science and Technology, Kattankulathur Campus, Chennai, Tamil Nadu, India
R. Brindha	Department of Computing Technologies, SRM Institute of Science and Technology, Kattankulathur, India
R. Deepalakshmi	Department of ECE, CARE College of Engineering, Tiruchirappalli, Tamil Nadu, India
R. Elanthirayan	Department of Electrical and Electronics Engineering, St. Joseph College of Engineering, Chennai, Tamil Nadu-600119, India
R. Sofia	Department of Electronics and Communication Engineering, Manakula Vinayagar Institute of Technology, Puducherry, India
Raji Rajmichael	Department of Bioinformatics (4th Floor), Science Block, Alagappa University, Karaikudi – 630003, Tamil Nadu, India

R. Nallakumar Department of Artificial Intelligence and Data Science, Karpagam Institute of Technology, Coimbatore, India

S. Mary Praveena Department of ECE, Sri Ramakrishna Institute of Technology, Coimbatore, India

S. Yazhinian Department of Computer Science, Vel Tech Rangarajan Dr. Sagunthala R&D Institute of Science & Technology, Chennai, India

Sabenabanu Abdulkadhar Department of Computer Science and Engineering, Koneru Lakshmaiah Education Foundation, Vaddeswaram, Guntur, Andhra Pradesh-522302, India
Department of Computer Applications, Faculty of Science and Humanities, SRM Institute of Science and Technology, Kattankulathur, Chennai-603203, Tamil Nadu, India

Saranya Jayapalan Department of Bioinformatics, Pondicherry University, Puducherry, India
current Affiliation SS TechLogix, C42, Centre of Excellence in Biotechnology, Tamil Nadu Agricultural University Campus, Coimbatore - 641003, India

Shijukumar K. Department of Computing Technologies, School of Computing, CET, SRM Institute of Science and Technology, Kattankulathur Campus, Chennai, Tamil Nadu, India

Sneha Subramaniyan Department of Bioinformatics (4th Floor), Science Block, Alagappa University, Karaikudi – 630003, Tamil Nadu, India

Sumit Govil School of Life and Basic Sciences, Jaipur National University, Jaipur, Rajasthan, India

T. Sayamsmruti Panda BRIC- Institute of Life Sciences, Bhubaneswar, Odisha, India

Tamilalagan S. Department of Computing Technologies, School of Computing, CET, SRM Institute of Science and Technology, Kattankulathur Campus, Chennai, Tamil Nadu, India

Telugu Maddileti Department of Electronics and Communication Engineering, Guru Nanak Institutions Technical Campus, Ibrahimpatnam, Ranga Reddy District, Telangana-501506, India

Uzma Patel School of Life and Basic Sciences, Jaipur National University, Jaipur, Rajasthan, India

Veerapandiyan Malaisamy Department of Bioinformatics (4th Floor), Science Block, Alagappa University, Karaikudi – 630003, Tamil Nadu, India

Yasmin Abdulkadhar Department of Artificial Intelligence and Data Science, Excel Engineering College (Autonomous), Pallakapalayam, Namakkal, Tamil Nadu-637303, India

CHAPTER 1

Introduction to Artificial Intelligence and Natural Language Processing in Healthcare

T. Sayamsmruti Panda[1,#], **Saranya Jayapalan**[2,#], **A. Shankar**[3] and **Basant K. Tiwary**[2,*]

[1] *BRIC- Institute of Life Sciences, Bhubaneswar, Odisha, India*

[2] *Department of Bioinformatics, Pondicherry University, Puducherry, India*

[3] *Department of ECE, Manakula Vinayagar Institute of Technology, Puducherry, India*

Abstract: The healthcare sector has rapidly evolved due to emerging trends. Integrating Artificial Intelligence (AI) and Natural Language Processing (NLP) within healthcare signifies a transformative shift in medical data analysis, interpretation, and utilization. The synergy of AI, with its ability to mimic human cognition and NLP, which empowers machines to comprehend and process human language, is essential to unlocking the hidden potential behind the vast amount of unstructured medical data. This chapter explores the fundamental concepts of AI and NLP and their applications in the healthcare sector. Various AI-enabled healthcare devices and their applications are described. The mechanism and applications of recently developed AI-powered wearable devices are also discussed. The ethical considerations of AI and NLP, as well as potential and future directions in revolutionizing healthcare delivery, are explained by examining current challenges, such as data privacy and domain-specific models. Also, this chapter describes the applications of AI and NLP in medical imaging as diverse and impactful, spanning early disease detection, workflow optimization, personalized medicine, and remote diagnostics. By automating complex processes and providing actionable insights, AI revolutionizes how medical images are analyzed and utilized. As advancements in AI continue, its potential to improve patient care, enhance diagnostic accuracy, and democratize healthcare access will only grow, making it an indispensable tool in modern medicine.

Keywords: Artificial Intelligence (AI), Machine Learning (ML), Healthcare, AI-powered wearables, AI-enabled healthcare devices, EHR.

* **Corresponding author Basant K. Tiwary:** Department of Bioinformatics, Pondicherry University, Puducherry, India; E-mail: basant@bicpu.edu.in.
Authors T. Sayamsmruti Panda and Saranya Jayapalan share equal contributions.
Current Affiliation of A. Shankar, Department of ECE, Hindustan College of Engineering and Technology, Coimbatore, India
Current Affiliation SS TechLogix, C42, Centre of Excellence in Biotechnology, Tamil Nadu Agricultural University Campus, Coimbatore - 641003, India

A. Shankar, Saranya Jayapalan, & Basant. K. Tiwary (Eds.)

INTRODUCTION

In today's world, technological advancements have become intensely woven into human life. New technological inventions have revolutionized human lifestyles through diverse applications. Artificial Intelligence (AI) has significantly transformed and simplified the challenges and obstacles associated with various day-to-day activities. It is undergoing rapid and significant growth across all domains, particularly within the medical and healthcare sectors [1, 2].

AI is the branch of computer science that creates decision-making entities, which are systems proficient in independently perceiving their environment, learning, reasoning, and taking actions to achieve desired outcomes. These actions may include problem-solving, object and word recognition, understanding and responding to natural language, making predictions, and making decisions in complex conditions [3, 4]. However, the roots of AI are deeply intertwined with various disciplines, including biology, mathematics, psychology, linguistics, and statistics. This interdisciplinary foundation is evident in the contributions of pioneers like Charles Babbage, Claude Shannon, Alan Turing, Richard Bellman, and Marvin Minsky, whose visionary work across these fields laid the foundation for countless essential AI concepts. Furthermore, significant advancements in computing, such as breakthroughs in hardware processing power and storage capacity, have provided the critical technological infrastructure that has fueled the rapid growth of AI in recent decades.

AI empowers machines to mimic human intelligence. It achieves different tasks through various Machine Learning (ML) algorithms, which are used to train them on relevant datasets to perform. Deep Learning (DL), a subfield of ML, has fueled numerous remarkable advancements, including self-driving cars. DL algorithms draw inspiration from the structure of the human brain. Natural Language Processing (NLP), another subfield of AI, utilizes ML algorithms to enable computers to comprehend and interact with human language. Fig. (**1**) depicts the schematic representation of AI and its subfields.

The advent of AI has impacted healthcare systems regarding disease diagnosis, treatment, and patient monitoring processes. AI technology is refining healthcare research and enhancing patient outcomes through greater diagnostic accuracy and personalized treatments. AI in healthcare excels at analyzing massive volumes of clinical data, enabling medical professionals to uncover hidden disease markers and identify novel disease associations that are difficult to detect through established conventional methods. The fusion of AI and healthcare offers immense potential for innovation and transformation while raising critical ethical concerns [5]. The continuous evolution of AI technologies drives significant transformations across the healthcare spectrum, impacting everything from diagnostic accuracy and treatment planning to developing novel therapies and future medicine.

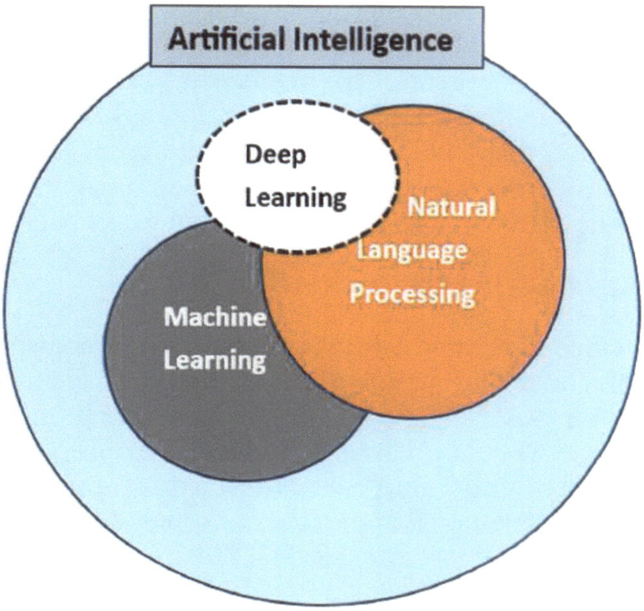

Fig. (1). Schematic representation of AI and its subfields.

Precision medicine, a keystone and one of the significant milestones of AI in healthcare, leverages ML algorithms trained on extensive and diverse datasets [6]. These datasets encompass a wide range of data formats, including biological information, medical images, and patient records, enabling the development of patient-specific therapies. Integrating AI into healthcare is advantageous in reducing the time taken for the treatment process in terms of diagnosis, timely care of the patient, and efficiency. By analyzing patient data with machine learning algorithms, healthcare providers can identify even subtle changes in patterns that may indicate an increased risk of adverse health outcomes [7].

A recent revolution in AI is the development of the AlphaFold2 [8] and AlphaFold3 [9] systems. AlphaFold3 expands upon the competencies of its predecessor, AlphaFold2, which predicts the structures of more diverse molecular assemblies. While AlphaFold2 primarily focuses on proteins and protein-protein complexes, AlphaFold3 can generate predictions encompassing proteins, DNA, RNA, ions, ligands, and chemical modifications. These enhanced models also demonstrate improved accuracy in predicting protein complex structures.

With AI tools and technology, healthcare providers and scientists can enhance the accuracy of deciphering complex genetic and image data and produce outcomes to address public health-related tasks efficiently. The past decade has been characterized by transformations across multiple sectors, including healthcare. The evolution of AI is evident in the execution of Electronic Health Records (EHR) [10], AI-driven wearable devices [11], medical robots [12], smart devices, and healthcare information systems. This drastic shift from conventional methods to AI technology was achieved and established through various ML tasks and algorithms. Ethical decision-making in public health crises, such as COVID-19, demands careful consideration of the trade-offs between maximizing intervention effectiveness and safeguarding economic and societal well-being [13].

Computational Advances in Clinical Practices

Computational methods are progressively recognized as indispensable tools in current medical practice. They involve a wide range of techniques, from data analysis and modeling to AI and ML for the application of healthcare informatics. Medical tools based on AI hold immense promise, but extensive validation studies are needed for incorporation into standard medical practice. This chapter illustrates AI-based computational approaches, AI tools for medical applications, and AI devices with their day-to-day usage [14].

Remote Patient Monitoring and Telehealth

AI-Powered Wearables and Sensors

The concept of wearable technology dates back to the 1960s, but it was not until the 2010s that wearables started gaining popularity. Early designed wearables were mainly focused on tracking physical activities and fundamental health measurements. nowadays, with ML and DL algorithms and techniques, wearables are more sophisticated, with multi-sensor systems that can track various physiological parameters, including blood oxygen level, sleep pattern, body temperature, heart rate, and blood pressure. Recently developed AI-wearable devices are advanced in detecting early signs of chronic diseases [15 - 18]. AI-enabled smart watches, AI smart glasses, belts, contact lenses, bands, and jackets show the different AI-powered devices and their uses.

AI in Heart Monitoring

Cardiovascular Diseases (CVDs) encompass the disease condition that disrupts the function of the heart and blood vessels, with a predominantly strong effect among patients with early records of diabetes mellitus, high cholesterol, and hypertension [19]. People with unhealthy diets, smoking, and a lack of exercise may also be affected by CVDs. Coronary artery disease is the most common CVD; it is defined as narrowed or blocked coronary arteries due to plaque formation, which leads to Myocardial Infarction (MI). Prevention, early diagnosis, and management of CVDs and MI are significant challenges in today's world. Electrocardiograms (ECGs) are mainly used for the early diagnosis of MI and heart rhythm changes when a patient comes with symptoms such as chest pain, sweating, shoulder pain, etc. However, receiving an ECG diagnosis will take some time, and the patients must reach the hospital on time. With the use of DL and ML applications, the AI-enabled ECG was invented. Scripps Research scientists developed an AI-generated Electrocardiogram (ECG) to detect heart attacks and heart rhythm disturbances; this work was reported in DPI Digital Medicine in August 2024. It employed DL algorithms with a massive dataset for constructing an AI-enhanced reconstruction of the 12-lead ECG rather than 3-leads with accurate clinical assessment, which overcomes the traditional ECG. This AI-enhanced ECG could be useful for emergency cases; it might be used even before acquiring an Electrocardiogram (ECG). This AI-based model can efficiently assess if a patient at triage needs an ECG [20]. The AI-equipped ECG data can produce accurate results once ECG data are available and also provide accurate interpretations, thus enabling comprehensive and clinical analysis and diagnosis. AI empowers clinicians by speeding up the data processing time. For instance, AI analyses of insertable cardiac-monitor-detected occurrences are related to effective classification, which reduces the technicians' workload through data curation.

AI in Predicting Women's Fertility

In recent days, infertility has become a global issue, and infertility rates are increasing steadily. There is a critical need for advanced methods and accurate assessments to overcome the various problems connected to infertility. AI has emerged as a growing supplementary tool for evaluating female reproductive function. AI-assisted *In Vitro* Fertilization (IVF) can enhance the outcomes and efficiency of the overall IVF process and streamline optimization [21, 22]. Using ML models to streamline ultrasound timing, ultrasound counts can be modulated, and the prediction of trigger time is helpful to avoid the risk of overresponse. Improved ML algorithms are widely used in various stages of the IVF process, such as follicular monitoring, oocyte retrieval, numbering, triggering, and ultrasound [23].

AI Wearables for the Blind and Visually Impaired

Smart glasses powered by AI are wearable for individuals with visual impairments. By combining AI, computer vision, and NLP, these wearable devices provide users with tasks like scanning, object identification, and scene perception. Envision glasses are innovative AI-powered smart glasses with cutting-edge applications specifically designed for those with vision issues. Among its many features, it enables users to use text-to-speech functions, allowing users to read mail, signage, recipes, and any text they encounter. 'Find Objects' and 'Describe Scene' features enhance users' understanding of their surroundings [24, 25]. The ARx AI headset is a talking camera that assists visually challenged people. Its dedicated app facilitates seamless connection to an Android or iOS smartphone to translate visual input into audio output.

Robotic Surgery and AI-Powered Surgical Robots

Robot-assisted surgery aids doctors in executing complex surgeries like orthopedics with more precision and control over complex procedures. Surgical robots are fully designed with automatic structures for disease diagnosis, treatment, and analytical study. AI-powered robotics significantly advances orthopedic surgery by developing preoperative planning, enhancing intraoperative accuracy, and improving postoperative results in hip, knee, and shoulder replacements [26 - 28].

FDA-Approved AI-driven Healthcare Devices

VBrain by Vysioneer speeds up the contouring process by achieving a 30% reduction in time and a 12% improvement in accuracy compared to manual methods. Its FDA-approved DL algorithm identifies the three most prevalent brain tumors: metastasis, meningioma, and acoustic neuroma [29].

GI Genius by Medtronic is an AI-powered "backup camera" that is FDA-approved to help find colon lesions during colonoscopy. Once integrated with existing endoscopy equipment, the tool immediately appears in the endoscopist's display monitor. It identifies suspected polyps in real time and marks them with green boxes [30].

LumineticsCore

LumineticsCore, with FDA approval, expedites the diagnosis of diabetic retinopathy and macular edema, resulting in increased patient engagement with ophthalmologists. Subsequently, a retinal camera captures images, and the system uses an AI-based and separate diagnostic algorithm to detect and analyze biomarkers. It provides a diagnosis at the same appointment, so patients can leave with a referral to an ophthalmologist [31].

NATURAL LANGUAGE PROCESSING (NLP) IN HEALTHCARE

Definition and Overview

NLP is a machine learning-based algorithm that allows text processing and analysis. It can help predict patient outcomes, improve hospital classification systems, and create diagnostic models that identify early-stage chronic disease when applied to medical notes [32]. This may be helpful in critical care, where there is more patient data to analyze and patient mortality prediction is frequent. The application of NLP in medicine has certain requirements, such as the presence of unbiased training data and clinicians' efficiency in getting training to implement NLP safely as part of everyday practice [33].

This chapter examines the advances and problems of NLP, emphasizing its significance, applications, and approaches. It divides NLP into two categories: Natural Language Understanding (NLU) and Natural Language Generation (NLG). It describes key components, such as phonology, morphology, syntax, semantics, and pragmatics. The chapter covers a variety of NLP tasks, including machine translation, summarization, sentiment analysis, and the datasets and models utilized in these applications. It also handles evaluation measures and obstacles like ambiguity and language barriers. The book emphasizes NLP's interdisciplinary nature, which includes linguistics, computer science, and psychology, and proposes future study areas, particularly in the healthcare industry. This book investigates the transformative impact of Natural Language Processing (NLP) on healthcare, specifically the extraction and processing of clinical data derived from multiple sources, including Electronic Health Records (EHRs). It emphasizes NLP's importance in improving patient care, illness detection, clinical decision-making, and medical transcription. It also examines various NLP techniques, such as rule-based methods, statistical approaches, and big language models that use transfer learning [34].

NLP Techniques in Healthcare

Text Mining

Despite its potential, language diversity and unstructured data limit adoption and require ongoing advancements in NLP techniques to improve accuracy and dependability in healthcare applications. NLP improves healthcare delivery through a variety of key factors. It allows for quick processing of Electronic Health Records (EHRs) [35] to extract crucial information regarding medicines, disease diagnoses, and symptoms, resulting in improved patient care and compliance [36]. In clinical decision support systems, NLP helps give evidence-based recommendations for treatment choices. Speech-to-text transcription technology improves clinical documentation by allowing clinicians to generate notes using voice instructions, leading to faster and higher-quality documentation [37]. NLP simplifies the processing of healthcare questionnaires and surveys for population screening that can handle vast amounts of medical data to detect adverse medication responses and probable disease outbreaks.Additionally, NLP aids in medical picture captioning, allowing physicians to study and describe medical images more rapidly.

Information Extraction

Extracting and analyzing the information include statistical techniques in NLP, providing valuable solutions to clinical data processing challenges. Statistical learning algorithms can extract useful information from EHRs, but require initial data preparation and structuring for optimal application [38]. These models contribute to overcoming the difficulty of unstructured clinical data by giving systematic approaches to data interpretation. Integrating statistical NLP techniques with medical expertise is critical, as the models require input from skilled medical personnel to annotate medical documents at appropriate accuracy levels. While these strategies [39] eliminate the need for substantial manual annotation, they nevertheless require the direct participation of medical practitioners to ensure data quality. These approaches help to overcome significant issues in the context of information extraction in healthcare, including implementing data processing, such as managing unstructured data, language diversity, and semantic ambiguity.

Question Answering

The following chapters of this book evaluate Question-answering (QA) systems created for healthcare professionals, analyzing their design, evaluation, and clinical usefulness. Previous studies showed that while machine learning breakthroughs have improved accuracy, most systems fail to address real-world clinical needs, frequently relying on simplistic or hypothetical inquiries. The main difficulties discovered are a lack of clinician input, insufficient communication of response dependability, and a significant risk of bias. Only a few systems meet the clinical utility criterion, emphasizing the need for more realistic datasets and improved techniques. To improve clinical practice adoption, the authors underline the necessity of building quality assurance systems that deliver trustworthy, contextually relevant answers and effectively express uncertainties using NLP. Most QA systems are constructed with little input from physicians and were intended to perform well on benchmark datasets rather than clinical scenarios. Studies frequently utilize straightforward questions or include too little information for widespread biological application. Specialized QA systems can offer advantages like automatic updates, reliable source filtering, and clustering of answers by medical themes. Additionally, general search engines may not adequately address healthcare-specific needs, such as answer verification, source reliability assessment, and clinical guidance provision. Research suggests that restricting searches to trustworthy medical sources increases answer relevance, something general search engines may not prioritize [40].

Machine Translation

Standardized medical terminology is a collection of linguistic standards and language to promote accurate and consistent information exchange. Examples include SNOMED Clinical Terms, ICD, RxNorm, and UMLS [41, 42]. However, the limited multilingual support for these terminologies is primarily available in English and a few other languages, which hampers research and automated medical data processing. NLP has been used to automate natural language translation into various languages, particularly in the medical field. NLP is frequently combined with Machine Translation (MT) to reduce the time and costs of manual translation while maintaining complete and accurate translations.

Sentiment Analysis

Sentiment analysis can improve clinical decision-making and patient care outcomes by studying patient interactions and feedback; healthcare practitioners can adjust their services to match patient requirements better, resulting in higher outcomes and satisfaction. The technology enables providers to pinpoint specific areas that require attention, such as communication or treatment techniques, allowing them to improve their procedures and care quality. Sentiment analysis also improves patient-provider communication by allowing healthcare personnel to better comprehend patients' problems, fears, and expectations, resulting in a more compassionate and responsive healthcare environment. In telehealth settings, sentiment analysis improves the management of chronic illnesses and mental health by assessing input for emotional indicators and allowing for more personalized treatment options. However, the limitations of sentiment analysis in healthcare closely reflect fundamental data privacy concerns in the broader healthcare ecosystem. Healthcare sentiment analysis necessitates processing sensitive patient data across multiple platforms and formats, requiring rigorous adherence to privacy and confidentiality regulations. The primary issue is balancing technological innovation with ethical considerations and data protection, which necessitates strong anonymization techniques and secure data management processes. Additionally, data confidentiality becomes critical as systems process large amounts of sensitive health information [43]. This entails installing strict data protection measures while maintaining transparency in data usage 24/7. Data sources, including social media, healthcare forums, and patient reviews, necessitate unique privacy considerations.

APPLICATIONS OF NLP IN HEALTHCARE

Electronic Health Record (EHR) Analysis

The advancement of AI for EHR processing and interpretation is a growing interest. Leveraging pre-trained language models, NLP provides a foundation for medical AI systems that analyze clinical narratives. EHR systems are increasingly being used to enhance healthcare delivery and outcomes. However, the increased paperwork burden on clinicians makes it challenging for medical AI systems to employ discrete data fields in clinical documentation. Natural language processing (NLP) is increasingly utilized to comprehend the rich, detailed patient information in clinical narratives. Most NLP systems are built on DL models that use neural network designs like Convolutional Neural Networks (CNN) and Recurrent Neural Networks (RNN). Transformer designs, such as Bidirectional Encoder Representations from Transformers (BERT), have shown cutting-edge results in named entity identification, Relation Extraction (RE), sentence similarity, natural language inference, and Question Answering. Large transformer models trained on vast text data performed better in emergence and homogeneity [44, 45]. Significant applications of AI and ML in the healthcare domain are illustrated in Fig. (**2**).

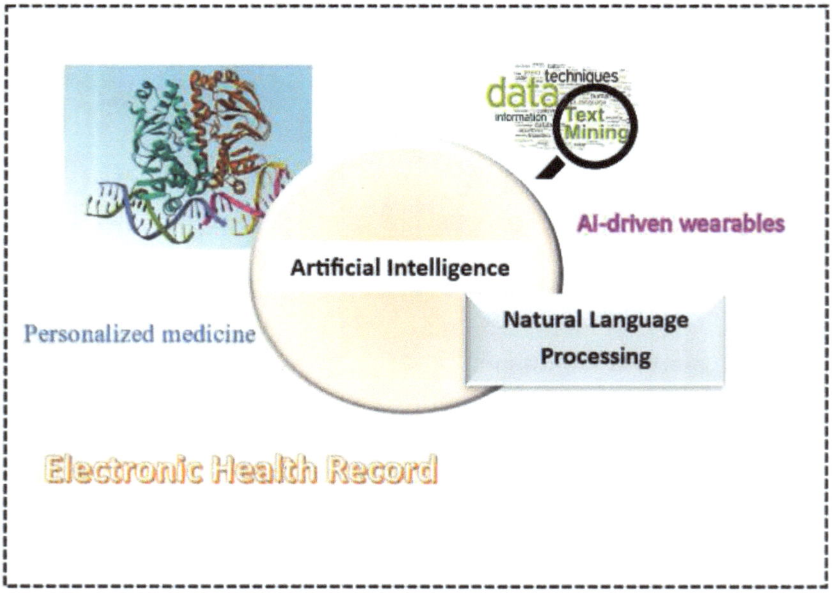

Fig. (2). Applications of AI and ML in healthcare.

Clinical Decision Support

Clinical Decision Support (CDS) tools help clinicians make decisions by connecting specific patient characteristics to a computerized knowledge base. A Clinical Decision Support (CDS) system's architecture can be likened to a neurological reflex arc, where patient data acts as the "receptor," decision rules and knowledge bases function as the "integration center," and the resulting patient-specific assessments or suggestions are the "effectors. NLP can extract the data required to actuate a variety of decision rules, possibly enriching all three key components of CDS systems. Over the past four decades, CDS systems have enhanced practitioner performance in roughly 60% of evaluated instances. NLP systems can provide automatic and proactive decision support as part of clinical workflow, making suggestions rather than assessments and giving decision support at the time and place of decision-making. NLP applications have been integrated into active and passive CDS, analyzing various textual sources, including clinical records, biomedical literature, web pages, and suicide notes. Active NLP CDS comprises alerting, monitoring, coding, and reminders, whereas passive NLP CDS focuses on information provision and patient population identification [46].

Medical Literature Mining

Biomedical Literature Mining (BLM) is the study of using text mining and Natural Language Processing (NLP) tools to extract and mine knowledge from biomedical literature automatically. Biomedical literature is more accessible because of the public database MEDLINE and free search engines like PubMed. It is written in professional language and can be lengthy and diverse. BLM combines NLP, Biomedical Informatics (BMI), and data mining, and it has been used successfully in applications such as biomedical literature retrieval, biomedical question/answering, and clinical decision support. Researchers from the BMI and Computer Science (CS) sectors have made essential contributions to BLM, with deep learning technologies demonstrating high potential in various disciplines, including NLP. BLM focuses on various deep learning techniques, divided into five sections: biomedical NER and normalization, biomedical text classification, RE, pathway extraction, and hypothesis generation [47]. These tasks are critical for enabling the execution of subsequent tasks, such as Relation Extraction. Identifying genotype-phenotype associations from biomedical literature is essential in precision medicine, with studies concentrating on relationships between human genes and phenotypes, disease, and gene correlations [48]. There are pattern-based and learning-based extraction strategies. Compound-target Interaction (CPI) is crucial in drug discovery and development, which makes automated extraction approaches appealing. Drug-drug Interaction

(DDI) detection is vital for post-market drug safety surveillance, and methods include co-occurrence, rule-based, and machine-learning approaches [49, 50]. Co-occurrence-based methods use co-occurrences to construct drug connections, whereas linguistic rule-based approaches combine shallow parsing and pattern matching. ML, intense neural networks, has gained popularity in DDI relation extraction tasks. Biomedical relation extraction can also help curate biomedical knowledge bases naturally assembled from biomedical NER and relation extraction.

Patient-Provider Communication

AI transforms patient-provider communication by enabling virtual health assistants to deliver timely information and support. These digital companions are available around the clock to answer questions, schedule appointments, and provide essential medical advice. AI-driven NLP is also excellent at customization, adapting communication to particular patient preferences and needs. It crosses linguistic barriers by providing real-time translation services and minimizing miscommunication in healthcare settings. AI also derives valuable information from patient-provider interactions, improving care quality and recognizing unique patient needs [51].

As a result, NLP effectively converts speech and free text in EHRs into structured data for clinical investigations, enhances hospital triage and prediction models, and addresses patient questions. Standardized medical terminology libraries enable NLP analysis of free-text notes, which improves patient care and allows for the development of assistant-like services such as chatbots to answer specific healthcare questions. Thus, the correct application of NLP technology can broaden the scope and ramifications of the healthcare industry.

Role of Artificial Intelligence in Medical Imaging Research

AI is transforming medical imaging research, redefining how medical images are analyzed, interpreted, and utilized in clinical and research settings. Integrating AI-driven technologies into medical imaging offers unprecedented opportunities to enhance diagnostic accuracy, streamline workflows, and improve patient outcomes.

Revolutionizing Image Analysis and Diagnosis

AI precisely possesses and analyzes vast amounts of imaging data. Dl and AI algorithms can detect subtle patterns and anomalies in medical images that may be imperceptible to human experts. For instance, AI systems have demonstrated remarkable accuracy in detecting conditions such as tumors, fractures, and other abnormalities in radiographic, Computed Tomography (CT), and Magnetic Resonance Imaging (MRI) scans [52].

These systems leverage Convolutional Neural Networks (CNNs), a deep learning model, to analyze image pixel-level details. By training on large datasets, AI models learn to recognize subtle features indicative of diseases, enabling earlier and more accurate diagnoses. This capability is especially critical in detecting life-threatening conditions like cancer at an early stage, where timely intervention can significantly improve survival rates [53].

Enhancing Efficiency and Reducing Errors

AI has the potential to revolutionize medical imaging workflows by automating repetitive and time-consuming tasks. Radiologists often face immense workloads, which increases the risk of diagnostic errors due to fatigue. AI tools can assist by pre-screening images and flagging areas of concern, allowing radiologists to focus their expertise on complex cases [54]. This collaborative approach reduces diagnostic turnaround times and minimizes the likelihood of missed diagnoses.

Additionally, AI algorithms excel in maintaining consistency in image interpretation. Unlike human experts, whose performance may vary due to experience and workload, AI models provide standardized assessments, ensuring uniformity in diagnostic outcomes. For example, AI-powered systems are increasingly being used to quantify lesion sizes, assess disease progression, and predict treatment responses with a high degree of reliability [55].

Applications in Personalized Medicine

AI's role in medical imaging research extends beyond diagnostics to personalized medicine. While merging imaging data with other clinical data, AI systems can provide insights into individual patient characteristics, enabling tailored treatment plans [56]. For instance, AI can analyze imaging data alongside genomic information in oncology to predict tumor behavior and recommend targeted therapies.

Furthermore, AI algorithms are being developed to simulate and predict the outcomes of various treatment modalities. This capability helps clinicians make informed decisions about the most effective interventions, reducing the trial-an--error approach often associated with complex medical conditions [57].

Supporting Remote and Resource-Limited Settings

AI is also essential in addressing healthcare disparities by enabling access to high-quality diagnostic services in remote areas. Cloud-based AI platforms can analyze medical images uploaded from rural clinics and provide expert-level interpretations, bridging the gap between underserved populations and advanced healthcare facilities [58 - 60]. These innovations can potentially democratize healthcare and ensure that patients in all regions receive timely and accurate diagnoses.

CONCLUSION

This chapter gives an overall introduction to AI and ML and their various techniques, algorithms, and applications in healthcare. Ongoing advancements in ML and the growing availability of high-quality datasets will likely drive the development of even more sophisticated AI models. These models will enhance diagnostic capabilities and play a pivotal role in drug discovery, disease prediction, and preventive healthcare. In addition, NLP is playing an increasingly important role in bioinformatics, with applications in deep learning, protein structure prediction, biological data mining, clinical decision-making, and EHR maintenance. NLP has a wide range of applications in the healthcare sector, including personalized medicine and targeted therapy. The integration of AI and NLP in the healthcare industry has the potential to provide more relevant insights into the vast quantity of data created and analyzed in the field. Thus, the future of AI research holds immense promise with tasks to deal with different data types and sizes. Despite its numerous advantages, integrating AI and ML into medical research involves challenges. Data privacy and security concerns are paramount, as AI systems rely on access to extensive datasets that may contain sensitive patient information. Thus, the next chapter describes the challenges of AI and ML in healthcare informatics.

ACKNOWLEDGEMENT

Authors, SJ and BKT, gratefully acknowledge the Indian Council of Medical Research (ICMR), New Delhi, for providing financial assistance through ICMR/RA Fellowship.

REFERENCES

[1] D. Chahal, and M.F. Byrne, "A primer on artificial intelligence and its application to endoscopy", *Gastrointest. Endosc.,* vol. 92, no. 4, pp. 813-820.e4, 2020. [http://dx.doi.org/10.1016/j.gie.2020.04.074] [PMID: 32387497]

[2] M. Kąpa, I. Koryciarz, N. Kustosik, P. Jurowski, and Z. Pniakowska, "Modern approach to diabetic retinopathy diagnostics", *Diagnostics (Basel),* vol. 14, no. 17, p. 1846, 2024. [http://dx.doi.org/10.3390/diagnostics14171846] [PMID: 39272631]

[3] A. Savino, E. Rondonotti, S. Rocchetto, A. Piagnani, N. Bina, P. Di Domenico, F. Segatta, and F. Radaelli, "GI genius endoscopy module: a clinical profile", *Expert Rev. Med. Devices,* vol. 21, no. 5, pp. 359-372, 2024. [http://dx.doi.org/10.1080/17434440.2024.2342508] [PMID: 38618982]

[4] E.V. Garcia, "Integrating artificial intelligence and natural language processing for computer-assisted reporting and report understanding in nuclear cardiology", *J. Nucl. Cardiol.,* vol. 30, no. 3, pp. 1180-1190, 2023.
[http://dx.doi.org/10.1007/s12350-022-02996-5] [PMID: 35725887]

[5] J.Y. Wang, V. Qu, C. Hui, N. Sandhu, M.G. Mendoza, N. Panjwani, Y.C. Chang, C.H. Liang, J.T. Lu, L. Wang, N. Kovalchuk, M.F. Gensheimer, S.G. Soltys, and E.L. Pollom, "Stratified assessment of an FDA-cleared deep learning algorithm for automated detection and contouring of metastatic brain tumors in stereotactic radiosurgery", *Radiat. Oncol.,* vol. 18, no. 1, p. 61, 2023.
[http://dx.doi.org/10.1186/s13014-023-02246-z] [PMID: 37016416]

[6] A.B. Lisacek-Kiosoglous, A.S. Powling, A. Fontalis, A. Gabr, E. Mazomenos, and F.S. Haddad, "Artificial intelligence in orthopaedic surgery", *Bone Joint Res.,* vol. 12, no. 7, pp. 447-454, 2023.
[http://dx.doi.org/10.1302/2046-3758.127.BJR-2023-0111.R1] [PMID: 37423607]

[7] B. Kayani, and F.S. Haddad, "Robotic total knee arthroplasty", *Bone Joint Res.,* vol. 8, no. 10, pp. 438-442, 2019.
[http://dx.doi.org/10.1302/2046-3758.810.BJR-2019-0175] [PMID: 31728181]

[8] C. Batailler, J. Shatrov, E. Sappey-Marinier, E. Servien, S. Parratte, and S. Lustig, "Artificial intelligence in knee arthroplasty: current concept of the available clinical applications", *Arthroplasty,* vol. 4, no. 1, p. 17, 2022.
[http://dx.doi.org/10.1186/s42836-022-00119-6] [PMID: 35491420]

[9] N. RaviChandran, Z.L. Teo, and D.S.W. Ting, "Artificial intelligence enabled smart digital eye wearables", *Curr. Opin. Ophthalmol.,* vol. 34, no. 5, pp. 414-421, 2023.
[http://dx.doi.org/10.1097/ICU.0000000000000985] [PMID: 37527195]

[10] A. Lavric, C. Beguni, E. Zadobrischi, A.M. Căilean, and S.A. Avătămăniţei, "A comprehensive survey on emerging assistive technologies for visually impaired persons: Lighting the path with visible light communications and artificial intelligence innovations", *Sensors (Basel),* vol. 24, no. 15, p. 4834, 2024.
[http://dx.doi.org/10.3390/s24154834] [PMID: 39123881]

[11] S. Hanassab, A. Abbara, A.C. Yeung, M. Voliotis, K. Tsaneva-Atanasova, T.W. Kelsey, G.H. Trew, S.M. Nelson, T. Heinis, and W.S. Dhillo, "The prospect of artificial intelligence to personalize assisted reproductive technology", *NPJ Digit. Med.,* vol. 7, no. 1, p. 55, 2024.
[http://dx.doi.org/10.1038/s41746-024-01006-x] [PMID: 38429464]

[12] V.S. Jiang, and C.L. Bormann, "Artificial intelligence in the *in vitro* fertilization laboratory: a review of advancements over the last decade", *Fertil. Steril.,* vol. 120, no. 1, pp. 17-23, 2023.
[http://dx.doi.org/10.1016/j.fertnstert.2023.05.149] [PMID: 37211062]

[13] D.J.X. Chow, P. Wijesinghe, K. Dholakia, and K.R. Dunning, "Does artificial intelligence have a role in the IVF clinic?", *Reprod. Fertil.,* vol. 2, no. 3, pp. C29-C34, 2021.
[http://dx.doi.org/10.1530/RAF-21-0043] [PMID: 35118395]

[14] F. Mason, A.C. Pandey, M. Gadaleta, E.J. Topol, E.D. Muse, and G. Quer, "AI-enhanced reconstruction of the 12-lead electrocardiogram *via* 3-leads with accurate clinical assessment", *NPJ Digit. Med.,* vol. 7, no. 1, p. 201, 2024.
[http://dx.doi.org/10.1038/s41746-024-01193-7] [PMID: 39090394]

[15] H.A.R.H. Khafaji, and J.M. Suwaidi, "Atypical presentation of acute and chronic coronary artery disease in diabetics", *World J. Cardiol.,* vol. 6, no. 8, pp. 802-813, 2014.
[http://dx.doi.org/10.4330/wjc.v6.i8.802] [PMID: 25228959]

[16] W.H. Wang, and W.S. Hsu, "Integrating artificial intelligence and wearable IoT system in long-term care environments", *Sensors (Basel),* vol. 23, no. 13, p. 5913, 2023.
[http://dx.doi.org/10.3390/s23135913] [PMID: 37447763]

[17] K.P. Seng, L.M. Ang, E. Peter, and A. Mmonyi, "Machine learning and AI technologies for smart

wearables", *Electronics (Basel),* vol. 12, no. 7, p. 1509, 2023.
[http://dx.doi.org/10.3390/electronics12071509]

[18] A. Ahmed, S. Aziz, A. Abd-alrazaq, F. Farooq, and J. Sheikh, "Overview of artificial intelligence–driven wearable devices for diabetes: scoping review", *J. Med. Internet Res.,* vol. 24, no. 8, 2022.e36010
[http://dx.doi.org/10.2196/36010] [PMID: 35943772]

[19] S. Shajari, K. Kuruvinashetti, A. Komeili, and U. Sundararaj, "The emergence of AI-based wearable sensors for digital health technology: a review", *Sensors (Basel),* vol. 23, no. 23, p. 9498, 2023.
[http://dx.doi.org/10.3390/s23239498] [PMID: 38067871]

[20] C.B. Collin, T. Gebhardt, M. Golebiewski, T. Karaderi, M. Hillemanns, F.M. Khan, A. Salehzadeh-Yazdi, M. Kirschner, S. Krobitsch, and L. Kuepfer, "Computational models for clinical applications in personalized medicine—guidelines and recommendations for data integration and model validation", *J. Pers. Med.,* vol. 12, no. 2, p. 166, 2022.
[http://dx.doi.org/10.3390/jpm12020166] [PMID: 35207655]

[21] Y. Shen, D. Guo, F. Long, L.A. Mateos, H. Ding, Z. Xiu, R.B. Hellman, A. King, S. Chen, C. Zhang, and H. Tan, "Robots under COVID-19 pandemic: a comprehensive survey", *IEEE Access,* vol. 9, pp. 1590-1615, 2021.
[http://dx.doi.org/10.1109/ACCESS.2020.3045792] [PMID: 34976569]

[22] A.A. Morgan, J. Abdi, M.A.Q. Syed, G.E. Kohen, P. Barlow, and M.P. Vizcaychipi, "Robots in healthcare: a scoping review", *Curr. Robot. Rep.,* vol. 3, no. 4, pp. 271-280, 2022.
[http://dx.doi.org/10.1007/s43154-022-00095-4] [PMID: 36311256]

[23] F. Sabry, T. Eltaras, W. Labda, K. Alzoubi, and Q. Malluhi, "Machine learning for healthcare wearable devices: the big picture", *J. Healthc. Eng.,* vol. 2022, pp. 1-25, 2022.
[http://dx.doi.org/10.1155/2022/4653923] [PMID: 35480146]

[24] J. Ye, D. Woods, N. Jordan, and J. Starren, "The role of artificial intelligence for the application of integrating electronic health records and patient-generated data in clinical decision support", *AMIA Jt. Summits Transl. Sci. Proc.,* vol. 2024, pp. 459-467, 2024.
[PMID: 38827061]

[25] J. Abramson, J. Adler, J. Dunger, R. Evans, T. Green, A. Pritzel, O. Ronneberger, L. Willmore, A.J. Ballard, J. Bambrick, S.W. Bodenstein, D.A. Evans, C.C. Hung, M. O'Neill, D. Reiman, K. Tunyasuvunakool, Z. Wu, A. Žemgulytė, E. Arvaniti, C. Beattie, O. Bertolli, A. Bridgland, A. Cherepanov, M. Congreve, A.I. Cowen-Rivers, A. Cowie, M. Figurnov, F.B. Fuchs, H. Gladman, R. Jain, Y.A. Khan, C.M.R. Low, K. Perlin, A. Potapenko, P. Savy, S. Singh, A. Stecula, A. Thillaisundaram, C. Tong, S. Yakneen, E.D. Zhong, M. Zielinski, A. Žídek, V. Bapst, P. Kohli, M. Jaderberg, D. Hassabis, and J.M. Jumper, "Accurate structure prediction of biomolecular interactions with AlphaFold 3", *Nature,* vol. 630, no. 8016, pp. 493-500, 2024.
[http://dx.doi.org/10.1038/s41586-024-07487-w] [PMID: 38718835]

[26] J. Jumper, R. Evans, A. Pritzel, T. Green, M. Figurnov, O. Ronneberger, K. Tunyasuvunakool, R. Bates, A. Žídek, A. Potapenko, A. Bridgland, C. Meyer, S.A.A. Kohl, A.J. Ballard, A. Cowie, B. Romera-Paredes, S. Nikolov, R. Jain, J. Adler, T. Back, S. Petersen, D. Reiman, E. Clancy, M. Zielinski, M. Steinegger, M. Pacholska, T. Berghammer, S. Bodenstein, D. Silver, O. Vinyals, A.W. Senior, K. Kavukcuoglu, P. Kohli, and D. Hassabis, "Highly accurate protein structure prediction with AlphaFold", *Nature,* vol. 596, no. 7873, pp. 583-589, 2021.
[http://dx.doi.org/10.1038/s41586-021-03819-2] [PMID: 34265844]

[27] F. Wang and A. Preininger, "AI in health: state of the art, challenges, and future directions," *Yearb. Med. Inform.,* vol. 28, no. 01, pp. 16–26, 2019.
[http://dx.doi.org/10.1055/s-0039-1677908]

[28] K.B. Johnson, W.Q. Wei, D. Weeraratne, M.E. Frisse, K. Misulis, K. Rhee, J. Zhao, and J.L. Snowdon, "Precision medicine, AI, and the future of personalized health care", *Clin. Transl. Sci.,* vol. 14, no. 1, pp. 86-93, 2021.

[http://dx.doi.org/10.1111/cts.12884] [PMID: 32961010]

[29] C.A. Kulikowski, "Beginnings of Artificial Intelligence in Medicine (AIM): computational artifice assisting scientific inquiry and clinical art – with reflections on present AIM challenges", *Yearb. Med. Inform.,* vol. 28, no. 1, pp. 249-256, 2019.
[http://dx.doi.org/10.1055/s-0039-1677895] [PMID: 31022744]

[30] P. Hamet, and J. Tremblay, "Artificial intelligence in medicine", *Metabolism,* vol. 69, pp. S36-S40, 2017.
[http://dx.doi.org/10.1016/j.metabol.2017.01.011] [PMID: 28126242]

[31] P. Amisha, P. Malik, M. Pathania, and V. Rathaur, "Overview of artificial intelligence in medicine", *J. Family Med. Prim. Care,* vol. 8, no. 7, pp. 2328-2331, 2019.
[http://dx.doi.org/10.4103/jfmpc.jfmpc_440_19] [PMID: 31463251]

[32] S. Locke, A. Bashall, S. Al-Adely, J. Moore, A. Wilson, and G.B. Kitchen, "Natural language processing in medicine: A review", *Trends Anaesth. Crit. Care,* vol. 38, pp. 4-9, 2021.
[http://dx.doi.org/10.1016/j.tacc.2021.02.007]

[33] A.P. Supriyono, A.P. Wibawa, Suyono, and F. Kurniawan, "Advancements in natural language processing: Implications, challenges, and future directions", *Telematics and Informatics Reports,* vol. 16, 2024.100173
[http://dx.doi.org/10.1016/j.teler.2024.100173]

[34] E. Hossain, R. Rana, N. Higgins, J. Soar, P.D. Barua, A.R. Pisani, and K. Turner, "Natural language processing in electronic health records in relation to healthcare decision-making: a systematic review", *Comput. Biol. Med.,* vol. 155, 2023.106649
[http://dx.doi.org/10.1016/j.compbiomed.2023.106649] [PMID: 36805219]

[35] S.V. Blackley, J. Huynh, L. Wang, Z. Korach, and L. Zhou, "Speech recognition for clinical documentation from 1990 to 2018: a systematic review", *J. Am. Med. Inform. Assoc.,* vol. 26, no. 4, pp. 324-338, 2019.
[http://dx.doi.org/10.1093/jamia/ocy179] [PMID: 30753666]

[36] Y. Wieland-Jorna, D. van Kooten, R.A. Verheij, Y. de Man, A.L. Francke, and M.G. Oosterveld-Vlug, "Natural language processing systems for extracting information from electronic health records about activities of daily living. A systematic review", *JAMIA Open,* vol. 7, no. 2, 2024.ooae044
[http://dx.doi.org/10.1093/jamiaopen/ooae044] [PMID: 38798774]

[37] A. Fong, N. Harriott, D.M. Walters, H. Foley, R. Morrissey, and R.R. Ratwani, "Integrating natural language processing expertise with patient safety event review committees to improve the analysis of medication events", *Int. J. Med. Inform.,* vol. 104, pp. 120-125, 2017.
[http://dx.doi.org/10.1016/j.ijmedinf.2017.05.005] [PMID: 28529113]

[38] D. Demner-Fushman, W.W. Chapman, and C.J. McDonald, "What can natural language processing do for clinical decision support?", *J. Biomed. Inform.,* vol. 42, no. 5, pp. 760-772, 2009.
[http://dx.doi.org/10.1016/j.jbi.2009.08.007] [PMID: 19683066]

[39] G. Kell, A. Roberts, S. Umansky, L. Qian, D. Ferrari, F. Soboczenski, B.C. Wallace, N. Patel, and I.J. Marshall, "Question answering systems for health professionals at the point of care—a systematic review", *J. Am. Med. Inform. Assoc.,* vol. 31, no. 4, pp. 1009-1024, 2024.
[http://dx.doi.org/10.1093/jamia/ocae015] [PMID: 38366879]

[40] R. Noll, L.S. Frischen, M. Boeker, H. Storf, and J. Schaaf, "Machine translation of standardised medical terminology using natural language processing: A scoping review", *N. Biotechnol.,* vol. 77, pp. 120-129, 2023.
[http://dx.doi.org/10.1016/j.nbt.2023.08.004] [PMID: 37652265]

[41] G. Cazzaniga, A. Eccher, E. Munari, S. Marletta, E. Bonoldi, V. Della Mea, M. Cadei, M. Sbaraglia, A. Guerriero, A.P. Dei Tos, F. Pagni, and V. L'Imperio, "Natural Language Processing to extract SNOMED-CT codes from pathological reports", *Pathologica,* vol. 115, no. 6, pp. 318-324, 2023.
[http://dx.doi.org/10.32074/1591-951X-952] [PMID: 38180139]

[42] A. Babu, and S.B. Boddu, "BERT-based medical chatbot: enhancing healthcare communication through natural language understanding", *Explor. Res. Clin. Soc. Pharm.,* vol. 13, 2024.100419 [http://dx.doi.org/10.1016/j.rcsop.2024.100419] [PMID: 38495953]

[43] X. Yang, A. Chen, N. PourNejatian, H.C. Shin, K.E. Smith, C. Parisien, C. Compas, C. Martin, A.B. Costa, M.G. Flores, Y. Zhang, T. Magoc, C.A. Harle, G. Lipori, D.A. Mitchell, W.R. Hogan, E.A. Shenkman, J. Bian, and Y. Wu, "A large language model for electronic health records", *NPJ Digit. Med.,* vol. 5, no. 1, p. 194, 2022. [http://dx.doi.org/10.1038/s41746-022-00742-2] [PMID: 36572766]

[44] X. Luo, Z. Deng, B. Yang, and M. Y. Luo, "Pre-trained language models in medicine: A survey", *Artificial Intelligence in Medicine.,* vol. 154, p. 102904, 2024. [http://dx.doi.org/10.1016/j.artmed.2024.102904]

[45] A. Rahali, and M. A. Akhloufi, "End-to-end transformer-based models in textual-based NLP", *AI,* vol. 4, no. 1, pp. 54-110, 2023. [http://dx.doi.org/10.3390/ai4010004]

[46] S. Zhao, C. Su, Z. Lu, and F. Wang, "Recent advances in biomedical literature mining", *Brief. Bioinform.,* vol. 22, no. 3, 2021.bbaa057 [http://dx.doi.org/10.1093/bib/bbaa057] [PMID: 32422651]

[47] W. Xing, J. Qi, X. Yuan, L. Li, X. Zhang, Y. Fu, S. Xiong, L. Hu, and J. Peng, "A gene–phenotype relationship extraction pipeline from the biomedical literature using a representation learning approach", *Bioinformatics,* vol. 34, no. 13, pp. i386-i394, 2018. [http://dx.doi.org/10.1093/bioinformatics/bty263] [PMID: 29950017]

[48] Y. Zhang, W. Zheng, H. Lin, J. Wang, Z. Yang, and M. Dumontier, "Drug–drug interaction extraction *via* hierarchical RNNs on sequence and shortest dependency paths", *Bioinformatics,* vol. 34, no. 5, pp. 828-835, 2018. [http://dx.doi.org/10.1093/bioinformatics/btx659] [PMID: 29077847]

[49] H. Poon, K. Toutanova, and C. Quirk, "Distant supervision for cancer pathway extraction from text," *Pac. Symp. Biocomput.,* pp. 120–131, 2015. [Online]. Available: https://pubmed.ncbi.nlm.nih.gov/25592574/

[50] P. N. Kumar Sarella and V. T. Mangam, "AI-driven natural language processing in healthcare: transforming patient-provider communication," Indian *J. Pharm. Pract.,* vol. 17, no. 1, pp. 21–26, Jan. 2024. [Online]. Available: http://dx.doi.org/10.5530/ijopp.17.1.4

[51] Shankar Arumugam and Saranya Jayapalan, *Medical Image Processing for Healthcare Applications.* Lambert Academic Publishing, 2024.

[52] T. Johnson, H. Li, and L. Zhao, "Multimodal pretraining with vision transformers for image-text alignment", *IEEE Trans. Vis. Comput. Graph.,* vol. 30, no. 8, pp. 2654-2668, 2023. https://github.com/chenllliang/DreamEngine

[53] K. Chen, S. Wang, and R. Lee, "Advancements in multimodal learning for image-text integration", *IEEE Trans. Pattern Anal. Mach. Intell.,* vol. 43, no. 6, pp. 1578-1589, 2023.

[54] H. Zhang, J. Li, and M. Park, "Image captioning with multimodal transformers: a review", *IEEE Trans. Multimed.,* vol. 25, no. 7, pp. 1805-1821, 2024.

[55] L. Wang, C. Zhou, and Y. Liu, "Visual question answering using cross-modal attention mechanisms", *IEEE Trans. Neural Netw. Learn. Syst.,* vol. 35, no. 2, pp. 654-669, 2024.

[56] F. Zhang, T. Xu, and X. Yang, "Improved image-text retrieval using deep learning techniques", *IEEE Access,* vol. 12, pp. 3942-3953, 2024.

[57] R. Gupta, P. Shah, and D. Kim, "Deep learning in multimodal AI systems for healthcare: a survey", *IEEE Trans. Biomed. Eng.,* vol. 72, no. 11, pp. 3124-3137, 2023.

[58] Y. Liu, J. Gao, and Z. Li, "Transformers for multimodal applications: image captioning and beyond",

IEEE Trans. Comput. Vis. Image Process., vol. 31, no. 9, pp. 1285-1301, 2022.

[59] M. Singh, N. Patel, and P. Wang, "BERT-based approaches for image and text fusion in AI models", *IEEE Trans. Neural Netw. Learn. Syst.,* vol. 36, no. 5, pp. 1937-1949, 2022.

[60] C. Huang, Q. Zhang, and S. Lee, "Bias and fairness in multimodal image-text datasets", *IEEE Trans. Artif. Intell.,* vol. 9, no. 3, pp. 673-687, 2023.

CHAPTER 2

Challenges in Natural Language Processing for Healthcare Informatics

R. Brindha[1,*], R. Elanthirayan[2], R. K. Pongiannan[1], Bharath Addepalli[1], K. Kyathisree[1], T. Y. S. Srihari[1] and **M. Harini Reddy[1]**

[1] *Department of Computing Technologies, SRM Institute of Science and Technology, Kattankulathur, India*

[2] *Department of Electrical and Electronics Engineering, St. Joseph College of Engineering, Chennai, Tamil Nadu-600119, India*

Abstract: This chapter addresses the challenge of adapting clinical Natural Language Processing (NLP) systems for diverse healthcare environments. We adapted an existing NLP system to evaluate colonoscopy quality using pathology and colonoscopy reports from four distinct clinical settings varying in geography, practice type, pay scale, and Electronic Health Record (EHR) systems between 2013 and 2015. Adaptation revealed significant obstacles, including heterogeneous report formats, specialized clinical language, and site-specific variability, which extended development time beyond initial expectations. Effective strategies involved leveraging local EHR expertise, setting realistic deadlines, and refining the iterative system. Our findings emphasize that adapting NLP tools to new clinical contexts remains a critical barrier to widespread adoption and highlight the need for research focused on simplifying this process.

Keywords: Multimodal generative AI, Natural Language Processing (NLP), Healthcare informatics, Transformer models, Named Entity Recognition (NER), Clinical Decision Support (CDS), Electronic Health Records (EHRs), Text classification, Sentiment analysis, Text generation.

INTRODUCTION

A branch of computational linguistics and Artificial Intelligence (AI) called Natural Language Processing (NLP) studies how computers and human languages interact. It entails the application of models and algorithms to provide machines the ability to meaningfully comprehend, interpret, produce, and react to human language. Massive volumes of natural language data can be processed and analyzed using NLP, combining computer science and linguistics methods. NLP

* **Corresponding author R. Brindha:** Department of Computing Technologies, SRM Institute of Science and Technology, Kattankulathur, India; E-mail: brindhar@srmist.edu.in

A. Shankar, Saranya Jayapalan, & Basant. K. Tiwary (Eds.)

improves many aspects of patient care, medical research, and administrative duties in the healthcare industry. NLP is used extensively in clinical documentation and data management, automating the transcription and organization of clinical notes, reducing workloads for medical staff, and enhancing the effectiveness of documentation. NLP also makes it easier to extract data from unstructured clinical documents, such as medical reports and Electronic Health Records (EHRs), which improves data management and retrieval. NLP systems are used in clinical decision support to evaluate enormous volumes of patient data and medical literature to give doctors pertinent information and recommendations based on solid evidence, assisting them in making well-informed decisions. NLP improves healthcare by using predictive analytics to analyze patient records for early diagnosis and individualized treatment strategies. Additionally, it enhances patient engagement *via* chatbots and virtual assistants, which increases patient satisfaction by offering information, resolving queries, and setting up appointments. By evaluating patient feedback and condensing medical research, NLP improves patient care even more, keeping researchers informed and expanding medical knowledge. Furthermore, by guaranteeing conformity to legal requirements, lowering risks, and spotting irregularities in patient data to advance safety and proactive risk management, NLP helps with compliance and risk management. By automating the extraction and structuring of data from unstructured sources like clinical notes and EHRs, NLP integration into healthcare systems greatly improves data management by increasing data accessibility and usability. The analysis of patient data and a wealth of medical literature facilitates better clinical decision-making by offering insightful analysis and suggestions based on solid evidence. By automating data input and documentation procedures, NLP also increases efficiency by lowering administrative responsibilities and freeing healthcare personnel to focus on patient care. Chatbots and virtual assistants with NLP capabilities coordinate appointments, provide information, and answer inquiries, improving patient engagement and increasing treatment plan adherence. NLP also advances research by analyzing large amounts of medical data to detect trends and insights, providing researchers with the most recent findings. Lastly, by guaranteeing regulatory compliance and identifying possible hazards and abnormalities in patient data, NLP supports proactive risk management and compliance while improving patient safety.

A large-scale, cross-sectional, machine-learning-based learning analytics method was applied to conduct a comparative study on neoadjuvant versus adjuvant immunotherapy for perioperative cancer patients. Through data-driven insights obtained *via* informatics analysis, knowledge was improved, treatments were optimized, and innovation was spurred within the medical industry.

Advanced informatics and machine-learning technologies were utilized to harness large-scale global clinical and research datasets, allowing for the extraction and synthesis of high-dimensional information. Neoadjuvant and adjuvant immunotherapy were analyzed in perioperative cancer patient cohorts, and foundational metrological parameters, inherent interrelationships, and temporal evolution across various immunotherapeutic modalities were identified. Key research indicators—such as treatment timing, immune response markers, survival outcomes, and biomarker dynamics—were systematically identified to inform a comparative framework. A data-driven scaffold was established to optimize therapeutic strategies and direct subsequent preclinical and clinical investigations by elucidating parallels and discrepancies among immunotherapy approaches. A large-sample, informatics-driven approach was employed, providing a robust foundation for the refinement of perioperative immunotherapy. Evidence-based optimization of treatment regimens was enabled, and future lines of inquiry in immuno-oncology were forecast [1].

Furthermore, a comprehensive informatics analysis was conducted to map the full scope of Liquid–Liquid Phase Separation (LLPS) research in the context of cancer. This study employed techniques such as hierarchical clustering, regression statistics, hotspot burst analysis, and the Walktrap algorithm to mine a decade of global scientific literature on LLPS in cancer. Informatics analysis in this context is as follows:

- Extracts and organizes unstructured scientific data to reveal research hotspots and development trends.
- Uses machine learning to classify research into dominant clusters and identify emerging areas.
- Highlights key molecular targets and under-explored but promising research directions.
- Maps global collaboration patterns and growth rates in this emerging field. This comprehensive informatics investigation provides a valuable reference for guiding future basic and clinical cancer research by uncovering latent knowledge and predicting promising avenues for exploration.
- Highlights how medical informatics analysis helps turn extensive, complicated biological data into information that can be put to use. Researchers may systematically map research landscapes, find necessary molecular and clinical fingerprints, and predict new trends by using data mining, machine learning, and network analysis methods on clinical and scientific information. This facilitates better decision-making while developing cancer treatments and setting priorities for research [2].

In this context, applying NLP and machine learning in medical informatics must be tailored to handle the unique linguistic complexity, unstructured formats, and privacy constraints. However, the following hypotheses and research questions are subsequently formulated.

How is the comparison of adjuvant and neoadjuvant immunotherapies enhanced by machine learning?

Which necessary research signatures will direct the development of new cancer therapy approaches?

How do informatics techniques highlight links between various immunotherapy modalities?

How can this extensive analysis impact clinical judgment in perioperative cancer care?

Background on NLP and Healthcare Informatics

A subfield of artificial intelligence called natural language processing, or NLP, concerns how computers and human language interact. Text classification, which uses methods like Bag of Words, TF-IDF, and deep learning to categorize text (*e.g.*, spam detection, sentiment analysis), is one of the key NLP technologies. Named Entity Recognition (NER) uses neural networks, statistical models, and rule-based systems to identify entities like names and dates. Text sentiment is measured by sentiment analysis, and text translation uses techniques ranging from rule-based to transformer models, such as GPT-3, to translate text between languages. Text generation uses sophisticated neural networks and transformers to produce coherent text from prompts, speech recognition uses them to translate spoken language into text, and question answering systems use them to answer questions automatically. NLTK, SpaCy, Hugging Face's Transformers, and Stanford NLP are notable Natural Language Processing (NLP) tools used in various applications, such as chatbots and translation services. Healthcare informatics is a field that combines information technology and healthcare to transform patient outcomes and treatment. Clinical Decision Support (CDS) systems assist with diagnosis and treatment decisions, Electronic Health Records (EHRs) assist with comprehensive patient data management, and Health Information Exchange (HIE) enables smooth data sharing amongst healthcare professionals. Remote consultations in telemedicine allow for the extension of care, and data analysis in health analytics provides insights into clinical and operational effectiveness. Patients are given tools to manage their health through Personal Health Records (PHRs), and interoperability ensures that different IT systems can communicate. Data security protects patient privacy and data integrity and is regulated by laws such as GDPR and HIPAA. When taken as a whole, these components improve the standard of treatment, simplify healthcare procedures, and encourage patient participation in their medical journey. Over the years, Natural Language Processing (NLP) in healthcare has changed dramatically. From basic text processing in the 1960s to rule-based systems like MYCIN in the 1970s, NLP has helped diagnose diseases. Statistical techniques like Conditional Random Fields and Hidden Markov Models gained popularity in the 1990s and increased accuracy in tasks like named entity recognition and medical coding. Integrating machine learning in the 21st century improved clinical decision support and the administration of electronic health records. NLP has undergone a revolution thanks to recent developments in deep learning and transformer models like BERT and GPT, which allow for creating and understanding medical language with greater nuance. These developments make automated coding, predictive analytics, and tailored medication possible. However, obstacles like data security, interoperability, and bias reduction must still be addressed if healthcare NLP advances.

Overview of NLP Technologies

Natural Language Processing (NLP), an essential branch of Artificial Intelligence (AI), aims to enable machines to understand, translate, and produce human language. Several significant advancements have defined the development of NLP technologies:

Text Classification: This involves categorizing text documents into predetermined categories. Previous techniques, such as Bag of Words (BoW) and Term Frequency-Inverse Document Frequency (TF-IDF), worked well for more manageable tasks like document classification and spam detection. However, advanced techniques like Convolutional Neural Networks (CNNs) and Recurrent Neural Networks (RNNs) have been developed with the advent of deep learning. These models greatly enhanced the accuracy and adaptability of text categorization tasks, especially when combined with word embeddings such as Word2Vec and GloVe.

Named Entity Recognition (NER): Entity recognition in text (NER) is an important NLP task that involves identifying entities such as people, places, dates, and organizations. Customized features and rule-based techniques were significant components of traditional NER systems. Modern NER systems, on the other hand, use deep learning techniques, such as transformer-based models like BERT, LSTM-CRF models, and Conditional Random Fields (CRFs), which may better capture the context and produce higher accuracy, especially in complicated areas like healthcare.

Sentiment Analysis: This method determines the text's sentiment, whether neutral, positive, or negative. Sentiment analysis is a popular tool for examining social media data about health and patient reviews. Sentiment analysis has evolved from lexicon-based methods to more advanced models that can understand complex linguistic elements like irony and sarcasm, thanks to deep learning models like bi-directional LSTM and attention processes.

Text Translation: Rule-based systems have given way to more complex neural networks, especially sequence-to-sequence models and transformers, in the evolution of machine translation. With its ability to translate text more fluently and accurately, Google's Neural Machine Translation (GNMT) and OpenAI's GPT series are noteworthy innovations. Precise translation of medical records and patient documentation is essential in the healthcare industry, particularly in multilingual and multicultural settings.

Text Generation: Transformer concepts have brought about a revolution in text generation models. GPT-3 and BERT-based text generation models can produce coherent and contextually relevant text based on a prompt. This is very helpful in the healthcare industry for creating patient education materials, clinical summaries, and automated paperwork.

Speech Recognition: The capacity to translate spoken language into text has completely changed clinical procedures. In voice-driven EHRs, Automatic Speech Recognition (ASR) systems driven by deep learning—specifically, RNNs and transformers like DeepSpeech and WaveNet—are utilized to improve clinical documentation efficiency and allow for hands-free operation.

Question Answering Systems: These systems are made to react to user queries automatically by using a provided text or knowledge base. These systems may extract pertinent information from literature or medical records using models like BERT and ALBERT, giving clinicians prompt, correct answers to their questions.

Key Healthcare Informatics Concepts

The multifaceted discipline of healthcare informatics combines computer science, information technology, and healthcare to enhance patient outcomes, simplify operations, and support research.

Electronic Health Records (EHRs): EHRs are electronic versions of paper patient charts. They include all of the patient's information, such as their medical history, diagnosis, prescriptions, plans of care, dates of vaccinations, allergies, radiological pictures, and laboratory test results [3]. The extraction of structured data from unstructured EHRs is a critical function of Natural Language Processing (NLP), which enhances the usability and accessibility of patient data for clinical decision-making.

Clinical Decision Support (CDS): CDS systems give healthcare professionals patient-specific evaluations or suggestions to support clinical decision-making. These systems process large volumes of clinical data using Natural Language

Processing (NLP), which provides insights into patient care, suggests diagnoses, and even proposes therapies based on the most recent research.

Health Information Exchange (HIE): HIE makes sharing patient data easier for various healthcare companies. By standardizing and analyzing data from several sources, NLP technology helps ensure that the data exchanged is accurate, relevant, and usable in multiple healthcare situations.

Telemedicine and Remote Consultations: The field of telemedicine has grown in significance, especially since the COVID-19 pandemic. By processing and analyzing data from online consultations, NLP technologies enable healthcare professionals to deliver high-quality care even when they are not physically present with the patient.

Health Analytics: Data analysis technologies extract knowledge from healthcare data. To assist population health management, operational effectiveness, and predictive analytics, natural language processing (NLP) is used to mine unstructured data, such as research papers and clinical notes [4].

Interoperability and Data Security: The capacity of various healthcare IT systems to successfully communicate and exchange data is called interoperability. NLP contributes to the compatibility and integration of data from several sources into a single system. In the meantime, patient privacy protection depends heavily on data security, which is regulated by laws like GDPR and HIPAA. NLP can help detect and reduce the risks of illegal access or data breaches.

Historical Context and Evolution of NLP in Healthcare

Several significant turning points have occurred in the history of NLP in healthcare:

1990s: A move toward data-driven methodologies was signaled by the advent of statistical models such as Conditional Random Fields (CRFs) and Hidden Markov Models (HMMs). These models made it possible to handle medical language more accurately, which is especially useful for activities where accuracy and consistency are crucial, like NER and medical coding.

2000s: NLP applications significantly advanced due to the integration of machine learning with NLP. During this time, increasingly advanced models that could learn from big datasets were developed, increasing the precision and dependability of NLP tools used in clinical decision-making and EHR management.

2010s: NLP in healthcare transformed with the emergence of transformer models and deep learning. Models such as BERT (Bidirectional Encoder Representations from Transformers) and GPT (Generative Pre-trained Transformer) introduced new levels of understanding and generating capabilities. Numerous healthcare activities, such as automated clinical coding, patient outcome prediction, and clinical text classification, have successfully used these models.

Present and Future: New applications in patient interaction, predictive analytics, and customized medicine are fueled by the continuous breakthroughs in natural language processing. There are still issues with protecting patient privacy, eliminating bias in natural language processing models, and incorporating NLP systems into current healthcare procedures. To overcome these obstacles and fully utilize NLP's potential to enhance patient care, healthcare professionals, legislators, and AI researchers will probably need to work together more closely.

DATA CHALLENGES

In healthcare, data challenges pose significant hurdles to effectively implementing Natural Language Processing (NLP) technologies. These challenges stem from the intrinsic complexity of healthcare data, encompassing issues of quality, privacy, availability, and standardization [5].

Data Quality and Standardization

Data quality and standardization are fundamental to successfully applying Natural Language Processing (NLP) in healthcare. However, the complexity and variability of healthcare data present significant challenges that can hinder the performance and reliability of NLP systems.

Inconsistencies in Medical Terminologies

Within the same facility, doctors frequently use different terms when referring to medical conditions. For instance, under certain situations, "myocardial infarction" may be referred to as "heart attack," "MI," or "acute coronary syndrome". From Fig. (**1**), these variances complicate the standardization and interpretation of medical data. Standardized vocabulary such as SNOMED CT, ICD-10, and LOINC has been extensively adopted to help with this, but consistent usage is still tricky.

The disparities in medical terminology used by different healthcare institutions and practitioners make documenting illnesses, treatments, and prescriptions more difficult. These variances present substantial hurdles for Natural Language

Processing (NLP) systems, which depend on reliable data to understand and analyze text correctly.

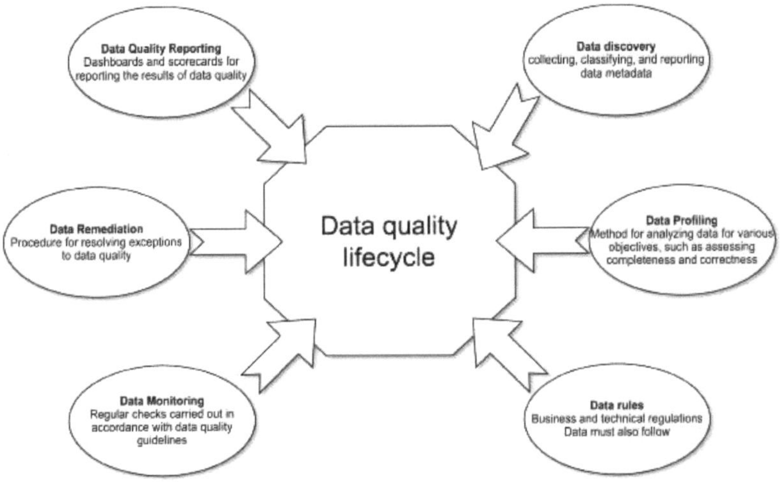
Data Quality Reporting
Dashboards and scorecards for reporting the results of data quality
Data discovery
collecting, classifying, and reporting data metadata
Data Remediation
Procedure for resolving exceptions to data quality
Data quality lifecycle
Data Profiling
Method for analyzing data for various objectives, such as assessing completeness and correctness
Data Monitoring
Regular checks carried out in accordance with data quality guidelines
Data rules
Business and technical regulations Data must also follow

Fig. (1). Data quality lifecycle.

Variability in Data Sources

Electronic Health Records (EHRs) contain structured and unstructured data, such as prescription lists, test results, physician notes, and discharge summaries. The lack of standard formats and differences in data recording procedures make integrating and assessing this data using Natural Language Processing (NLP) tools difficult.

Specifically, the free-text nature of clinical notes can pose significant issues due to the prevalence of acronyms, misspellings, and vocabulary not commonly used by practitioners. "N/V," for example, may indicate "nausea and vomiting," but it can also mean something else depending on the situation. Numerous sources provide healthcare data, such as Electronic Health Records (EHRs), clinician notes, lab results, imaging reports, and patient-reported outcomes. The structure, format, and content of these sources might vary greatly, which makes it difficult for NLP systems to handle and integrate data efficiently.

Normalization: It is crucial to employ strategies like translating disparate terminologies to standardized medical vocabulary. Techniques like the Unified Medical Language System (UMLS) Metathesaurus can help bring disparate medical concepts into one common vocabulary.

Data Quality assessment: To ensure that NLP outputs are reliable, it is essential to implement strong data quality evaluation tools to find and fix inconsistencies in real-time [5].

Data Privacy and Security

Data privacy and security are paramount in healthcare due to the sensitive nature of patient information. Natural Language Processing (NLP) systems, which often process large volumes of personal health data, must navigate a complex landscape of regulatory requirements and technical challenges to protect patient privacy and health data security [6].

Regulatory Requirements

To ensure data security and patient privacy, NLP systems must be designed to handle, store, and share patient data in accordance with these stringent guidelines. This includes safeguarding against unauthorized access and breaches through rigorous security protocols.

Strict privacy regulations apply to healthcare data, such as the Health Insurance Portability and Accountability Act (HIPAA) in the US and the General Data Protection Regulation (GDPR) in Europe. Patient information must be protected according to these standards, and breaking them can have serious consequences.

NLP systems must be built to handle, store, and distribute patient data in compliance with these strict criteria to guarantee data security and patient privacy. Protecting sensitive patient data entails putting strong security measures in place, like encryption and access limits [7].

NLP systems can ensure compliance with privacy regulations and secure patient information by implementing strict security mechanisms that prevent unwanted access and breaches.

Anonymization and De-Identification Challenges

To ensure data security and patient privacy, NLP systems must be designed to handle, store, and share patient data according to these stringent guidelines. This includes safeguarding against unauthorized access and breaches through rigorous security protocols.

To safeguard patient privacy, healthcare data must frequently be anonymized or de-identified before being used for NLP research and applications. Names, addresses, and social security numbers are personal identifiers that must be eliminated or obscured during this process. From Fig. (**2**), even de-identified data can occasionally be re-identified *via* inference attacks or linking to other databases. For example, cases with rare diseases may still be traceable even after using normal anonymization techniques, which makes ensuring total privacy very difficult.

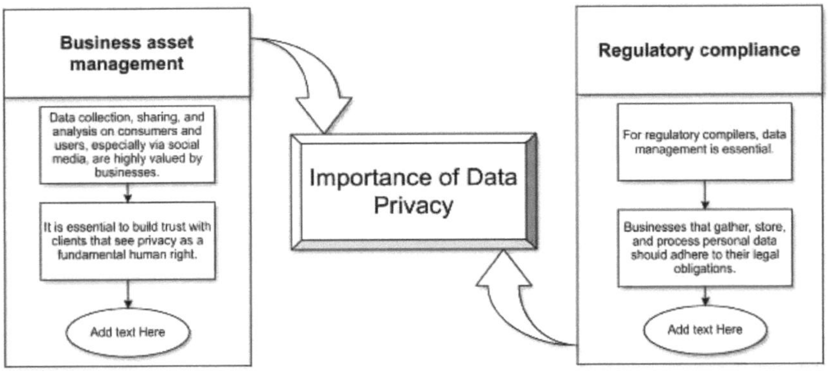

Fig. (2). Importance of data quality.

Advanced De-Identification Methods: Using methods like k-anonymity and differential privacy can reduce the likelihood of re-identification.

A Legal and Ethical Perspective: It is essential to create standards and norms for the moral use of data and regulatory compliance. Speaking with ethicists and legal professionals can help you navigate these obstacles.

Data Availability

Data availability refers to the ease and extent to which data can be accessed, used, and shared by authorized individuals or systems when needed. The following terms are defined in the context of healthcare and NLP:

Accessibility: It refers to whether datasets, particularly large and annotated ones, are available for researchers, developers, and clinicians to use. This includes having access to the right kind of data that is relevant and suitable for the intended NLP tasks.

Sharing: It involves the ability to share data across different institutions, systems, or research teams. Data sharing is often complicated by legal, ethical, and technical barriers, especially when it involves sensitive patient information.

From Fig. (**2**), this aspect refers to the capacity to combine data from different sources, such as various healthcare providers or different types of data (structured and unstructured), into a unified dataset that can be used for analysis.

Limited Access to Large, Annotated Datasets

For NLP systems to train and validate models efficiently, large amounts of annotated data are required. For the purpose of creating precise models, these datasets—which contain text analyzed with important details like relationships, medical entities, and classifications—are crucial. But when it comes to healthcare, these datasets are frequently constrained by strict privacy laws and the high expense of manual annotation.

Although freely accessible datasets such as the MIMIC-III clinical database provide useful information, they might not include all of the real-world clinical data needed for a thorough NLP model construction. The model's capacity to generalize across various patient demographics and medical circumstances may be impacted by this constraint. For NLP applications in healthcare to advance, continued efforts must be made to build more varied and representative annotated datasets.

Issues with Data Sharing and Integration:

Healthcare data is frequently siloed across various institutions and systems, making data sharing and integration challenging. Different Electronic Health Record (EHR) systems often use disparate data formats and standards, complicating merging data from multiple sources [8]. For instance, integrating data from a hospital's EHR system with information from wearable devices or patient-reported outcomes requires extensive efforts in data cleaning, normalization, and standardization. These steps ensure the data is compatible and usable for comprehensive analysis and decision-making.

Interoperability Standards: Promoting the adoption of interoperability standards, such as HL7 FHIR, can facilitate data sharing across different systems and institutions.

Collaborative Data Sharing Initiatives: Encouraging collaborative efforts among healthcare organizations, research institutions, and government agencies can help overcome data availability and sharing challenges. Initiatives like data consortia and public-private partnerships can play a significant role.

LINGUISTIC CHALLENGES

Linguistic challenges are significant in applying Natural Language Processing (NLP) within healthcare. These challenges arise from the complexity and variability of language used in medical contexts, which can significantly impact the performance and reliability of NLP systems. Addressing these challenges requires a deep understanding of the nuances in medical language, ambiguity, and the variability of language across different regions and populations.

Domain-Specific Language

Natural Language Processing (NLP) has particular difficulties when dealing with domain-specific terminology in industries like healthcare, law, finance, and engineering. Some of these difficulties include specialized terminology, acronyms with several meanings, and the ambiguity of terms like "lead" in several settings. Furthermore, traditional NLP techniques cannot effectively comprehend the complicated syntax and semantics of technical descriptions and compound phrases, which call for nuanced comprehension [8]. From Fig. (**3**), the lack of data and the dynamic nature of domain-specific language add to the complexity, requiring constant updates to Natural Language Processing (NLP) models and modifications to new terminologies such as those originating from developing diseases. Named Entity Recognition (NER), essential for healthcare diagnostics applications, struggles to distinguish between concepts with identical names but different meanings.

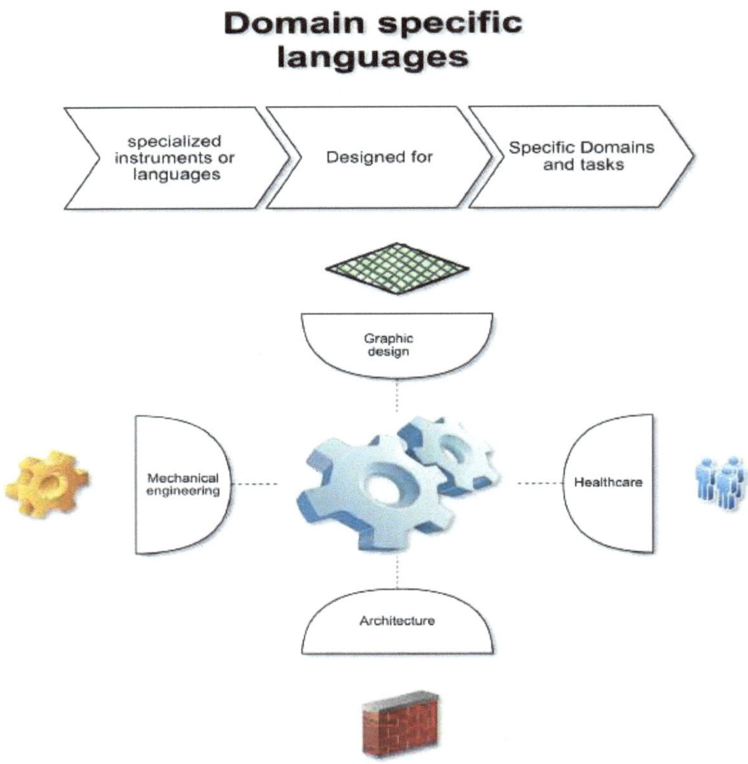

Fig. (3). Domain-specific languages in healthcare.

Specialized Medical Terminology and Jargon

Medical professionals frequently speak in highly technical terms that are unique to both medicine and specific fields of medicine, like neurology, cardiology, or cancer. This terminology is necessary for clear communication, but obstacles may arise when they are translated into other languages or understood differently by professionals from other cultural backgrounds. There could be miscommunication when a term frequently used in one specialization has a different meaning or use in another.

Variability in Language Use Among Different Specialties

Different specialties can use medical terms differently, even within the same language. For example, in dermatology, "lesion" may refer to a different kind of condition than in neurology. The previously mentioned variability may be increased in cross-cultural settings, as disparate linguistic and cultural circumstances impact the interpretation and utilization of medical terminology.

Ambiguity and Polysemy

Due to the difficulty of comprehending words and phrases having numerous meanings, ambiguity and polysemy provide substantial linguistic hurdles for Natural Language Processing (NLP). When a term or phrase has many meanings, such as "bank," which can refer to both a financial organization and the side of a river, ambiguity occurs. Semantic ambiguity refers to different meanings of phrases in context, whereas syntactic ambiguity, such as "I saw the man with the telescope," contains several potential sentence constructions. Polysemy, in which a single word has two or more related meanings (for example, "bat" might refer to a flying animal or a piece of sporting equipment), makes interpretation even more difficult. Advanced contextual knowledge is needed to address these problems, and contemporary NLP models that include contextual embeddings from transformers like BERT and GPT frequently make this possible [9]. Enhancing accuracy requires semantic knowledge bases, domain-specific training, and disambiguation algorithms. To improve NLP systems' capacity to precisely interpret and comprehend human language in various circumstances, ambiguity and polysemy management must be handled effectively.

Challenges with Ambiguous Terms and Phrases

Fig. (**3**) shows several terminologies in medical jargon that can be confusing depending on the context. For instance, in everyday speech, the term "positive" can denote a desirable result. Still, in medical contexts, it frequently denotes sickness, as in the case of a "positive test result." When medical literature is translated or when practitioners with various linguistic backgrounds interpret these phrases, this confusion may cause difficulty.

Contextual Understanding in Medical Texts

Context has a significant role in how medical terminology is understood. A phrase may have more than one meaning (polysemy), and the correct interpretation depends on the context of the surrounding text and the particular medical setting. This can be especially difficult in cross-cultural contexts since cultural differences might affect how words and context are understood. Treatment options may change depending on how the term "crisis" is interpreted in different cultural contexts.

Language Variability

Because language is utilized differently in different circumstances, populations, and geographical areas, linguistic variety poses serious issues for Natural Language Processing (NLP) [9]. Regional slang and dialectal distinctions, such as those between British and American English, bring new vocabulary and idioms that NLP systems might be unable to understand. Interpretation is further complicated by sociolects, which are influenced by social factors such as age and occupation, and distinct registers such as formal and informal language. Complexity is increased, particularly in multilingual settings, by code-switching, the practice of speakers switching between languages or dialects. Furthermore, NLP models must be updated because language changes over time with the emergence of new words and linguistic trends. Adaptive NLP systems are necessary due to the various text formats in many media, including official papers and social media. Although difficult, building representative and diverse annotated corpora is crucial. Using multiple training data, implementing adaptation strategies, creating multilingual models, and routinely upgrading systems to account for linguistic change are some strategies to deal with these problems. By managing language variability well, NLP systems can analyze and comprehend the vast diversity of human language more accurately and inclusively.

Multilingual and Multicultural Issues

It is common for doctors and patients in cross-cultural medical settings not to speak the same first language. This multilingual setting can make communication difficult because medical terminology may not have direct translations in other languages or because cultural variations may affect how medical information is understood and communicated. Communication can be made more difficult by the influence of artistic traditions and beliefs on how symptoms are expressed and treatments are viewed.

Variations in Language Use Across Regions and Populations

How medical vocabulary and concepts are employed varies significantly throughout communities and areas, even within the same language. These differences might cause misconceptions or misinterpretations, primarily when practitioners work across cultural boundaries and may not know local linguistic quirks. Errors in diagnosis or treatment may occur when a phrase regularly used in one location to represent a specific symptom or illness is unfamiliar or has a different meaning in another region [10].

COMPUTATIONAL CHALLENGES

Computational challenges in NLP for healthcare informatics involve the technical difficulties in designing, implementing, and maintaining systems that can efficiently process and analyze vast amounts of complex medical data. These challenges can be broadly categorized into three main areas:

Model Training and Evaluation

Model training and evaluation are central to successfully deploying NLP systems in healthcare. Yet, they present intricate challenges due to the unique characteristics of medical data and tasks. As shown in Fig. (**4**), these challenges include the limitations of existing models for specific medical tasks and the complexity of evaluating model performance in healthcare settings.

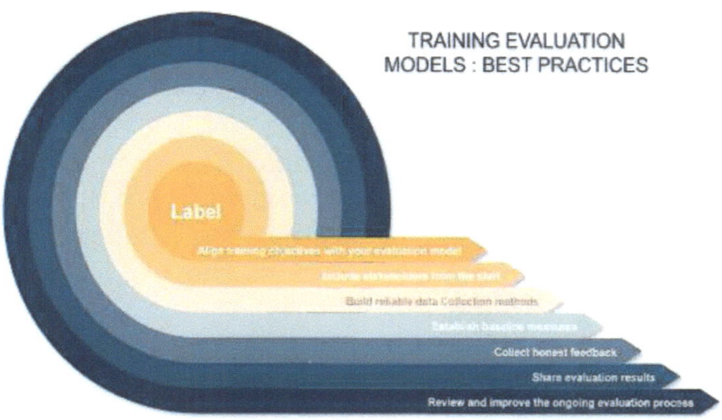

Fig. (4). Training evaluation modules.

Limitations of Existing Models for specific Medical Tasks

General language databases are the leading training source for many Natural Language Processing (NLP) models, including the well-known BERT and GPT models. As a result, they can require extra fine-tuning to function well on particular medical duties. Models must be trained on big, domain-specific datasets that capture every aspect of medical language and context to accurately comprehend and interpret medical texts.

Task-Specific Complexity: Many of the NLP models that are now in use are general-purpose and might not work well for specific medical tasks like reading clinical notes, spotting uncommon illnesses, or forecasting patient outcomes. Medical terminology and domain-specific jargon are complicated, and models need a rich domain knowledge base. For example, a model trained on standard English text would find it difficult to understand a clinical document with many medical jargon, abbreviations, and professional language used by healthcare providers [10].

Scarcity of Annotated Data: The lack of massive, structured data sets in the medical field is another significant barrier that makes it challenging to train high-quality models. In contrast to other domains where labeled data is plentiful, healthcare data is sensitive and frequently unavailable for study owing to privacy issues, making it difficult to build reliable NLP models suited for medical use.

Bias and Generalization Issues: Because of the distinctive features of clinical trials or patient demographics, medical data is frequently skewed, which makes it difficult for models to generalize effectively across various patient populations (Fig. **4**). For instance, because of differences in patient demographics or medical practices, a model trained on data from a particular hospital or region might not function correctly when applied to a different healthcare setting.

Example: Think about the term “cold.” It could refer to a prevalent illness or a low body temperature. A generic NLP model would find it difficult to determine between these meanings in a medical setting. Nevertheless, medical-specific models trained on biomedical literature—such as BioBERT—are more suited to handle these kinds of distinctions with accuracy.

Challenges in Evaluating Model Performance in Healthcare

Because of the complexity and importance of the tasks involved, evaluating NLP models in the healthcare sector presents special challenges. Traditional measurements, such as accuracy, precision, recall, and F1 score, might not fully capture the model's effectiveness in clinical settings.

Defining Appropriate Metrics

Evaluating model performance in the healthcare industry is more complicated and context-specific than typical NLP jobs. The efficacy of a model may not always be fully captured by accuracy, precision, recall, or F1-score in a clinical situation, where false positives and negatives might have serious consequences. It is necessary to consider metrics like cost-effectiveness, patient safety, and improvements in clinical outcomes.

Interpretability and Explainability

Models used in healthcare must be understood in addition to being accurate. Clinicians and other healthcare professionals must comprehend how a model comes to its findings, particularly when those conclusions impact patient care. A significant obstacle in this area is the "black box" character of many deep learning models, which calls for creating interpretable models or tools that may clarify intricate model decisions [11].

Validation and Testing

Thorough validation and testing in actual clinical situations are necessary yet complex. Clinical environments are highly varied, as shown in Fig. (**4**), so to assure reliability and safety, models must be evaluated across various institutions, patient demographics, and clinical scenarios. Furthermore, post-deployment monitoring and updates are necessary to keep models effective over time.

Example: A model may show excellent recall and precision when recognizing medicine names. It can still be insufficient for clinical applications if it lacks crucial details regarding dosage and administration.

Scalability and Efficiency

Scalability and efficiency are critical factors in developing and deploying NLP models in healthcare. These factors directly influence the feasibility of implementing NLP solutions across different healthcare settings, ranging from small clinics to large hospital networks. However, achieving scalability and efficiency presents significant challenges due to the resource-intensive nature of NLP models, the computational requirements, and the need for optimization.

Resource-Intensive Nature of NLP Models

Modern NLP models, intensive learning models, demand significant computing power for training and inference. Their application in real-time clinical settings, where resources may be few, may be hampered by this demand [11, 12].

Computational Costs

Primary computational resources are needed for training big NLP models, intense learning models like BERT or GPT. These resources include enormous memory, storage capabilities, and high-performance GPUs or TPUs. Because of this, many healthcare organizations—especially the smaller ones—find it challenging to create or implement cutting-edge NLP solutions.

Time and Energy Consumption

Large models may require weeks or even months to train, using a lot of energy that is expensive and environmentally problematic. This difficulty is exacerbated by the requirement for regular model updates to incorporate fresh data and medical knowledge, making repetitive, computationally intensive training procedures necessary.

Example: Not every healthcare facility has the financial means to set aside several days for the intensive training of a BERT model on high-end GPUs. From Fig. (**5**), the substantial resource requirements further impact energy usage and operating costs.

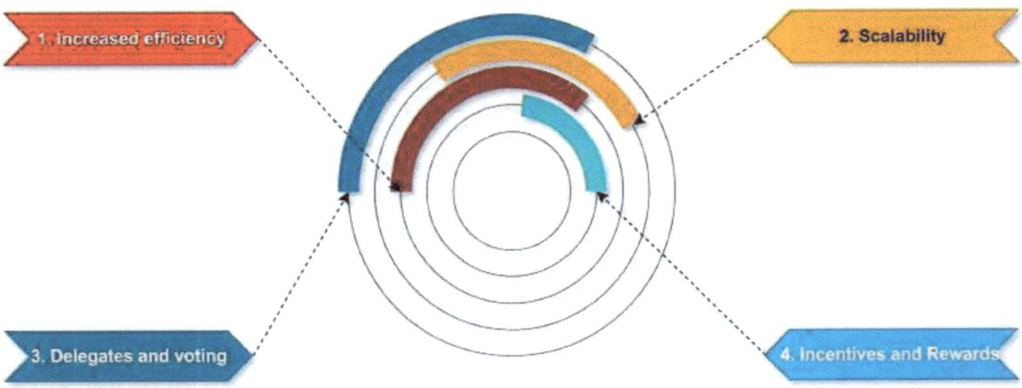

Fig. (5). Enhancing efficiency and scalability.

Computational Requirements and Optimization

A careful trade-off between accuracy and computing efficiency must be made when optimizing NLP models for healthcare applications. From Fig. (**5**), model-pruning, quantization, and distillation are popular methods for increasing speed and reducing model size without significantly compromising performance.

Efficient Algorithms

More effective algorithms that can provide comparable performance with less computing cost are required to solve the scalability problem. Model pruning, quantization, and distillation are a few methods being investigated to help minimize the size and complexity of models without compromising their accuracy.

Distributed Computing

Distributed computing frameworks can help manage the computational load by parallelizing tasks across multiple machines. Nevertheless, this methodology presents novel obstacles concerning synchronization, data consistency, and the effective management of extensive datasets dispersed among various nodes.

Cloud-Based Solutions

By providing a scalable substitute, cloud computing enables healthcare providers to have on-demand access to high-performance computing resources. However, caution must be exercised when handling issues with data protection, HIPAA compliance, and possible reliance on outside service providers.

Example: From Fig. (**5**), model pruning can reduce model size and increase inference speed by eliminating less essential neurons from a neural network. This technique is helpful when implementing NLP models on mobile devices or edge servers in healthcare settings.

Integration with Existing Systems

Integrating Natural Language Processing (NLP) solutions into existing healthcare systems presents several challenges that can affect the success and efficiency of these technologies. While NLP has the potential to revolutionize healthcare by improving clinical decision-making, automating administrative tasks, and enhancing patient care, integrating these solutions into the complex ecosystem of healthcare technology is a significant undertaking.

Challenges in Incorporating NLP Solutions into Clinical Workflows

Electronic Health Record (EHR) systems and other healthcare IT infrastructure must seamlessly integrate NLP technologies into current clinical procedures. This entails ensuring that NLP tools are compatible with the many workflow protocols, user interfaces, and data formats that healthcare practitioners employ.

Workflow Disruption

Integrating NLP technology into clinical workflows without interfering with day-to-day operations is a significant difficulty. From Fig. (**6**), healthcare workers are notoriously resistant to change, especially when implementing new technologies that necessitate substantial alterations to their well-established practices. It is imperative to ensure that NLP technologies enhance current procedures rather than make them more difficult.

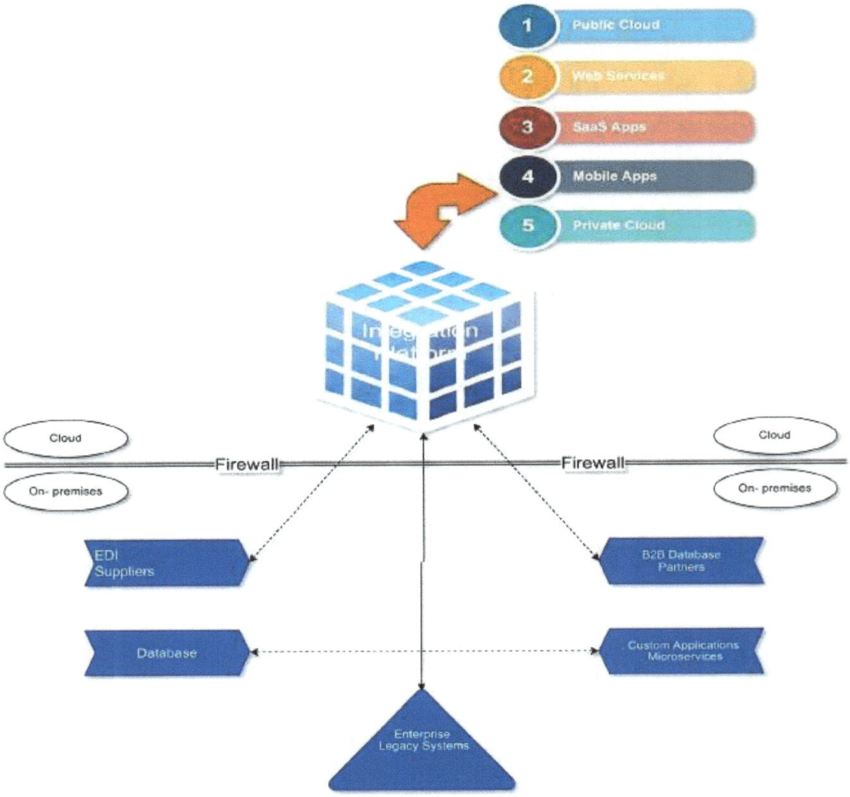

Fig. (6). Integration with existing systems.

Training and Adoption

Healthcare providers must have sufficient training to utilize NLP technologies effectively. In addition to technical training, this entails ensuring providers know the advantages and constraints of NLP systems. Furthermore, adoption rates can be sluggish, particularly when the benefits are not immediately apparent.

Example: An NLP tool intended to help with clinical documentation must link with the hospital's EHR system to automatically extract and input pertinent data from clinicians' notes. This integration must guarantee data consistency and an intuitive interface to prevent clinician workflow interference.

Interoperability with Other Healthcare Technologies

Achieving interoperability between diverse healthcare technologies is essential to effectively implementing NLP systems. This entails following guidelines like HL7 FHIR (Fast Healthcare Interoperability Resources) for easy data transfer across various devices and systems.

Data Standardization and Compatibility

Maintaining interoperability with many Clinical Decision Support Systems (CDSS), Electronic Health Record (EHR) systems, and other healthcare IT infrastructure is one of the most challenging tasks when combining NLP with current technology. From Fig. (**6**), Seamless integration is complex because various systems frequently employ disparate coding standards, vocabularies, and data formats.

APIs and Middleware

It is crucial to provide reliable middleware and APIs (Application Programming Interfaces) that may connect NLP applications to current healthcare systems. These tools must process data in real time and ensure NLP outputs are contextualized and correctly written for use in other systems.

Regulatory Compliance

All systems, including the NLP solutions, must comply with the GDPR and HIPAA standards about healthcare as part of integration efforts. This also entails secure data transfer, storage, and access controls to preserve patient confidentiality and data integrity.

Example: To link textual data with lab findings, an NLP system that extracts patient information from clinical notes needs to integrate with the hospital's Laboratory Information System (LIS). Respecting interoperability standards is necessary to guarantee accurate and fast data sharing. By resolving these computational obstacles, NLP systems can be more successfully used in healthcare settings, increasing their usefulness and influence on clinical outcomes and patient care.

ETHICAL AND SOCIAL IMPLICATIONS

Though applying Natural Language Processing (NLP) to information technology for healthcare presents promising new opportunities, it also raises moral and social problems that require careful thought. The essential topics of bias and justice, openness and explainability, and the effect on medical professionals are all covered in this section.

Bias and Fairness

Healthcare could change thanks to Natural Language Processing (NLP), which can automate processes including decision support, patient communication, and clinical documentation. However, NLP integration into healthcare systems brings up serious issues with fairness and prejudice that may harm patient treatment. This research examines the concerns of biased results in NLP applications and how they affect different patient populations.

Risks of Biased Outcomes in NLP applications

When biased Natural Language Processing (NLP) models are trained on datasets that do not fairly reflect a range of demographic groups, it can lead to significant discrepancies in diagnosis and treatment. A model may find it difficult to diagnose patients who do not fit into that demographic appropriately or to understand symptoms when it is mainly based on data from that cohort. When members of underrepresented groups receive either ineffective or unsuitable care for their particular requirements, it can result in unequal healthcare outcomes. For instance, a symptom frequently linked to a specific ailment in one population may be disregarded or misread in another, resulting in inaccurate diagnosis and perhaps detrimental treatment regimens. These discrepancies are especially alarming in the medical field, where a proper diagnosis and course of treatment can mean the difference between life and death.

Furthermore, the misunderstanding issue may be made worse by the biases included in the training data and the intrinsic intricacy of medical terminology. There are significant differences in medical terminology among various linguistic or cultural groupings; therefore, it is not universal. For example, terms or expressions widely used in one community may be utterly foreign to another. An NLP model may misread the symptoms or diseases reported by patients from different backgrounds if trained on a broad enough dataset to identify these variations. This misconception can harm a patient's health and well-being, including inaccurate diagnoses, postponed treatment, or even disregarding the patient's complaints.

The existence of bias in NLP models presents serious ethical and legal issues in addition to technical and therapeutic ones. Ethically, the essential values of justice and equality in medical practice are compromised by the employment of biased models. The justice of the healthcare system as a whole is called into question when biased algorithms routinely disadvantage particular groups. Furthermore, these prejudices may put healthcare organizations and practitioners at legal jeopardy. Legal difficulties, including litigation and regulatory fines, may befall healthcare providers if biased NLP systems lead to discriminatory behaviors or injure patients. This emphasizes how crucial it is to guarantee that NLP models used in healthcare are equitable, transparent, and accountable in addition to being technically sound. To safeguard patient rights and provide fair healthcare outcomes for all people, regardless of their origin or features, addressing bias in NLP is not only a technical problem but also a moral and legal responsibility.

Impact on Diverse Patient Populations

Biased Natural Language Processing (NLP) applications in the medical field significantly affect several essential domains. First of all, when NLP models ignore language variety, underrepresented groups' access to high-quality healthcare is jeopardized. For example, models not sufficiently trained to comprehend variants such as African American Vernacular English (AAVE) may misread patients' symptoms, resulting in treatment errors or delays.

Second, when prejudiced NLP systems reinforce unjust treatment judgments, patient-provider trust is weakened. For historically oppressed populations already on the defensive against healthcare inequities resulting from historical injustices, this erosion of trust is particularly harmful [9].

Thirdly, by possibly overlooking early indicators of illnesses common in particular communities, biased NLP models worsen health inequities. Over time, this oversight may lead to worse health outcomes and more significant public health issues.

Furthermore, patients may experience psychological and social suffering if biased NLP outputs reinforce stereotypes or stigmas. Inaccurate correlations between diseases or habits and specific demographic groups might lower patient self-esteem and discourage people from getting the care they need.

Finally, biased NLP has important policy and public health ramifications. Biased data-driven decision-making can reinforce structural injustices by resulting in insufficient resource allocation and actions that fall short of meeting the varied needs of communities, especially those already marginalized.

To address these problems, NLP models must be rigorously tested for biases and made inclusive, accurate, and morally sound to support fair healthcare outcomes and patient care.

Transparency and Explainability

Transparency and explainability are crucial aspects of NLP in healthcare informatics, as they address how models make decisions and ensure that their outputs are trustworthy and actionable. Here is how these challenges fit into the broader computational challenges section:

Need for Interpretability of NLP Systems in Healthcare

Interpretability is essential to promote openness and confidence in using Natural Language Processing (NLP) systems in the healthcare industry. Healthcare professionals evaluate the validity and applicability of these insights in clinical decision-making by comprehending how NLP systems produce diagnostic and therapy suggestions. Transparency in healthcare facilitates the effective communication of complex medical information to patients, which is crucial for patient-centered treatment and improves clinical accuracy. Interpretable Natural Language Processing (NLP) technologies enable patients to actively engage in their treatment plans and respect their right to understand the process through which healthcare decisions are made [10].

Furthermore, interpretability is necessary for healthcare systems to meet strict regulatory requirements that demand accountability and openness from medical decision support technologies. Healthcare organizations comply with these regulations, protecting patient welfare and upholding their procedures' legal integrity by ensuring comprehensible NLP systems. Therefore, as shown in Fig. (**5**), adding interpretability to NLP systems improves clinical processes and patient interaction while guaranteeing ethical and legal compliance, raising the standard and reliability of healthcare delivery overall.

Balancing Automation with Human Oversight

To minimize dangers and optimize possible advantages, a careful balance between automation and human oversight is required to effectively deploy Natural Language Processing (NLP) in the healthcare industry. Tasks like clinical documentation and information extraction from Electronic Health Records (EHRs) are made much more efficient by Natural Language Processing (NLP) because of its capacity to automate the study of massive amounts of unstructured medical data. While this automation makes data processing more efficient, clinical validation still requires human monitoring. To guarantee that NLP-generated insights are correctly suited to patient-specific circumstances and are in line with accepted medical procedures, healthcare professionals are essential. The ability of doctors to recognize and address biases or mistakes in NLP outputs that can harm patient care makes this supervision crucial to risk management as well.

Furthermore, human oversight guarantees that patient privacy, consent, and other ethical requirements are respected in NLP-driven healthcare solutions. Moral issues are of the utmost importance. Clinicians must handle equity, prejudice, and patient autonomy concerns, ensuring these systems function within ethical bounds. Finally, because algorithm development is iterative and driven by clinician feedback, this balance supports the ongoing enhancement of NLP systems. Automation and human knowledge continue to work together to improve NLP's interpretability, accuracy, and general efficacy in healthcare, guaranteeing that these technologies improve clinical effectiveness and protect patient safety and moral integrity.

Impact on Healthcare Professionals

The impact of NLP technologies on healthcare professionals is multifaceted, influencing their workflow, decision-making, and interactions with patients. Here is how the challenges in NLP, including transparency and explainability, affect healthcare professionals:

Effects on Clinical Decision-Making

Natural language processing, or NLP, can change clinical decision-making by improving healthcare delivery's efficacy, precision, and efficiency. The speed and efficiency with which NLP can process enormous volumes of medical data are among its most important applications. Healthcare workers can now access, evaluate, and understand vast amounts of unstructured data—including patient records, clinical notes, and medical literature—much more quickly than done manually. NLP has the potential to significantly increase diagnostic accuracy and aid in the development of more successful treatment programs by offering detailed insights and recommendations derived from this extensive study. This is especially helpful when combining many data sources in complicated circumstances, which can help doctors make more accurate and well-informed recommendations.

Additionally, NLP makes healthcare facilities more efficient by automating repetitive procedures that would otherwise take much time. NLP, for example, may automatically extract pertinent data from Electronic Health Records (EHRs), saving clinicians the laborious task of manually sorting through patient data. In addition to streamlining processes, this automation relieves healthcare providers of some of their administrative workload, freeing them up for patient care. Consequently, mundane and repetitive duties are done by NLP systems, allowing physicians to concentrate on the human elements of healthcare, such as patient engagement, empathy, and individualized treatment.

Beyond effectiveness and precision, NLP has a direct impact on patient outcomes. The application of NLP contributes to evidence-based medicine, which bases clinical choices on the most up-to-date and comprehensive data possible, by enabling faster and more dependable access to pertinent patient information. This lowers the possibility of medical errors and raises the standard of care overall by allowing more accurate and prompt interventions. For instance, in an emergency, NLP's quick analysis and presentation of vital information can save lives by empowering medical professionals to act quickly and intelligently. When these advances in decision-making are combined, patient outcomes can be considerably improved over time. Treatment plans can be customized to meet patients' unique requirements and circumstances.

In summary, by enhancing decision support, optimizing processes, and enhancing patient outcomes, incorporating Natural Language Processing (NLP) into healthcare systems revolutionizes clinical decision-making. Natural Language Processing (NLP) is expected to play a more significant role in healthcare as technology advances. NLP will drive innovations that improve care effectiveness, efficiency, and customization across various medical specialties.

NLP systems can significantly impact healthcare decision-making by offering appropriate data and insights gained from massive volumes of data. But there is a chance that doctors will become overly dependent on these tools, which could impair their ability to think critically and diagnose patients. NLP systems must be designed to supplement, not to replace, clinical judgment.

Potential Shifts in Job Roles and Responsibilities

The introduction of Natural Language Processing (NLP) in healthcare significantly reshapes job roles and responsibilities among healthcare professionals. As NLP tools become more integrated into clinical practice, healthcare providers must adapt to and utilize these technologies effectively. This involves understanding how to interpret NLP-generated insights and integrating them into established clinical workflows. Despite the automation of data analysis by NLP systems, human oversight remains crucial for interpreting results and validating them against clinical expertise. This shift necessitates more engagement from clinicians in reviewing and verifying NLP outputs for accuracy and relevance. Furthermore, adopting NLP underscores the need for continuous learning and professional development, as healthcare professionals must stay updated with technological advancements and best practices.

A new professional path may be opened for those specializing in NLP-driven analytics or supporting the use of these technologies in clinical settings. Given the growing reliance on NLP, a greater understanding of ethical guidelines and their implications for patient care and professional responsibilities is also necessary for healthcare professionals. These moral considerations include patient privacy, consent, and responsible technology use.

Work roles and responsibilities may also be modified using NLP in the healthcare industry. There are worries about job displacement due to the potential automation of several functions that healthcare professionals have historically undertaken. However, NLP can also provide doors for professionals to take on more challenging and fulfilling work. For instance, doctors may devote more time to direct patient treatment, teaching, and research, and less time to administrative tasks.

CASE STUDIES

Through case studies, we explore practical uses of Natural Language Processing (NLP) in the healthcare industry in this section. These illustrations show how NLP can revolutionize clinical documentation, provider-patient communication, and medical research.

NLP in Clinical Documentation

The application of Natural Language Processing (NLP) is growing to improve the accuracy and efficiency of clinical documentation. An outline of NLP's use in this field is provided below, along with instances of systems that are used to analyze and transcribe clinical notes:

Example of NLP Systems for Transcribing and Interpreting Clinical Notes

Automated Clinical Note Transcription: Dragon Medical One

Nuance Communications' well-known NLP technology, Dragon Medical One, automatically transcribes clinical notes. Instead of transcribing their notes by hand, healthcare workers can now dictate their notes thanks to this system that translates spoken words into text.

Features

Speech Recognition: Dragon Medical One precisely translates physician speech into text using cutting-edge speech recognition technology, picking up on subtleties in medical jargon and intricate expressions.

Customization: It improves transcription accuracy by providing vocabulary and templates that may be adjusted to suit particular medical specialties and practice requirements.

Integration: The technology allows for the direct entry of transcribed notes into patient records by smoothly integrating them with Electronic Health Records (EHRs).

Advantages

Efficiency: Frees up more time for patient treatment by minimizing the time professionals must spend on documentation.

Preserves consistency in the structure of clinical notes and reduces errors.

NLP for Patient-Provider Communication

By utilizing chatbots and AI-powered assistants to expedite encounters, boost patient engagement, and optimize healthcare delivery, Natural Language Processing (NLP) is transforming communication between patients and providers [10]. An overview of how these technologies are being used in healthcare settings is provided here:

Use Cases of Chatbots and Virtual Assistants in Healthcare Settings

<u>Checking and Prioritizing Symptoms: Ada Health</u>

Ada Health offers a chatbot that checks symptoms and walks users through the triage procedure using Natural Language Processing (NLP).

Qualities

Symptom Assessment: Ada Health's chatbot inquires about its users' symptoms and medical background, then uses Natural Language Processing (NLP) to analyze the answers to generate a preliminary assessment.

Advice: The chatbot provides suggestions for the next course of action based on the evaluation. These suggestions may include calling a doctor, visiting a clinic, or caring for symptoms at home.

Integration: Ada Health integrates with other healthcare systems to assist patients toward the best course of care.

Advantages

Accessibility: Offers patients prompt support in comprehending their signs and possible ailments.

Efficiency: Facilitates efficient patient flow management and case prioritization for healthcare practitioners by streamlining the triage process.

NLP in Medical Research

Through its ability to make scientific literature and research data easier to analyze, natural language processing, or NLP, is a vital component of medical research advancement. An outline of its uses in different domains is provided below:

Applications in Analyzing Scientific Literature and Research Data

<u>NLP Tools in PubMed for the Analysis of Scientific Literature</u>

Researchers may navigate and evaluate many scientific publications using Natural Language Processing (NLP) technologies using PubMed, a premier medical literature database.

Applications

Literature mining: From millions of academic papers, NLP algorithms extract pertinent data, including crucial discoveries, techniques, and trends.

Research topics and emerging trends are identified and categorized using topic modeling tools, which help researchers find pertinent studies. These tools examine textual data.

Semantic search: Natural Language Processing (NLP) improves search performance by interpreting the meaning and context of user questions, leading to more accurate literature searches.

Advantages

Efficiency: Organizes and extracts pertinent data automatically, which expedites the literature review process.

Finding hidden patterns and trends in scientific literature through insight generation helps researchers make informed decisions about their next course of study.

FUTURE DIRECTIONS AND RESEARCH OPPORTUNITIES

Emerging technologies and trends in Natural Language Processing (NLP) are opening up new avenues for creative applications in the medical field. Several potential future directions and study areas are becoming more and more pertinent as the subject develops. Below is a summary of these elements:

Emerging Trends and Technologies in NLP

Emerging trends and technologies in NLP are rapidly advancing the field, offering new possibilities and addressing existing challenges.

Advances in Deep Learning and Transformer Models

The performance of NLP systems has been dramatically enhanced by recent developments in deep learning, especially the creation of transformer models such as BERT (Bidirectional Encoder Representations from Transformers) and GPT (Generative Pre-trained Transformer). These models are excellent at understanding context and meaning, which makes them perfect for complex tasks like automatic patient record summarization, clinical language comprehension, and the extraction of relevant information from unstructured data.

Integration of Multimodal Data

Integrating multimodal data—text combined with additional data types, including photos, genetic information, and physiological signals—will probably be a significant component of NLP in the healthcare industry in the future. A comprehensive approach helps improve the precision of diagnoses and individual treatment programs. For instance, NLP systems could provide complete insights into patient situations by correlating clinical notes with genomic sequences or imaging data.

Explainable AI (XAI) and Trustworthy NLP

Explainable AI (XAI) is becoming increasingly critical as NLP systems become more complex, ensuring that healthcare practitioners can understand and depend on the judgments and predictions made by these systems.

This characteristic will help NLP models become more widely used in clinical settings by producing clear, easy-to-understand outputs.

Potential Areas for Further Research

Identifying potential areas for further research in NLP, especially within the context of healthcare informatics, can guide the development of new technologies and methodologies.

Handling Bias and Ensuring Fairness

It is still essential to conduct research in the field of selectivity in NLP systems. Developing techniques to identify and reduce biases in training data and algorithms should be the main emphasis of future research. Scholars may investigate methods like bias reviews, adversarial training, and fairness-aware learning to develop more equitable NLP systems that function effectively for various patient populations.

Enhancing Contextual Understanding

Enhancing NLP systems' understanding of context is yet another crucial area for research. This involves developing models that can precisely understand clinical language quirks, including informal phrases, acronyms, and distinct terminology employed by various medical professionals. Improving contextual comprehension will raise the precision and dependability of NLP uses in medical settings.

Personalization and Adaptability

Another potential research area is developing NLP systems that are customized and adaptive to specific patients and healthcare environments. To improve the relevance and efficacy of NLP models, personalization involves adapting them to particular patient demographics, medical specializations, and clinical workflows. Adaptive systems constantly learn and update their knowledge base with fresh information to stay up to speed on the newest medical findings and procedures.

Collaborations Between NLP Researchers and Healthcare Professionals

Collaboration between NLP researchers and healthcare professionals is essential for developing effective and practical NLP solutions in healthcare.

Interdisciplinary Research Teams

Researchers studying Natural Language Processing (NLP) and healthcare practitioners must work closely to apply NLP in healthcare successfully. NLP specialists, data scientists, and clinicians working together in interdisciplinary research teams can guarantee that the creation and application of NLP systems align with clinical requirements and procedures. These groups can collaborate to find pertinent clinical issues, select excellent training data, and confirm the effectiveness of NLP applications in practical contexts.

Shared Datasets and Open Research

Large-scale annotated dataset creation and sharing are essential to advancing NLP research in the medical field. The research community benefits from initiatives such as the National NLP Clinical Challenges (n2c2) and the Medical Information Mart for Intensive Care (MIMIC) database. Through collaborative efforts, open research, and data sharing can accelerate the development of robust NLP systems and promote innovation.

Continuous Education and Training

Healthcare practitioners must participate in ongoing education and training programs regarding the applications and constraints of NLP technologies. Healthcare professionals can more effectively use NLP technologies in their workflows by being aware of how they operate and how they might affect clinical practice. Furthermore, continuing education can assist professionals in staying current with NLP best practices and breakthroughs.

CONCLUSION

For healthcare informatics, NLP has transforming power; it improves clinical documentation, simplifies patient-provider interactions, and speeds medical research. Healthcare systems can significantly reduce the administrative load on medical practitioners and free them to concentrate more on patient care by including NLP technologies to automate the transcription of clinical notes and extract relevant information from extensive unstructured data. Moreover, by offering real-time, practical insights, NLP helps to promote clinical decision-making and advanced patient involvement. However, if NLP is to be completely fair and effective, it is imperative to solve issues of bias, justice, and the inclusion of new technologies in current healthcare systems. Harnessing the full potential of NLP in transforming healthcare practices depends on coordinated efforts by NLP academics and healthcare practitioners, together with continuous developments in explainable artificial intelligence.

REFERENCES

[1] S.B. Guo, L.S. Hu, W.J. Huang, Z.Z. Zhou, H.Y. Luo, and X.P. Tian, "Comparative investigation of neoadjuvant immunotherapy *versus* adjuvant immunotherapy in perioperative patients with cancer: a global-scale, cross-sectional, and large-sample informatics study", *Int. J. Surg.,* vol. 110, no. 8, pp. 4660-4671, 2024.
[http://dx.doi.org/10.1097/JS9.0000000000001479] [PMID: 38652128]

[2] S.B. Guo, X.Z. Feng, W.J. Huang, Z.Z. Zhou, and X.P. Tian, "Global research hotspots, development trends and prospect discoveries of phase separation in cancer: a decade-long informatics investigation", *Biomark. Res.,* vol. 12, no. 1, p. 39, 2024.
[http://dx.doi.org/10.1186/s40364-024-00587-9] [PMID: 38627840]

[3] A.L. Beam, and I.S. Kohane, "Big data and machine learning in health care", *JAMA,* vol. 319, no. 13, pp. 1317-1318, 2018.
[http://dx.doi.org/10.1001/jama.2017.18391] [PMID: 29532063]

[4] I.Y. Chen, S. Joshi, M. Ghassemi, and K.P. Liao, "Ethical machine learning in health care", *Annu. Rev. Biomed. Data Sci.,* vol. 3, pp. 123-144, 2020.
[http://dx.doi.org/10.1146/annurev-biodatasci-092820-114757]

[5] J. Devlin, M.W. Chang, K. Lee, and K. Toutanova, "BERT: Pre-training of deep bidirectional transformers for language understanding", *Proceedings of the 2019 Conference of the North American Chapter of the Association for Computational Linguistics: Human Language Technologies,* vol. Volume 1, 2019pp. 4171-4186

[6] K. Ferryman, and M. Pitcan, *Fairness in Precision Medicine.,* 2018. https://datasociety.net/output/fairness-in-precision-medicine/

[7] M.A. Gianfrancesco, S. Tamang, J. Yazdany, and G. Schmajuk, "Potential biases in machine learning algorithms using electronic health record data", *JAMA Intern. Med.,* vol. 178, no. 11, pp. 1544-1547, 2018.
[http://dx.doi.org/10.1001/jamainternmed.2018.3763] [PMID: 30128552]

[8] F. Jiang, Y. Jiang, H. Zhi, Y. Dong, H. Li, S. Ma, Y. Wang, Q. Dong, H. Shen, and Y. Wang, "Artificial intelligence in healthcare: past, present and future", *Stroke Vasc. Neurol.,* vol. 2, no. 4, pp. 230-243, 2017.
[http://dx.doi.org/10.1136/svn-2017-000101] [PMID: 29507784]

[9] A.E.W. Johnson, T.J. Pollard, L. Shen, L.H. Lehman, M. Feng, M. Ghassemi, B. Moody, P. Szolovits, L. Anthony Celi, and R.G. Mark, "MIMIC-III, a freely accessible critical care database", *Sci. Data,* vol. 3, no. 1, 2016.160035
[http://dx.doi.org/10.1038/sdata.2016.35] [PMID: 27219127]

[10] Y. Liu, P.H.C. Chen, J. Krause, and L. Peng, "How to read articles that use machine learning", *JAMA,* vol. 322, no. 18, pp. 1806-1816, 2019.
[http://dx.doi.org/10.1001/jama.2019.16489] [PMID: 31714992]

[11] S.M. McKinney, M. Sieniek, V. Godbole, J. Godwin, N. Antropova, H. Ashrafian, T. Back, M. Chesus, G.S. Corrado, A. Darzi, M. Etemadi, F. Garcia-Vicente, F.J. Gilbert, M. Halling-Brown, D. Hassabis, S. Jansen, A. Karthikesalingam, C.J. Kelly, D. King, J.R. Ledsam, D. Melnick, H. Mostofi, L. Peng, J.J. Reicher, B. Romera-Paredes, R. Sidebottom, M. Suleyman, D. Tse, K.C. Young, J. De Fauw, and S. Shetty, "International evaluation of an AI system for breast cancer screening", *Nature,* vol. 577, no. 7788, pp. 89-94, 2020.
[http://dx.doi.org/10.1038/s41586-019-1799-6] [PMID: 31894144]

[12] E.J. Topol, "High-performance medicine: the convergence of human and artificial intelligence", *Nat. Med.,* vol. 25, no. 1, pp. 44-56, 2019.
[http://dx.doi.org/10.1038/s41591-018-0300-7] [PMID: 30617339]

CHAPTER 3

Deep Learning Techniques for Medical Text Analysis

L. Sankar Ganesh[1,*] and **P. Mohan Kumar**[1]

[1] *School of Computer Science and Engineering, Vellore Institute of Technology, Vellore, India*

Abstract: Medical text analysis is critical to healthcare delivery because it allows for extracting important data from electronic health records, clinical notes, and medical literature. Traditional NLP techniques are frequently limited by the complexity and volume of medical language. Because deep learning techniques offer sophisticated methods that outperform conventional approaches, they have revolutionized this field. Models such as convolutional neural networks and recurrent neural networks play a key role. These models' capacity to concentrate on pertinent text is further improved by attention mechanisms. This paper examines these methods, emphasizing their uses and advantages for enhancing patient care and furthering medical research. Along with these issues, the chapter also discusses the difficulties specific to medical text analysis, including protecting patient privacy, enhancing model interpretability, and utilizing domain expertise. By looking at these areas, we show how important deep learning is for advancing medical text analysis and overcoming conventional constraints.

Keywords: Deep learning, Electronic health records, Healthcare informatics, Medical text analysis, Natural language processing.

INTRODUCTION

The healthcare industry has recently experienced an explosion of data in the form of electronic health records, clinical notes, and medical publications. EHRs may contain structured data, such as diagnoses, lab reports, *etc*. While clinical notes are essentially unstructured, text-based documents created by physicians, they contain narrative text, which introduces challenges mainly because of variations in medical terminology and abbreviations and the lack of semantic meaning [1]. The complexity of medical language makes expressions more challenging as they use many abbreviations with different definitions for the same abbreviation. Traditional methods, such as rule-based NLP, struggle with these challenges and produce inefficiencies while extracting valuable insights from that data [1, 2].

* **Corresponding author L. Sankar Ganesh:** School of Computer Science and Engineering, Vellore Institute of Technology, Vellore, India; E-mail: sankarganesh.l2023@vitstudent.ac.in

Deep learning techniques have emerged as a more advanced solution, capable of identifying complex patterns and understanding context more effectively than traditional models, which often struggle with these limitations. This would enhance accuracy in interpreting medical text and thus support clinical decisions, research, and health management [3]. Recent DL research has dramatically transformed NLP, opening up possibilities to analyze large-scale unstructured text more effectively. Approaches like CNNs, RNNs, and transformer-based models such as BERT have shown exceptional effectiveness in medical text analysis, enhancing accuracy and processing efficiency. In this chapter, we review these DL methods and their applications in medical text analysis with experimental validation of their effectiveness.

Background

Natural Language Processing in Healthcare

Natural language processing has become an essential tool in healthcare, addressing the challenges associated with unstructured medical data and improving data analysis and interpretation. By enabling computers to comprehend and interpret human language, NLP bridges the gap between traditional data analysis methods and the vast, unstructured information in patient records, clinical notes, and research articles. Applications of NLP in healthcare are far-reaching. It can automate administrative tasks like coding and abstracting medical records, reducing the burden on healthcare providers and improving documentation accuracy [4]. Additionally, NLP aids in clinical decision-making by analyzing patient data to identify patterns, predict outcomes, and inform diagnosis and treatment. Furthermore, NLP enhances biomedical research by retrieving valuable insights from medical literature, discovering new drug targets, and deepening the understanding of disease mechanisms. The healthcare industry has traditionally relied on statistical machine-learning techniques and rule-based systems for NLP applications [3]. However, these approaches face challenges due to the ambiguity, specialized terminology, and context-dependence of medical language. The complexity and nuances of medical language often hinder the accuracy of traditional NLP systems.

Deep Learning Approaches

Deep learning, a subset of machine learning that utilizes artificial neural networks, has contributed significantly to advancements in artificial intelligence, particularly in NLP. Unlike traditional techniques that require manual feature extraction, deep learning models can automatically identify and learn intricate data patterns. Initially, neural networks such as *"RNNs," "LSTMs,"* and *"CNNs"* were implemented for medical text analysis, providing a foundation for more advanced deep learning models [5]. However, transformer models like BERT have revolutionized the field by delivering contextualized word embeddings that understand the meaning and structure of medical language. BioBERT and ClinicalBERT are BERT-based models. They are particularly successful in specific medical terminology because they are pre-trained in biomedical and clinical texts. These models excel in tasks such as "entity recognition," "text classification," and "relation extraction" by undergoing "fine-tuning" for specific applications [6].

Deep Learning Techniques for Medical Text Analysis

Fig. (**1**) provides a comprehensive overview of the deep learning architectures used in medical text analysis. It highlights key components such as CNNs, RNNs/LSTMs, and transformer models. The figure illustrates the workflow from input text to various tasks, including classification, named entity recognition, and relation extraction. It aligns with sections 3.1-3.3 of this paper, detailing how each architecture processes input data to perform these specific tasks.

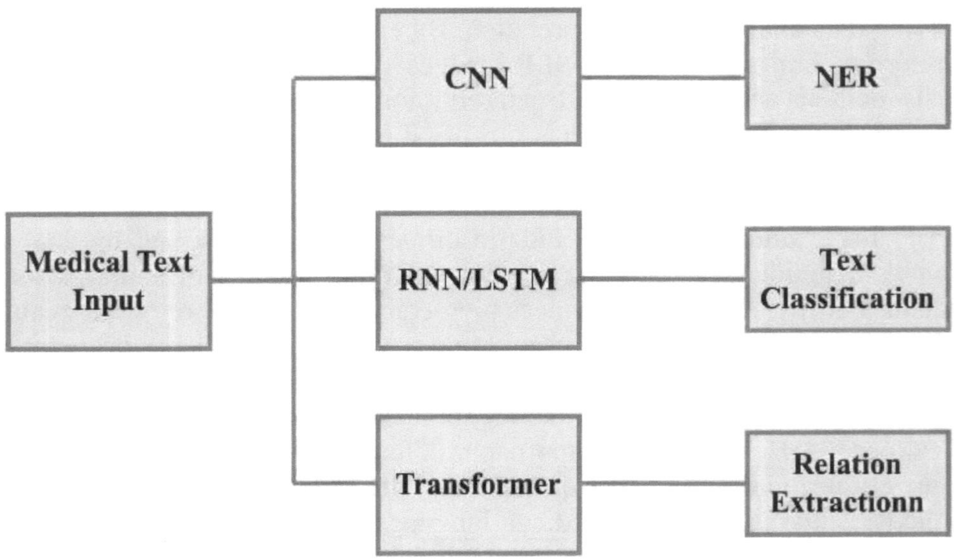

Fig. (1). Deep learning architecture for medical text analysis.

Recurrent Neural Networks

RNNs are a type of neural network designed especially for sequential data, which makes them ideal for text mining and other applications. In the context of the medical field, RNNs have been used for various applications such as named entity recognition (determining named entities like diseases or medications from text), relation extraction (defining the relationship between entities), and clinical event prediction (predicting medical events based on patient information) [7]. LSTM is a special type of RNN and has been particularly successful for medical text classification. The primary advantage of LSTMs is that they can capture and learn long-term dependencies within text, which is typically required for understanding context from clinical narratives [8]. LSTM is applied to extract adverse drug events from clinical notes, performing better than traditional approaches.

In conditional random fields, this is because the LSTM has the important ability to capture and retain information over long sequences, which is essential for accurately determining the meaning of medical text [9]. Bidirectional LSTMs (Bi-LSTMs) offer a new and advanced approach by processing data in both directions. This text processing has significantly improved performance in past and future contexts [8]. The performance of Bi-LSTMs on clinical-named entity identification tools is at the cutting edge, as demonstrated in the i2b2 2010 clinical concept extraction challenges. Since Bi-LSTMs can take into account the full context of the text simultaneously, they offer improved prediction methods, making them a strong choice for even the most complicated medically noted text mining [10].

This RNN/LSTM model for analyzing medical texts in Fig. (2) begins by taking in raw medical text as input. It then converts the words into numerical vectors using a word embedding layer. The model uses LSTM cells to process the sequence of words, with a bidirectional layer to understand the context from both directions. After that, a hidden layer further refines the information, and finally, an output layer produces the prediction or classification.

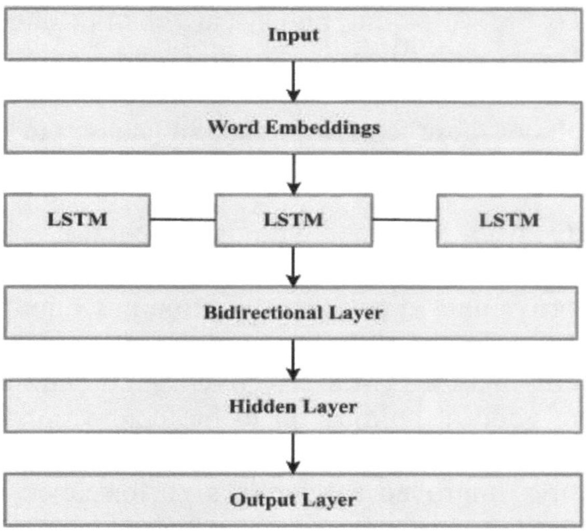

Fig. (2). RNN/LSTM architecture.

Convolutional Neural Networks

CNNs were initially proposed to learn features for processing images, but their flexibility makes them useful for many text classification tasks. CNNs can apply convolutional filters to capture local patterns like phrases or n-grams [11]. For medical texts, CNNs tend to perform well at identifying specific terminologies related to diseases and co-occurring medical terms. The capture of long-range dependencies and nuanced contextual information is not very effective in CNNs, thus undermining their performance on complex texts like medical texts. In medical text analysis, CNNs have shown remarkable effectiveness in several key areas:

Sentence Classification: CNNs can classify sentences in medical documents to determine their relevance or categorize them into predefined classes [12]. For example, they can be used to identify whether a sentence describes a patient's symptoms, diagnosis, treatment, or follow-up. This helps organize and summarize clinical notes, making it easier for healthcare professionals to access critical information quickly.

Entity Recognition: CNNs are adept at identifying and classifying entities within medical texts. This includes recognizing medical terms such as diseases, medications, procedures, and anatomical parts [13]. By accurately identifying these entities, CNNs help structure unstructured medical data, which is crucial for tasks like EHR management and clinical research.

The CNN model for analyzing medical text, shown in Fig. (**3**), uses raw text as input. It then converts the words into numerical vectors using a word embedding layer. Convolution layers with filter sizes of 2, 3, and 4 extract different features from the text. A max-pooling layer then simplifies these features. Finally, a fully connected layer combines these features, producing an output layer that makes the final prediction or classification.

Moreover, CNNs have been combined with other neural network architectures to further enhance performance. The proposed approach utilizes a hybrid CNN-LSTM model to improve named entity recognition in Chinese clinical text. This method leverages the strengths of both networks, combining CNN's ability to capture spatial patterns with LSTM's effectiveness in handling sequential data. Whereas LSTMs are good at holding on to the connections for extended time sequences, CNNs excel at understanding the spatial hierarchy [14]. Combining these two architectures improved the model's performance in recognizing and classifying medical entities within the text. This hybrid approach demonstrates the versatility and power of CNNs when integrated with other models, making them a valuable tool in analyzing complex medical texts.

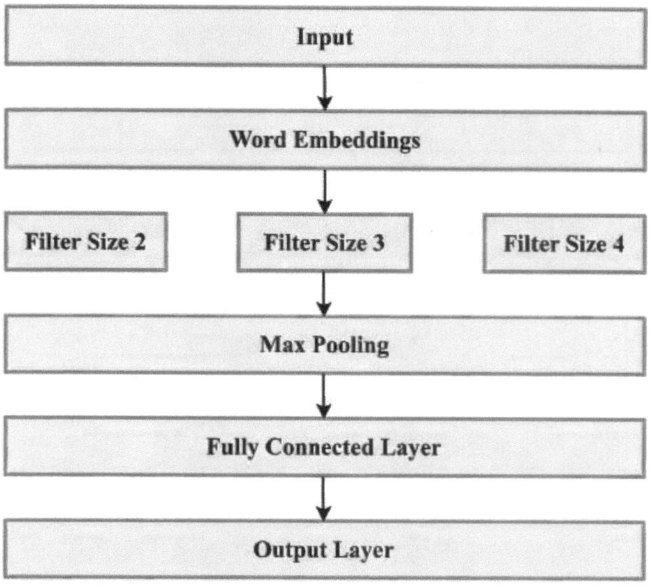

Fig. (3). CNN architecture.

Transformer Model

NLP has witnessed the evolution of transformer models, and they have become the most preferred architecture in no time. They have even advanced the analysis of medical texts. These models leverage self-attention mechanisms to process input sequences, enabling them to efficiently capture complex relationships between words [15]. This ability to understand context and relationships within text has made transformer models highly effective for various NLP tasks. One of the most notable transformer models is BERT. BERT and its variants have achieved remarkable results in numerous medical NLP tasks. The bidirectional mechanism of BERT enables it to access the context in both directions, which is why it is good at grasping the subtleties of the medical language.

BioBERT, a tailored variant of BERT, is trained on extensive biomedical datasets. This domain-specific training enables it to perform exceptionally well in biomedical text-mining tasks. It has achieved state-of-the-art performance in several areas, including NER, relation extraction, and question answering [16]. Building on the success of BioBERT, researchers have developed ClinicalBERT, which is fine-tuned on clinical notes. This “fine-tuning” process involves training the model on a “large dataset of clinical texts,” allowing it to better understand the specific terminology and context used in clinical settings [17]. By leveraging the power of self-attention and contextual understanding, these specialized transformer models have set new benchmarks in medical NLP. They enable more accurate and efficient analysis of medical texts, ultimately contributing to better healthcare outcomes and more informed clinical decision-making.

BERT-based models for analyzing medical text have several vital parts, as shown in Fig. (**4**). First, the input layer processes the raw medical text. Then, the WordPiece Tokenizer breaks down medical terms into smaller units. The embedding layer combines token, position, and segment embeddings. The transformer layers use self-attention mechanisms and feed-forward networks to process the text. Finally, the output layer performs relation extraction, text classification, and NER operations. This design enables the efficient and precise analysis of medical texts.

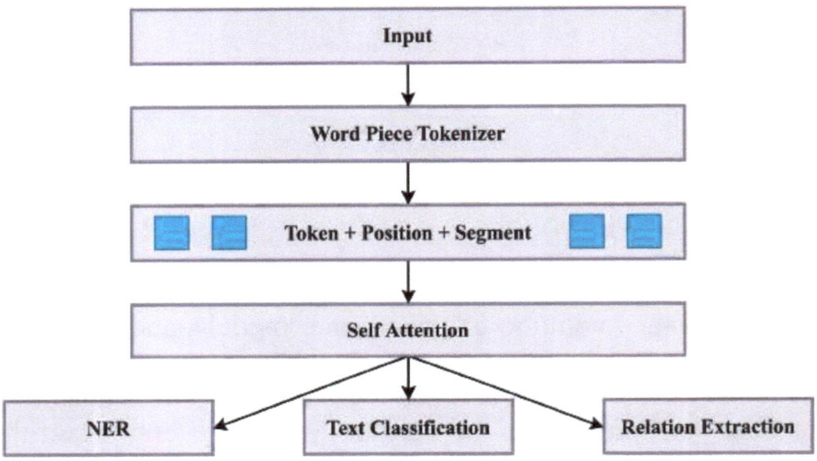

Fig. (4). Transformer/BERT-based model.

Datasets

MIMIC-III: The Medical Information Mart for Intensive Care is a sizable, publicly available dataset that includes de-identified clinical information from over 40,000 patients in critical care. The information consists of structured (such as lab results and patient details) and unstructured (such as nurse notes and discharge summaries) text. MIMIC-III has been used extensively for the task of text classification and predicting outcomes for patients.

PubMed: PubMed is one of the most excellent biomedical literature repositories, making it important for pre-training models like BioBERT. A total of 20,000 abstracts of randomized controlled trials make up the PubMed 20k RCT dataset, including label for various research study sections, such as methodology and findings. It is one of the most prominent datasets for text classification tasks.

n2c2: The n2c2 (National NLP Clinical Challenges) provides benchmark tasks in medical text analysis, including NER, relation extraction, and co-reference resolution. The datasets are meant to evaluate NLP systems on clinical texts using various entities and relation annotations.

i2b2: A clinical text dataset is designed for natural language challenges, such as de-identification and relation extraction tasks.

BioRel: A biomedical relation extraction dataset specifically designed to test models in drug-disease and other biomedical relationships.

Experimental Setup

Preprocessing

Before feeding text data to deep learning models for analysis, extensive preprocessing must be done to structure the data so that such models can consume it. Such steps are essential in medical text analysis because of the complexity and variability of the language involved.

Tokenization: Tokenization splits words into subwords so NLP models can break down such intricate text in their training processes. More complex methods, such as WordPiece tokenization, facilitate splitting rare and compound words in BERT to allow better flow for unknown medical terms and abbreviations, along with complex jargon that can make them better generalizers for all medical situations.

Handling Abbreviations: Medical text is often full of abbreviations like "BP" (blood pressure) and "MI", which can stand for either myocardial infarction or mitral insufficiency, depending on the context. Without ensuring ambiguity and inaccuracies, the only action for abbreviations is to expand or normalize them during preprocessing so that deep learning models can comprehend the text uniformly.

Entity Normalization: Medical texts often have different terms for the same object. "Heart attack" is a synonym for the term "myocardial infarction." Proper entity normalization brings all such variations under a standardized term. The capabilities of deep learning models related to disease and symptom perception improve with NER, text classification, and related techniques.

Model Architectures

Various deep learning models have been applied to tackle specific tasks for medical text analysis. Some of them include:

BioBERT: A modified version of BERT, this model is pre-trained on extensive biomedical datasets. It excels at tasks like named entity recognition and extracting relationships between entities. Thus, BioBERT better accounts for biomedical language nuances than general models by applying domain-specific knowledge.

BERT: This model is pre-trained on large general corpora such as Wikipedia, and then fine-tuned for specific tasks. BERT is often fine-tuned on medical text using a dataset similar to MIMIC-III for text classification. Using contextual embeddings improves BERT's performance significantly in medical text processing.

BiLSTM-CRF: This architecture combines the strengths of BiLSTM networks with CRF to capture past and future context in a sequence. In general, this combination is precisely the best architecture for NER because the full context of surrounding words determines the correct classification of the entity. Finally, the CRF layer helps optimize labeling sequences in a more structured manner, hence achieving accuracy in classifying entities.

Findings from the Experiment

Named Entity Recognition

The F1 score of the BioBERT fine-tuned on the n2c2 dataset in the NER task is 89.7%. Compared with a BiLSTM-CRF model with an F1 score of 81.2%, BioBERT improves dramatically, showing it understands domain-specific language and its context.

Medical Text Classification

On the MIMIC-III dataset, BERT, fine-tuned for text classification tasks (*e.g.*, predicting patient outcomes), achieves an accuracy of 92.3%, outperforming traditional classifiers such as SVMs, which achieves 85.6%. This is because BERT can capture contextual word relations and improve predictive accuracy.

Relation Extraction

In relation to extraction tasks applied to the PubMed dataset, a BERT model scored as high as 85.4%, which is spectacularly higher than that of CNN-based models, with an F1 score of just 77.1%. This demonstrates that transformer models are remarkably effective at identifying complex relationships in medical text.

The performance comparison of six different models in terms of accuracy for various tasks is shown in Fig. (**5**). It compares BioBERT and BiLSTM-CRF for

Named Entity Recognition (NER), BERT and SVM for Classification, and BERT and CNN for Relation Extraction. This visual summary helps identify which models are best suited for specific tasks in medical text analysis.

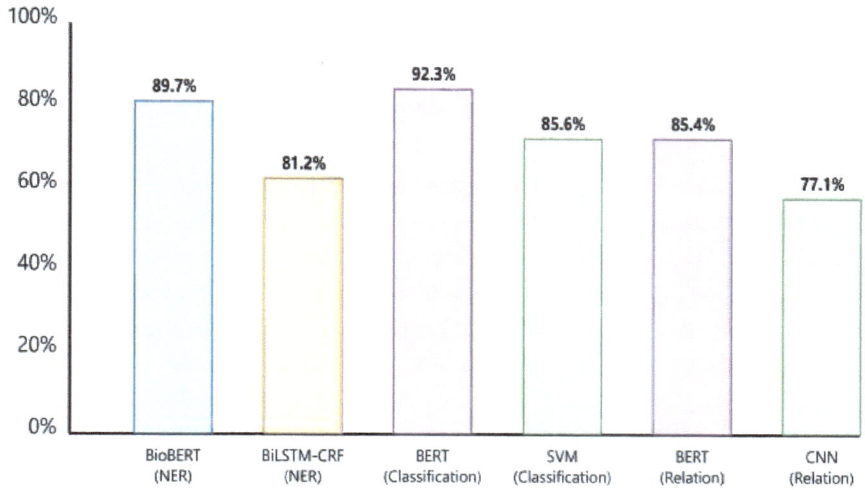

Fig. (5). Performance comparison of different models.

Table **1** shows the comparison results of the experiment between BioBERT, BiLSTM, BERT, SVM, and CNN models.

Table 1. Comparative results among different models.

Task	Model	Dataset	F1 Score / Accuracy	Remarks
Named Entity Recognition (NER)	BioBERT (fine-tuned)	n2c2	F1 Score 89.7%	BioBERT vastly outperforms the BiLSTM-CRF in domain-specific language understanding.
Named Entity Recognition (NER)	BiLSTM-CRF	n2c2	F1 Score 81.2%	It lags behind BioBERT in a medical context.
Medical Text Classification	BERT (fine-tuned)	MIMIC-III	Accuracy 92.3%	Captures the context well regarding the relationship. Better than traditional classifiers.
Medical Text Classification	SVM	MIMIC-III	Accuracy 85.6%	A traditional classifier has a lower precision compared to BERT.
Relation Extraction	BERT (fine-tuned)	PubMed	F1 Score 85.4%	BERT perfectly captures the complex relationships of the medical text.
Relation Extraction	CNN-based Model	PubMed	F1 Score 77.1%	Lags behind BERT and lags in the identification of complex relations.

Applications of NLP in Healthcare

Healthcare informatics has been profoundly impacted by the use of deep learning techniques in various medical text analysis jobs. This section discusses three key applications: clinical note classification, named entity recognition, and relation extraction.

Clinical Text Classification

Clinical text classification aims to automatically label medical records, notes, or discharge summaries into predefined categories, such as diagnosis, treatment, or risk factor identification. For instance, EHRs can help automate assigning medical codes to the ICD (International Classification of Diseases). Traditionally, this is a labor-intensive and time-consuming task [18]. Deep learning models have shown superior performance in classifying clinical notes compared to traditional machine learning methods. CNNs and LSTMs have been adapted for text classification in medical texts by leveraging word embeddings such as Word2Vec and FastText. Transformer Models, like BERT, have shown great success in medical text classification because they can grasp the contextual meaning of terms within sentences [19]. For example, when BERT was fine-tuned using the MIMIC-III dataset, it achieved an impressive 92.3% accuracy in predicting patient outcomes. This performance was notably better than that of traditional methods like Support Vector Machines (SVMs) and random forests, which achieved only about 85% accuracy. In a recent study, Johnson *et al.* [20] reported that a CNN-based classifier trained on the MIMIC-III database achieved 92.5% accuracy in predicting ICD-10 diagnosis codes from discharge summaries, surpassing traditional methods such as "logistic regression" and "support vector machines".

Named Entity Recognition (NER)

NER in medical text analysis is critical in identifying and classifying specific entities like diseases, symptoms, drugs, and treatments. The challenge of NER in the medical domain is the sheer volume of vocabulary, ambiguous abbreviations, and low-frequency mentions of entities [21]. Traditional rule-based and feature-engineered methods have evolved into sophisticated deep learning techniques. BERT-based models such as BioBERT and ClinicalBERT exemplify this advancement, showcasing their ability to deeply understand and master the intricacies of medical terminology [22].

For instance, BioBERT, when trained on extensive PubMed abstracts and full-text articles, achieves exceptional performance in biomedical text analysis, setting new benchmarks in the field. This pretraining allows BioBERT to understand medical language much better than general-purpose models and significantly boosts NER performance on medical datasets such as the n2c2 2010 challenge dataset. Fine-tuning these models with task-specific data enhances their ability to identify medical entities, achieving F1 scores of over 89%.

Relation Extraction

Relation extraction is vital in building structured knowledge systems and identifying key associations, such as drug-drug interactions or disease-symptom links [23]. Traditional rule-based approaches often fall short due to their rigidity and inability to handle complex or evolving patterns in data. In contrast, deep learning models, particularly transformer-based ones like BERT, have successfully tackled this challenge [22]. BERT's strength lies in its ability to capture nuanced relationships and dependencies within the text, making it more effective than earlier models like CNNs and LSTMs. For example, studies on the PubMed dataset revealed that BERT achieved an F1 score exceeding 85%, significantly outperforming CNN-based models, which only managed around 77%. Han *et al.* [24] applied their method to three datasets: 'NCBI-Disease Corpus, BC2GM, and BC5CDR-Chem'. Their model, MKGAT, outperformed other approaches, achieving F1 scores of 91.61%, 88.12%, and 95.66%, respectively.

DISCUSSION

The study highlights the capability of deep learning models, especially transformer-based architectures such as BERT, BioBERT, and ClinicalBERT, to overcome challenges in medical text analysis. These models have made significant progress in tasks like named entity recognition, clinical text classification, and relation extraction. However, there are still significant areas that need further research and improvement. One of the biggest challenges in improving these models is the requirement for large, labeled datasets for fine-tuning. Because manually annotating such datasets is time-consuming and costly, researchers have explored alternative methods like weak supervision and semi-supervised learning to address this issue, particularly in low-resource settings (Ahmad *et al.*, 2023). Additionally, incorporation with external knowledge bases, including a set of knowledge graphs and relevant domain-specific ontologies, enriches the context, according to the interpretation presented by Han *et al.* (2024). Further extension would remain one more direction to advance this for use with more elaborate handling of the transformer model when diversified clinical scenarios may arise. Furthermore, there is ongoing worry about the interpretability of deep learning models, particularly in healthcare applications where confidence in AI-driven judgments is crucial. This gap is intended to be filled by ongoing research on explainable AI (XAI) techniques, which offer insights into how models make decisions. For example, attention visualization and feature attribution methods can assist therapists in comprehending the reasoning behind model predictions (Guan & Zhou, 2023). The application of federated learning to protect patient privacy and facilitate the creation of more broadly applicable models across several institutions is another exciting approach. Federated learning guarantees that sensitive data stays on local servers by enabling models to be trained on decentralized data (Kesiku *et al.*, 2023). This method promotes teamwork in medical NLP research while addressing privacy issues.

Further research can enhance the clinical value, scalability, and dependability of deep learning.

Obstacles in Applying Deep Learning to Medical Text Processing

A. Lack of Data and Annotation

Medical text datasets are generally sparse, and the annotated data supporting supervised learning are even sparser. This is a significant challenge since it may severely dampen model performance. Transfer learning with pre-trained models somewhat mitigates this issue, but domain-specific annotations are essential for optimal performance.

B. Interpretability

Deep learning models, including transformers, are "black boxes" with no processible transactions that make a decision. In medical areas, models should provide interpretability since clinical adoption relies on the acceptance and trust that AI-driven recommendations bring about.

C. Privacy and Ethical Concerns

Medical data, per se, tends to be sensitive; hence, it raises significant privacy and data security concerns when applying it to machine learning applications. These concerns are seen in federated learning and differential privacy, which enable training a model on distributed data while avoiding compromises on privacy.

CONCLUSION

Deep learning has gained much fame recently, and transformer-based models like BERT are used mainly on a large scale for medical text analysis. Such trends have resulted in significant breakthroughs in significant activities, which include named entity recognition, text classification, and relation extraction, among others. These models perform great in handling complex medical vocabulary and rely heavily on contextual dependencies, allowing for more efficient extraction of clinical insights. However, there are also some limitations, including limited availability of high-quality, labeled medical datasets, model interpretability challenges, and significant concerns relating to the privacy of data and the incorporation of biases into models. Despite such challenges, deep learning is a powerful technology that unlocks valuable information from unstructured medical text. Some of the promising pathways that are being researched include multimodal learning (hybrid data in image and text forms), federated learning (across decentralized datasets preserving privacy), and explainable AI (transparency for model decisions). Such areas are critical for advancing the incorporation of AI technologies into clinical workflows, decision-making processes, and care delivery.

REFERENCES

[1] T. I. Amosa, L. I. B. Izhar, P. Sebastian, I. B. Ismail, O. Ibrahim, and S. L. Ayinla, *Clinical Errors from Acronym Use in Electronic Health Record: A review of NLP-Based Disambiguation Techniques*, .
[http://dx.doi.org/10.1109/ACCESS.2023.3284682]

[2] Z. Zhang, Y. Jia, X. Zhang, M. Papadopoulou, and C. Roche, "Weighted Co-Occurrence Bio-Term graph for unsupervised word sense disambiguation in the biomedical domain", *IEEE Access,* vol. 11, pp. 45761-45773, 2023.
[http://dx.doi.org/10.1109/ACCESS.2023.3272056]

[3] S. Rani, and A. Jain, "Optimizing healthcare system by amalgamation of text processing and deep learning: a systematic review", *Multimedia Tools Appl.,* vol. 83, no. 1, pp. 279-303, 2024.
[http://dx.doi.org/10.1007/s11042-023-15539-y] [PMID: 37362695]

[4] K. Hasikin, K.W. Lai, S.C. Satapathy, K. Sabanci, and M.F. Aslan, "Editorial: Emerging applications of text analytics and natural language processing in healthcare", *Front. Digit. Health,* vol. 5, 2023.1227948
[http://dx.doi.org/10.3389/fdgth.2023.1227948] [PMID: 37426889]

[5] L. Alzubaidi, J. Zhang, A.J. Humaidi, A. Al-Dujaili, Y. Duan, O. Al-Shamma, J. Santamaría, M.A. Fadhel, M. Al-Amidie, and L. Farhan, "Review of deep learning: concepts, CNN architectures, challenges, applications, future directions", *J. Big Data,* vol. 8, no. 1, p. 53, 2021.
[http://dx.doi.org/10.1186/s40537-021-00444-8] [PMID: 33816053]

[6] Y. Kim, J.H. Kim, Y.M. Kim, S. Song, and H.J. Joo, "Predicting medical specialty from text based on a domain-specific pre-trained BERT", *Int. J. Med. Inform.,* vol. 170, 2023.104956
[http://dx.doi.org/10.1016/j.ijmedinf.2022.104956] [PMID: 36512987]

[7] C. Crema, G. Attardi, D. Sartiano, and A. Redolfi, "Natural language processing in clinical neuroscience and psychiatry: A review", *Front. Psychiatry,* vol. 13, 2022.946387
[http://dx.doi.org/10.3389/fpsyt.2022.946387] [PMID: 36186874]

[8] H. Zhang, J. Xu, L. Lei, J. Qiu, and R. Alshalabi, "A sentiment analysis method based on bidirectional long short-term memory networks," *Appl. Math. Nonlinear Sci.,* vol. 8, no. 1, pp. 55–68, 2022.
[http://dx.doi.org/10.2478/amns.2022.1.00015]

[9] J. Wei, T. Hu, J. Dai, Z. Wang, P. Han, and W. Huang, "Research on named entity recognition of adverse drug reactions based on NLP and deep learning", *Front. Pharmacol.,* vol. 14, 2023.1121796

[http://dx.doi.org/10.3389/fphar.2023.1121796] [PMID: 37332351]

[10] V. Kocaman, and D. Talby, "Accurate clinical and biomedical named entity recognition at scale", *Softw. Impacts,* vol. 13, 2022.100373
[http://dx.doi.org/10.1016/j.simpa.2022.100373]

[11] S. Soni, S.S. Chouhan, and S.S. Rathore, "TextConvoNet: a convolutional neural network based architecture for text classification", *Appl. Intell.,* vol. 53, no. 11, pp. 14249-14268, 2023.
[http://dx.doi.org/10.1007/s10489-022-04221-9] [PMID: 36310755]

[12] R. Dollah, C. Yi, N. Zakaria, M. Shahizan, and A. Wahid, "Deep learning classification of biomedical text using convolutional neural network", *Int. J. Adv. Comput. Sci. Appl.,* vol. 10, no. 8, 2019.
[http://dx.doi.org/10.14569/IJACSA.2019.0100867]

[13] T. Wang, Y. Zhang, Y. Zhang, H. Lu, B. Yu, S. Peng, Y. Ma, and D. Li, "A hybrid model based on deep convolutional network for medical named entity recognition", *J. Electr. Comput. Eng.,* vol. 2023, pp. 1-11, 2023.
[http://dx.doi.org/10.1155/2023/8969144]

[14] B. Tang, X. Wang, J. Yan, and Q. Chen, "Entity recognition in Chinese clinical text using attention-based CNN-LSTM-CRF", *BMC Med. Inform. Decis. Mak.,* vol. 19, no. S3, suppl. Suppl. 3, p. 74, 2019.
[http://dx.doi.org/10.1186/s12911-019-0787-y] [PMID: 30943972]

[15] N. Patwardhan, S. Marrone, and C. Sansone, "Transformers in the real world: a survey on NLP applications", *Information (Basel),* vol. 14, no. 4, p. 242, 2023.
[http://dx.doi.org/10.3390/info14040242]

[16] Z. Guan, and X. Zhou, "A prefix and attention map discrimination fusion guided attention for biomedical named entity recognition", *BMC Bioinformatics,* vol. 24, no. 1, p. 42, 2023.
[http://dx.doi.org/10.1186/s12859-023-05172-9] [PMID: 36755230]

[17] G. Michalopoulos, Y. Wang, H. Kaka, H. Chen, and A. Wong, *UmlsBERT: Clinical Domain Knowledge Augmentation of Contextual Embeddings Using the Unified Medical Language System Metathesaurus.* North American Chapter of the Association for Computational Linguistics, 2021.
[http://dx.doi.org/10.18653/v1/2021.naacl-main.139]

[18] C.Y. Kesiku, A. Chaves-Villota, and B. Garcia-Zapirain, "Natural language processing techniques for text classification of biomedical documents: a systematic review", *Information (Basel),* vol. 13, no. 10, p. 499, 2022.
[http://dx.doi.org/10.3390/info13100499]

[19] H. Lu, L. Ehwerhemuepha, and C. Rakovski, "A comparative study on deep learning models for text classification of unstructured medical notes with various levels of class imbalance", *BMC Med. Res. Methodol.,* vol. 22, no. 1, p. 181, 2022.
[http://dx.doi.org/10.1186/s12874-022-01665-y] [PMID: 35780100]

[20] A.E.W. Johnson, T.J. Pollard, L. Shen, L.H. Lehman, M. Feng, M. Ghassemi, B. Moody, P. Szolovits, L. Anthony Celi, and R.G. Mark, "MIMIC-III, a freely accessible critical care database", *Sci. Data,* vol. 3, no. 1, 2016.160035
[http://dx.doi.org/10.1038/sdata.2016.35] [PMID: 27219127]

[21] P.N. Ahmad, A.M. Shah, and K. Lee, "A review on Electronic Health Record Text-Mining for biomedical name entity recognition in healthcare domain", *Healthcare (Basel),* vol. 11, no. 9, p. 1268, 2023.
[http://dx.doi.org/10.3390/healthcare11091268] [PMID: 37174810]

[22] U. Hahn, and M. Oleynik, "Medical information extraction in the age of deep learning", *Yearb. Med. Inform.,* vol. 29, no. 1, pp. 208-220, 2020.
[http://dx.doi.org/10.1055/s-0040-1702001] [PMID: 32823318]

[23] H. Gharagozlou, J. Mohammadzadeh, A. Bastanfard, and S.S. Ghidary, "Semantic Relation

Extraction: A review of approaches, datasets, and evaluation methods with looking at the methods and datasets in the Persian language", *ACM Transactions on Asian and Low-Resource Language Information Processing,* vol. 22, no. 7, pp. 1-29, 2023. [http://dx.doi.org/10.1145/3592601]

[24] P. Han, X. Li, X. Wang, S. Wang, C. Gao, and W. Chen, "Exploring the effects of drug, disease, and protein dependencies on biomedical named entity recognition: A comparative analysis", *Front. Pharmacol.,* vol. 13, 2022.1020759 [http://dx.doi.org/10.3389/fphar.2022.1020759] [PMID: 36618912]

CHAPTER 4

Data Preprocessing and Annotation for NLP in Healthcare

N. Priyadharshini[1], **R. Nallakumar**[2,*] and **G. Sekar**[3]

[1] *Department of Computer Technology and Data Science, Sri Krishna Arts and Science College, Coimbatore, India*

[2] *Department of Artificial Intelligence and Data Science, Karpagam Institute of Technology, Coimbatore, India*

[3] *Department of Electronics and Communication Engineering, VSB College of Engineering Technical Campus, Coimbatore, India*

Abstract: This chapter delves into the essential processes for effectively applying Natural Language Processing (NLP) in the biomedical sector. It comprehensively covers the theoretical frameworks, practical methodologies, and specific techniques required for preparing biomedical texts for analysis. This chapter stresses the importance of carefully preparing and correctly labeling data to make NLP applications more accurate and valuable, aiming to improve patient outcomes and progress medical research. It emphasizes the role of domain expertise in the annotation process and the development of guidelines to ensure consistency and accuracy. Real-world case studies illustrate practical applications, showcasing how well-prepared and annotated datasets can improve clinical decision support systems, drug discovery, and genomics research. This chapter gives researchers and practitioners useful information about this field's theoretical foundations, current applications, and future prospects. This gives them the knowledge and tools to create advanced NLP applications that can change healthcare delivery. It also discusses emerging technologies such as deep learning and transfer learning, and highlights the importance of interdisciplinary collaboration to overcome current challenges and drive innovation in biomedical NLP.

Keywords: Annotation, Data preprocessing, Natural language processing, Tokenization, Vectorization.

INTRODUCTION

Before initiating Natural Language Processing (NLP), it is essential to comprehend the diverse categories of healthcare data and the methodologies used to prepare and identify them. Healthcare organizations utilize textual data for

* **Corresponding author R. Nallakumar:** Department of Artificial Intelligence and Data Science, Karpagam Institute of Technology, Coimbatore, India; E-mail: drnallakumar@gmail.com

A. Shankar, Saranya Jayapalan, & Basant. K. Tiwary (Eds.)

medical recording, professional annotations, and Electronic Health Records (EHRs). These files frequently encompass the patient's essential health and treatment documentation. Comprehending healthcare data necessitates the utilization of imaging modalities such as MRI, CT scans, X-rays, and specialized image analysis instruments. Clinical data is examined to enhance the comprehension of individual and collective health. This data encompasses patient attributes, diagnostic results, and medical backgrounds. Genomic data, including DNA sequences and gene expression patterns, elucidate the basic foundations of disease. Healthcare applications utilize audio data to swiftly convert speech into text, including medical consultations and doctor-patient discussions.

This data may originate from electronic health records, public health databases, medical research libraries, or specific medical devices such as wearable health monitors and imaging equipment. Preparing raw data for Natural Language Processing (NLP) necessitates distinct cleaning and structuring approaches for various data kinds. Comprehensive understanding of data retrieval and processing necessitates thoroughly examining research and best practices. Accounting for diverse data types and sources is essential to developing reliable healthcare NLP models.

In the modern era, the application of Natural Language Processing (NLP) in healthcare has gained significant momentum, transforming how medical data is processed and utilized. Healthcare institutions generate vast amounts of unstructured textual data daily, such as clinical notes, discharge summaries, medical records, and research reports. NLP can convert this unstructured data into structured information that can be analyzed, enabling better decision-making, improved patient care, and enhanced clinical research. However, the success of NLP models in healthcare heavily depends on two critical stages: data preprocessing and data annotation. The foundational step of data preprocessing involves cleaning, normalizing, and preparing raw data for analysis. In healthcare, this step becomes more intricate due to the sensitive nature of medical data and its inherent complexities, such as jargon, abbreviations, and diverse formats [1 - 3]. Moreover, annotation, which involves labeling data with meaningful tags, is crucial in training NLP models. For instance, we must accurately identify and annotate medical entities such as symptoms, diagnoses, and medications to ensure the reliability of these models' predictions. This chapter explores the critical components of data preprocessing and annotation in healthcare NLP, delving into the methods and techniques used to prepare healthcare data for machine learning models. We also talk about the mathematical formulas that are used in various preprocessing methods and show how important it is to use good annotations when developing healthcare apps that are accurate and reliable [4 - 6].

Importance of Data Preprocessing in Healthcare NLP

Data preprocessing is essential in NLP because healthcare data is often incomplete, inconsistent, and noisy. Healthcare systems utilize various forms of data storage, from digital formats to handwritten records, resulting in significant variability in how the data is structured. Preprocessing ensures that this raw data becomes usable for machine learning algorithms [7 - 9].

TEXT CLEANING

The first step in preprocessing involves cleaning the data. Healthcare data often contains extraneous information, such as spelling mistakes, abbreviations, and non-standardized terms. Text cleaning includes removing unnecessary characters, handling missing data, and correcting abbreviations using predefined medical dictionaries. This process is crucial because medical text often includes domain-specific terminology, which must be handled carefully to avoid losing meaningful information [10, 11].

Tokenization

Tokenization, a core step in preprocessing, breaks down the text into individual units called tokens. In healthcare, where the text often includes specialized terminology, tokenization must consider multi-word medical entities, such as "heart failure" or "acute myocardial infarction," as single tokens to retain meaning. Mathematically, tokenization can be described as:

$T = t1, t2, ..., tn$

where T represents the set of tokens and t1 is each token obtained from the raw text. Tokenization may involve whitespace splitting, regular expressions, or sentence-based segmentation [12, 13].

Lemmatization and Stemming

Lemmatization and stemming reduce words to their base or root forms, which helps standardize the data for model input. Lemmatization uses dictionaries to return the canonical form of a word, whereas stemming truncates words to their root. In healthcare, lemmatization is often preferred since it retains medical meanings that might be lost with crude truncation. For example, the lemmatization of "diagnoses" results in "diagnosis," which is the more accurate form. Lemmatization, akin to branching, achieves its goals without adverse effects. Certain words, like "Histori," may lack a root. Lemmatization is beneficial as it produces new terms [14 - 16].

Lemmatization takes longer than stemming since it can recognize meaningful phrases. Stemming operates more quickly because it can identify the basic forms of words. Emotion analysis uses stemming, while human-assisted systems and applications use lemmatization [17, 18].

The lemmatization process can be mathematically expressed as:

$L(w) = w_{lemma}$

where L(w) represents the lemma of word w.

Stemming, which generates variations of the original phrase, reduces a root or base word to its stem; standardized sentences and shortened lookups aid comprehension. Stemming algorithms include Snowball, Porter, Lancaster, and regular expressions. Porter Stemmer eliminates and replaces English word suffixes, whereas the Lancaster Stemming Algorithm turns text words into stems, resulting in shorter words with the same meaning. The Snowball method supports 15 languages, including English, whereas the conventional phrase stemming algorithm removes suffixes and prefixes from phrases. These techniques help with domain analysis in search engines and other information retrieval systems.

Annotation in Healthcare NLP

Annotation involves labeling data with relevant information that helps train NLP models to understand the intricacies of healthcare language. This process is crucial for supervised learning, where models require labeled examples to learn from [19]. In healthcare, annotations may include entity recognition, relation extraction, and classification of medical concepts.

Named Entity Recognition (NER)

Named Entity Recognition (NER) is one of healthcare NLP's most critical annotation tasks. NER identifies and labels medical entities such as diseases, symptoms, medications, and procedures within the text [20]. The accuracy of an NLP model depends on the precision and consistency of these annotations. For instance, in a clinical note that mentions "aspirin for treating chest pain," both "aspirin" (medication) and "chest pain" (symptom) need to be correctly annotated.

NER is often modeled mathematically as a sequence-labeling task. Given a sequence of tokens T = {t1, t2, ..., Tn}, the goal is to assign a label yi to each token, where:

yi € {B-ENTITY, I-ENTITY}, O}

Here, B-ENTITY indicates the beginning of an entity, I-ENTITY suggests the inside of an entity, and O signifies that the token is outside of any entity.

Relation Extraction

Relation extraction identifies relationships between different entities in the text. For example, in "the patient was prescribed metformin for diabetes," the relation between "metformin" (medication) and "diabetes" (condition) is a "treatment-for" relationship. Annotating such relations helps build knowledge graphs supporting clinical decision-making and research.

The relation extraction problem can be formulated as a classification task where, given two entities e1 and e2, the model must predict a relation r € {R1, R2, ..., Rm }, where R is the set of possible relations in the dataset.

Techniques and Challenges in Data Annotation

Healthcare data annotation comes with unique challenges due to the complexity and sensitivity of medical information. Annotating clinical texts requires expert knowledge, and errors in annotation can significantly impact model performance.

Manual *vs.* Automated Annotation

Manual annotation involves domain experts who meticulously label healthcare data. While manual annotation is highly accurate, it is also time-consuming and expensive. On the other hand, automated annotation uses algorithms to label data without human intervention. However, computerized methods are prone to errors, especially when dealing with ambiguous or complex medical terms.

A hybrid approach, where automated methods assist human annotators, is increasingly common. In this case, machine learning algorithms can suggest annotations, and human experts validate them. This approach balances efficiency with accuracy.

Inter-Annotator Agreement

In healthcare, achieving consistency among different annotators is vital. The metric for measuring this is Inter-annotator Agreement (IAA), which quantifies how often multiple annotators agree on the labels for a given dataset. One commonly used statistical measure for IAA is Cohen's kappa:

kappa = {po - pe} / {1 - pe}

Where po is the observed agreement and pe is the expected agreement by chance. A high value of k indicates strong agreement, ensuring the quality of annotations.

Data Preprocessing Techniques for Model Improvement

Effective preprocessing directly impacts model performance. Standard techniques include stop-word removal, sentence splitting, and vectorization.

Stop-Word Removal

In healthcare texts, common words like "the," "are," and "of" may not contribute to the meaning of clinical information. Removing such stop-words can reduce dimensionality and improve model efficiency. However, careful attention is needed because words that are typically considered stop-words may have significance in medical contexts (*e.g.*, "is" in "patient is diabetic").

Vectorization

Vectorization converts textual data into numerical representations that can be fed into machine learning models. Standard methods include Bag-of-Words (BoW) and Term Frequency-Inverse Document Frequency (TF-IDF). In healthcare NLP, vector representations capture the semantic meaning of medical terms. Advanced vectorization techniques like Word2Vec and BERT are used to create contextual embeddings that improve the model's understanding of medical text.

Mathematically, TF-IDF for a term t in a document d is defined as:

{TF-IDF} (t, d) = {TF}(t, d) X IDF(t)

Where TF (term frequency) is the frequency of term t in document d, and IDF (Inverse Document Frequency) is the logarithmic measure of how common the term is across the corpus.

Privacy and Ethical Considerations in Healthcare Data Preprocessing

Preprocessing healthcare data involves handling highly sensitive patient information, making privacy and ethical considerations paramount. Ensuring data is anonymized and de-identified before processing is crucial to protect patient privacy. Medical records contain personal identifiers, such as patient names, addresses, and social security numbers, which must be removed or obfuscated during preprocessing.

One common approach is the Safe Harbor Method, which removes 18 identifiers from the dataset as defined by the Health Insurance Portability and Accountability

Act (HIPAA). An alternative method, statistical de-identification, uses algorithms to minimize the risk of re-identifying patients in large datasets.

From a mathematical perspective, de-identification can be achieved by applying differential privacy techniques, where noise is added to the data to obscure individual records. The formula for differential privacy is expressed as:

P(f(D) = t) < e€P(f(D') = t)

Where D and D' are datasets that differ by one record, f(D) is the output of the data analysis function, and € controls the amount of privacy. By adding this layer of privacy protection, data preprocessing workflows in healthcare must ensure compliance with ethical guidelines while retaining data utility.

Evaluation Metrics for Preprocessing and Annotation Quality

Ensuring the quality of data preprocessing and annotation is crucial for building adequate healthcare NLP models. Various evaluation metrics are used to assess the accuracy and efficiency of preprocessing techniques and the reliability of annotation tasks.

Preprocessing Evaluation Metrics

To measure the impact of preprocessing, we evaluate how well the resulting processed data improves model performance. Common metrics include:

Accuracy: This measures how accurately a model performs after preprocessing. It compares the model's predictions against the ground truth.

Perplexity: A measure of how well a probabilistic model predicts a sample. It is used in language models to evaluate the efficacy of preprocessing steps like tokenization and stop-word removal.

Mathematically, perplexity is defined as:

Perplexity (P) = 2{H(P)

where (H(P)) is the entropy of the model distribution.

ANNOTATION QUALITY METRICS

For annotations, metrics like precision, recall, and F1 score are essential for evaluating how well the entities and relationships have been identified. These metrics provide insights into the annotation process's accuracy and completeness.

Precision: Measures the proportion of correct annotations out of all the annotations made by the model. Mathematically:

Precision = {TP}/ {TP + FP}

where TP is the true positives, and FP is the false positives.

Recall: Measures the proportion of actual annotations that were correctly identified by the model:

Recall = {TP}/ {TP + FN}

FN is the false negatives.

F1 Score: The harmonic mean of precision and recall, providing a balanced evaluation:

F1 Score = 2 X {Precision} X{Recall}}/ {Precision} + {Recall}

These metrics ensure that both preprocessing and annotation phases are optimized for accuracy, ensuring robust healthcare NLP models that can make reliable predictions and support clinical decision-making.

CONCLUSION

Data pre-processing and annotation are indispensable for applying NLP in healthcare. Healthcare organizations can make more reliable and accurate models for predicting diagnoses, patient outcomes, and clinical decision support by carefully cleaning, normalizing, and annotating medical data. Despite challenges like complex medical language and high annotation costs, advancements in automated techniques and hybrid human-machine systems continue improving data preparation efficiency and scalability.

The future of healthcare will be the integration of advanced pre-processing pipelines, transforming the process. Innovations like sophisticated annotation tools and cutting-edge NLP models will enable more accurate data analysis, improve model training, and enhance the ability to extract meaningful insights from unstructured medical data. As a result, healthcare providers will be better equipped to optimize diagnoses, deliver personalized treatments, and ultimately improve patient outcomes, driving the next generation of personalized medicine.

REFERENCES

[1] C. Zong, R. Xia, and J. Zhang, "Data annotation and preprocessing," in Text Data Mining, Singapore: Springer, 2021.
[http://dx.doi.org/10.1007/978-981-16-0100-2_2]

[2] A. Noori, C. Magdamo, X. Liu, T. Tyagi, Z. Li, A. Kondepudi, H. Alabsi, E. Rudmann, D. Wilcox, L. Brenner, G.K. Robbins, L. Moura, S. Zafar, N.M. Benson, J. Hsu, J. R Dickson, A. Serrano-Pozo, B.T. Hyman, D. Blacker, M.B. Westover, S.S. Mukerji, and S. Das, "Development and evaluation of a natural language processing annotation tool to facilitate phenotyping of cognitive status in electronic health records: diagnostic study", *J. Med. Internet Res.,* vol. 24, no. 8, 2022.e40384
[http://dx.doi.org/10.2196/40384] [PMID: 36040790]

[3] A. Rajput, "Natural language processing, sentiment analysis, and clinical analytics", *Innovation in Health Informatics,* no. Jan, pp. 79-97, 2020.
[http://dx.doi.org/10.1016/B978-0-12-819043-2.00003-4]

[4] G.K. Thakur, A. Thakur, N. Khan, and H. Anush, "The role of natural language processing in medical data analysis and healthcare automation", *2024 International Conference on Knowledge Engineering and Communication Systems (ICKECS),* vol. vol. 37, 2024pp. 1-5
[http://dx.doi.org/10.1109/ICKECS61492.2024.10616749]

[5] B. Zhou, G. Yang, Z. Shi, and S. Ma, "Natural language processing for smart healthcare", *IEEE Rev. Biomed. Eng.,* vol. 17, pp. 4-18, 2024.
[http://dx.doi.org/10.1109/RBME.2022.3210270] [PMID: 36170385]

[6] E. Hossain, "Use of AI/ML-enabled state-of-the-art method in electronic medical records: A systematic review", *Comput. Biol. Med.,* vol. 155, 2023.106649
[http://dx.doi.org/10.1016/j.compbiomed.2023.106649] [PMID: 36805219]

[7] J. Stolp, C. Weber, D. Ammon, A. Scherag, C. Fischer, C. Kloos, G. Wolf, P.C. Schulze, U. Settmacher, M. Bauer, A. Stallmach, M. Kiehntopf, and B. Betz, "Automated sample annotation for diabetes mellitus in healthcare integrated biobanking", *Comput. Struct. Biotechnol. J.,* vol. 24, pp. 724-733, 2024.
[http://dx.doi.org/10.1016/j.csbj.2024.10.033] [PMID: 39668942]

[8] A. Marcello Nesca, "Katz, C. K. Leung, and L. M. Lix, “A scoping review of preprocessing methods for unstructured text data to assess data quality", *PubMed,* vol. 7, no. 1, pp. 1757-1757, 2022.
[http://dx.doi.org/10.23889/ijpds.v6i1.1757]

[9] W. Sun, Z. Cai, Y. Li, F. Liu, S. Fang, and G. Wang, "Data processing and text mining technologies on electronic medical records: a review", *J. Healthc. Eng.,* vol. 2018, pp. 1-9, 2018.
[http://dx.doi.org/10.1155/2018/4302425] [PMID: 29849998]

[10] A. Mustafa, and M. Rahimi Azghadi, "Automated machine learning for healthcare and clinical notes analysis", *Computers,* vol. 10, no. 2, p. 24, 2021.
[http://dx.doi.org/10.3390/computers10020024]

[11] J.S. Grosman, P.H.T. Furtado, A.M.B. Rodrigues, G.G. Schardong, S.D.J. Barbosa, and H.C.V. Lopes, "Eras: Improving the quality control in the annotation process for Natural Language Processing tasks", *Inf. Syst.,* vol. 93, 2020.101553
[http://dx.doi.org/10.1016/j.is.2020.101553]

[12] G.M. Silverman, H.S. Sahoo, N.E. Ingraham, M. Lupei, M.A. Puskarich, M. Usher, J. Dries, R.L. Finzel, E. Murray, J. Sartori, G. Simon, R. Zhang, G.B. Melton, C.J. Tignanelli, and S.V.S. Pakhomov, "NLP methods for extraction of symptoms from unstructured data for use in prognostic COVID-19 analytic models", *J. Artif. Intell. Res.,* vol. 72, pp. 429-474, 2021.
[http://dx.doi.org/10.1613/jair.1.12631]

[13] I. Li, J. Pan, J. Goldwasser, N. Verma, W.P. Wong, M.Y. Nuzumlalı, B. Rosand, Y. Li, M. Zhang, D. Chang, R.A. Taylor, H.M. Krumholz, and D. Radev, "Neural Natural Language Processing for unstructured data in electronic health records: A review", *Comput. Sci. Rev.,* vol. 46, 2022.100511

[http://dx.doi.org/10.1016/j.cosrev.2022.100511]

[14] A. Bhatia, R. Titus, J.G. Porto, J. Katz, D.M. Lopategui, R. Marcovich, D.J. Parekh, and H.N. Shah, "Application of Natural Language Processing in Electronic Health Record data extraction for navigating prostate cancer care: A narrative review", *J. Endourol.,* vol. 38, no. 8, pp. 852-864, 2024. [http://dx.doi.org/10.1089/end.2023.0690] [PMID: 38613805]

[15] N. Tvardik, I. Kergourlay, A. Bittar, F. Segond, S. Darmoni, and M.H. Metzger, "Accuracy of using natural language processing methods for identifying healthcare-associated infections", *Int. J. Med. Inform.,* vol. 117, pp. 96-102, 2018. [http://dx.doi.org/10.1016/j.ijmedinf.2018.06.002] [PMID: 30032970]

[16] M. Siino, I. Tinnirello, and M. La Cascia, "Is text preprocessing still worth the time? A comparative survey on the influence of popular preprocessing methods on Transformers and traditional classifiers", *Inf. Syst.,* vol. 121, pp. 102342-102342, 2024. [http://dx.doi.org/10.1016/j.is.2023.102342]

[17] A. Maoliniyazi, C. Ma, X. Meng, and Y. Peng, "LEAF: a less expert annotation framework with active learning", *Lect. Notes Comput. Sci.,* vol. 14647, no. Jan, pp. 369-384, 2024. [http://dx.doi.org/10.1007/978-981-97-2259-4_28]

[18] X. Ming, S. Li, M. Li, L. He, and Q. Wang, "AutoLabel: automated textual data annotation method based on active learning and large language model", *Lect. Notes Comput. Sci.,* vol. 14887, no. Jan, pp. 400-411, 2024. [http://dx.doi.org/10.1007/978-981-97-5501-1_30]

[19] L. Colucci Cante, S. D'Angelo, B. Di Martino, and M. Graziano, "Text annotation tools: A comprehensive review and comparative analysis," in Complex, Intelligent and Software Intensive Systems (CISIS 2024), Lecture Notes on Data Engineering and Communications Technologies, vol. 87, L. Barolli, Ed. Cham, Switzerland: Springer, 2024. [http://dx.doi.org/10.1007/978-3-031-70011-8_33]

[20] A. Sbei, K. ElBedoui, and W. Barhoumi, "Synergistic text annotation based on rule-based expressions and distilbert", *Lect. Notes Comput. Sci.,* vol. 14796, pp. 408-422, 2024. [http://dx.doi.org/10.1007/978-981-97-4985-0_32]

CHAPTER 5

Evaluating Large Language Models for RNA Interaction Extraction: A Comparative Study on Biomedical Research

Balu Bhasuran[1,*], **Forhan Bin Emdad**[1] and **Mohammad Ishtiaque Rahman**[2]

[1] *eHEALTH Lab, College of Communication and Information, Florida State University, TallahasseeFL, 32306-2100, USA*

[2] *Department of Information Systems, University of Maryland - Baltimore County, USA*

Abstract: RNA interactions are pivotal in a wide range of biological functions, including gene regulation, cellular differentiation, and the development of diverse pathological conditions (such as cancer, cardiovascular issues, and neurological disorders). Gaining insight into these interactions is key to unraveling disease pathways and pinpointing promising therapeutic avenues. Nevertheless, extracting such information efficiently from the extensive scholarly literature poses a considerable obstacle. In this work, we conducted an in-depth appraisal of Large Language Models (LLMs) to accurately identify RNA-related interactions in scientific texts. We evaluated the effectiveness of multiple cutting-edge systems, including GPT-4o and Gemini, in detecting these interactions. Our assessment centered on precision, recall, F1 scores, and ROC curve metrics in zero-shot settings, using two recognized datasets—miRNA–mRNA Interaction Corpus (MMIC) and lncRNA–protein interaction corpus (LPInsider). Among the tested LLMs, GPT-4o achieved the best accuracy, F-score, precision, and recall (0.63, 0.60, 0.66, and 0.55, respectively) for miRNA–mRNA interactions. Meanwhile, Gemini led the lncRNA–protein interaction analysis with top accuracy, F-Score, precision, and recall (0.69, 0.66, 0.74, and 0.59, respectively). These findings illuminate both the advantages and drawbacks of current LLMs for extracting RNA interactions, offering valuable guidance for future refinements in precision and overall performance within biomedical research.

Keywords: Biomedical text mining, Relation extraction, Large language models, RNA, Genes.

INTRODUCTION

RNA interactions are central to a wide range of biological processes, including gene regulation, cellular differentiation, and the emergence of multiple

* **Corresponding author Balu Bhasuran:** eHEALTH Lab, College of Communication and Information, Florida State University, Tallahassee FL, 32306-2100, USA; E-mail: bb23u@fsu.edu

A. Shankar, Saranya Jayapalan, & Basant. K. Tiwary (Eds.)

pathological conditions (including, but not limited to, cancer, cardiovascular complications, and neurological disorders). Understanding these interactions is crucial for advancing biomedical research and identifying potential therapeutic targets. However, extracting RNA-related interactions from the vast, ever-growing body of scientific literature presents significant challenges. Traditional methods of manually curating these interactions are time-consuming and often impractical given the sheer volume of published studies. The border area commonly referred to as Biomedical Text Mining (BTM) involves extracting information about biological entities and their relationships, including genes, proteins, diseases, drugs, cell types, miRNAs, phenotypes, and even broader concepts such as biological events and pathways, from scientific texts [1 - 5]. Various methods have been developed for these tasks, including dictionary matching, rule-based approaches, machine learning, deep learning, and transformer-based techniques [6 - 12]. Such approaches strive to improve both the accuracy and efficiency of information extraction in the biomedical domain, supporting research and clinical applications. The three major steps in BTM include information retrieval, information extraction, and knowledge discovery. Various studies have reported the discovery of new knowledge using BTM techniques [13 - 15].

Recently, the rise of Large Language Models (LLMs) has had a transformative effect on Natural Language Processing (NLP) and its applications in biomedical research [16 - 19]. LLMs, such as GPT-4 [20], LLaMA3 [21], Gemini [22], and Mixtral [23], have demonstrated considerable promise in various NLP tasks, including relation extraction. By leveraging massive amounts of training data, these models can comprehend and generate human language with notable sophistication. Their potential to automate the extraction of complex biological interactions from scientific texts has garnered significant interest among researchers.

This study focuses on the application of LLMs for the extraction of RNA-related interactions from scientific literature. RNA plays a pivotal role in numerous biological processes, and effectively identifying its interactions is essential for research in genomics, transcriptomics, and other related fields. Our work evaluates the performance of two state-of-the-art LLMs in extracting RNA interactions to assess their suitability for different biomedical research contexts. Specifically, we analyze these models' precision, recall, and F1 scores, along with ROC curves, to determine their effectiveness in handling the complexity and specificity of RNA-related terminology.

By offering a comprehensive comparative evaluation of these two robust LLMs, this study strives to enrich the broadening scholarly discourse regarding the utilization of artificial intelligence in biomedical research. The insights gained from this evaluation will offer valuable guidance to researchers seeking to leverage LLMs for relation extraction tasks, ultimately enhancing the efficiency and accuracy of RNA-focused research workflows.

MATERIALS AND METHODS

This study evaluates the effectiveness of LLMs in extracting RNA-related interactions from scientific literature. Unlike traditional approaches, this study focuses exclusively on using pre-existing relation corpora and large language models, eliminating the need for entity recognition and manual annotation processes. The primary goal is to assess the performance of several state-of-the-art LLMs, including GPT-4o and Gemini, in accurately extracting and categorizing RNA interactions from curated datasets.

The study utilized pre-existing relation extraction corpora, namely the miRNA–mRNA Interaction Corpus (MMIC) [24] and the lncRNA–protein interaction corpus (LPInsider) [25], which contain annotated RNA interactions. These corpora were selected based on their relevance to RNA-related studies and widespread use in the biomedical NLP community. The datasets included annotations of RNA interactions with other RNA entities, proteins, and genes, providing a comprehensive basis for evaluating the performance of the LLMs. Fig. (**1**) depicts the schematic architecture of the study pipeline, illustrating the Corpus Selection process, which involves identifying and curating relevant datasets based on predefined inclusion criteria to ensure comprehensive and high-quality source material for analysis, followed by LLM-based prediction and evaluation.

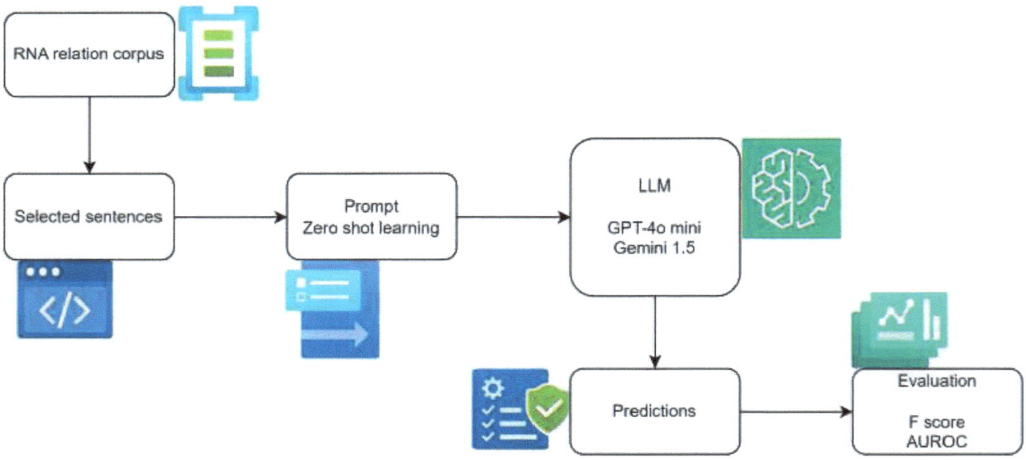

Fig. (1). Schematic architecture of the study pipeline, corpus selection.

The selected corpora were preprocessed to ensure compatibility with the input requirements of the LLMs. This preprocessing included standardization of text formats, removal of extraneous metadata, and segmentation of text into manageable units for input into the models. We selected 200 disease-specific sentences (100 positive and 100 negative) from each corpus, focusing specifically on major cancer types—breast, lung, colon, and prostate—to create a final evaluation set totaling 400 RNA interaction sentences.

LARGE LANGUAGE MODELS

This study focused exclusively on using large language models and evaluating their performance in extracting RNA interactions directly from preprocessed corpora. All LLMs were accessed via the AI-based bot interaction platform Poe [26].

The LLMs used in this study were:

- GPT-4o: An optimized version of GPT-4 designed to deliver faster and more efficient processing.
- Gemini: A versatile and efficient language model designed for both general-purpose and specialized NLP tasks, delivering fast and accurate performance across a wide range of applications. Its optimized architecture ensures adaptability in handling open-domain challenges while excelling at specific, complex problem-solving.

MODEL CONFIGURATION AND TRAINING

Given the study's reliance on existing corpora, the models were evaluated for their out-of-the-box configurations and with minimal fine-tuning to adjust for domain-specific terminology. The fine-tuning process involved exposing the models to a small subset of the corpora to familiarize them with the specific patterns and structures of RNA interactions.

Zero-shot Learning: The models were tasked with extracting RNA interactions without any prior exposure to examples from the corpora. This method tests the models' inherent ability to generalize and accurately predict interactions based solely on their pre-trained knowledge.

EVALUATION METRICS

The performance of each model was assessed using standard NLP metrics:

Precision: The proportion of correctly identified RNA interactions out of all interactions predicted by the model.

Recall: The proportion of actual RNA interactions that were correctly identified by the model.

F1-Score: The harmonic mean of precision and recall, providing a balanced measure of the model's performance.

Accuracy=(TP + TN)(TP + TN + FP + FN) (1)

Precision=TP (TP + FP) (2)

Recall=TP (TP + FN) (3)

F1 Score =2 * (Precision * Recall)(Precision+ Recall) (4)

Where: TP = True Positives, TN = True Negatives, FP = False Positives, FN = False Negatives

ROC curve directly uses True Positive Rate (TPR) and False Positive Rate (FPR) to visualize the trade-offs between true positives and false positives. The closer the curve is to the top-left corner, the better the model performs across different thresholds.

These metrics were calculated for zero-shot learning scenarios to provide a comprehensive assessment of each model's capabilities.

COMPARATIVE ANALYSIS

After obtaining the results, a comparative analysis was conducted to identify the strengths and weaknesses of each model in the context of RNA interaction extraction. The analysis focused on understanding the trade-offs among precision, recall, and overall efficiency, helping to determine the most suitable models for specific biomedical research tasks.

RESULTS

Table (**1**) presents the performance metrics of two models, GPT-4o and Gemini, for extracting interactions between RNA molecules and proteins. Specifically, the table focuses on miRNA-mRNA and lncRNA-Protein interactions, evaluated using accuracy, F1-score, precision, and recall. For the miRNA-mRNA task, GPT-4o demonstrates higher performance across all metrics compared to Gemini. It achieves an accuracy of 0.63 and an F1-score of 0.60, indicating better overall predictive power, while Gemini shows lower values with an accuracy of 0.45 and an F1-score of 0.40. Similarly, GPT-4o's precision (0.66) and recall (0.55) surpass Gemini's precision (0.44) and recall (0.37).

Table 1. Overall model performance for RNA interaction extraction.

Model	Size	Accuracy	F1-Score	Precision	Recall
miRNA-mRNA					
GPT-4o	unknown	0.63	0.60	0.66	0.55
Gemini	8b	0.45	0.40	0.44	0.37
lncRNA-Protein					
GPT-4o	unknown	0.67	0.71	0.64	0.80
Gemini	7b	0.69	0.66	0.74	0.59

In the lncRNA-Protein task, both models perform comparably but with slight variations. GPT-4o achieves an accuracy of 0.67 and an F1-score of 0.71, which is marginally different from Gemini's accuracy of 0.69 and F1-score of 0.66. Notably, GPT-4o has a higher recall (0.80) compared to Gemini's (0.59), suggesting that GPT-4o captures more true interactions, whereas Gemini shows a slightly better precision of 0.74 compared to GPT-4o's 0.64. Overall, GPT-4o tends to be more consistent across both interaction types, especially in terms of recall, while Gemini shows relatively better precision for lncRNA-Protein extraction.

The comparison of GPT-4o and Gemini across different RNA interaction extraction tasks reveals notable differences in their strengths. For miRNA-mRNA extraction, GPT-4o outperforms Gemini in every performance metric, showing a significant lead in accuracy (0.63 *vs.* 0.45), precision (0.66 *vs.* 0.44), recall (0.55 *vs.* 0.37), and F1-score (0.60 *vs.* 0.40). This indicates that GPT-4o is generally more reliable in capturing the number of correct interactions (as seen in the higher precision) and ensuring fewer relevant interactions are missed (as evidenced by the higher recall). Gemini, on the other hand, struggles with both precision and recall, leading to an overall lower F1-score, suggesting that its predictions are less consistent for miRNA-mRNA interactions compared to GPT-4o.

The performance gap between the two models is narrower for the lncRNA-Protein interaction task. Both models achieve comparable accuracy (0.67 for GPT-4o and 0.69 for Gemini), but the individual strengths differ. GPT-4o shows a considerably higher recall (0.80), which implies it is better at detecting true interactions and reducing false negatives. Conversely, Gemini demonstrates a higher precision (0.74), suggesting that it makes fewer false-positive predictions, albeit at the expense of potentially missing more interactions (as indicated by its lower recall of 0.59). The F1-score results (0.71 for GPT-4o and 0.66 for Gemini) reflect these trade-offs: GPT-4o provides a better balance overall, especially when it is crucial not to miss potential interactions. These differences highlight that

GPT-4o may be preferable when completeness is prioritized, while Gemini may be more suitable when minimizing incorrect interactions is essential. Figs. (**2** and **3**) present the confusion matrices for the miRNA-mRNA and lncRNA-Protein corpora, respectively, for both LLMs.

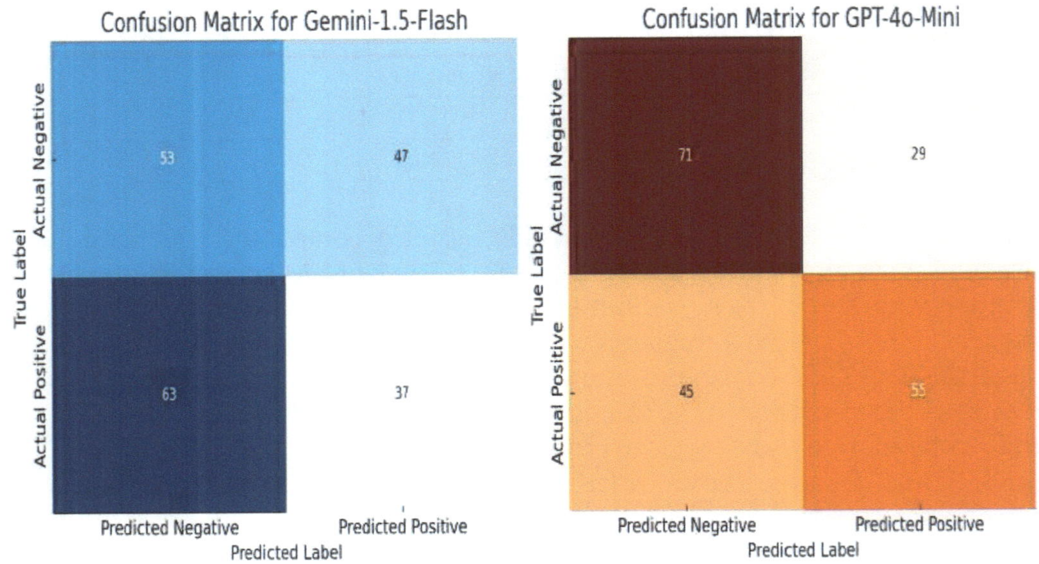

Fig. (2). Confusion matrix for the miRNA-mRNA corpus test set.

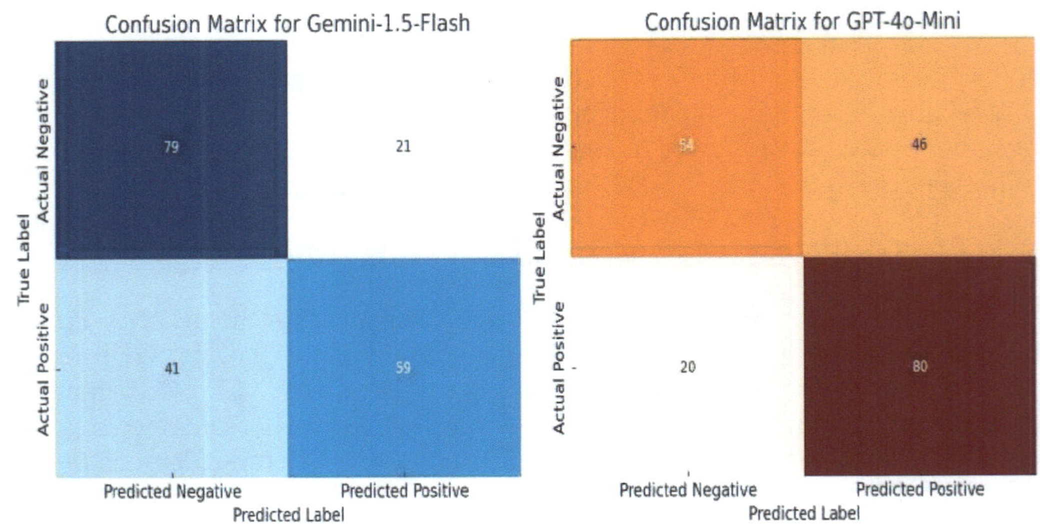

Fig. (3). Confusion matrix for the lncRNA-Protein corpus test set.

From the Fig. (**4**) ROC curve, GPT-4o-mini shows a significantly higher AUC of 0.63 compared to Gemini 1.5 Flash's AUC of 0.45, which indicates superior performance for GPT-4o-mini in extracting interactions. The curve for GPT-4--mini lies above the curve for Gemini 1.5 Flash, which suggests that GPT-4o-mini has a better balance between sensitivity and specificity, making fewer incorrect predictions overall. Gemini's lower AUC value indicates its performance is closer to random guessing, while GPT-4o-mini demonstrates a clear advantage in distinguishing between the two classes. Fig. (**5**) shows that the Area Under the Curve (AUC) is used to summarize the overall performance of the models. The Gemini 1.5 Flash model has an AUC of 0.69, while the GPT-4o-mini has an AUC of 0.67.

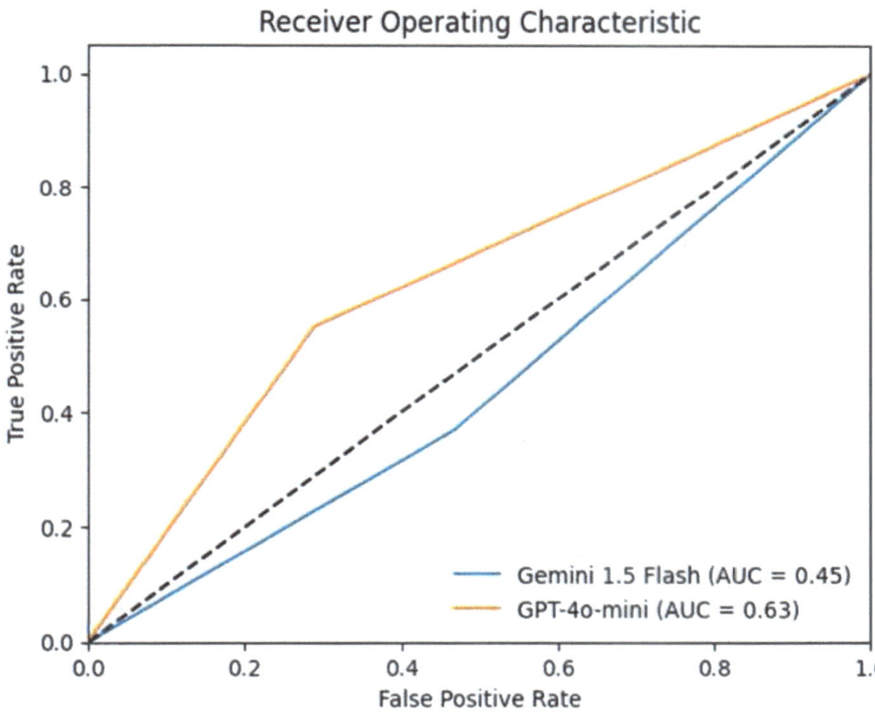

Fig. (4). ROC curve for LLMs on miRNA-mRNA interaction corpus.

Although both models perform similarly, Gemini 1.5 Flash has a slight advantage in terms of AUC, indicating that it is better at distinguishing between true positive and false positive cases than GPT-4o-mini. However, the difference in AUC values is not substantial, suggesting that both models have comparable overall performance, with slight variations in their ability to balance sensitivity (TPR) and specificity (FPR).

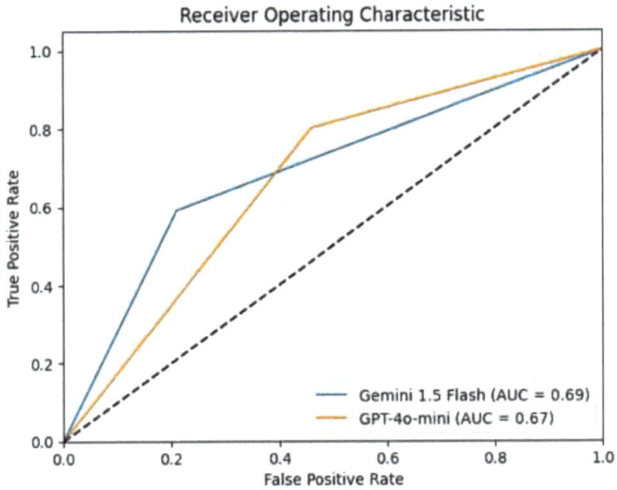

Fig. (5). ROC curve for LLMs on lncRNA-Protein interaction corpus.

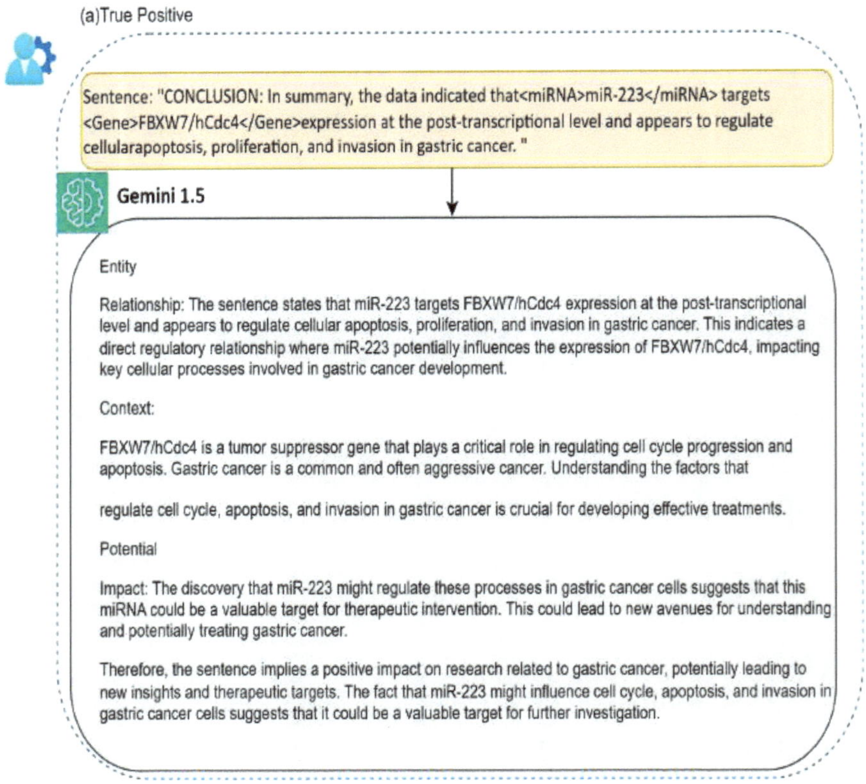

Fig. (6a). Snapshot of accurate positive prediction by Gemini on miRNA-mRNA interaction corpus.

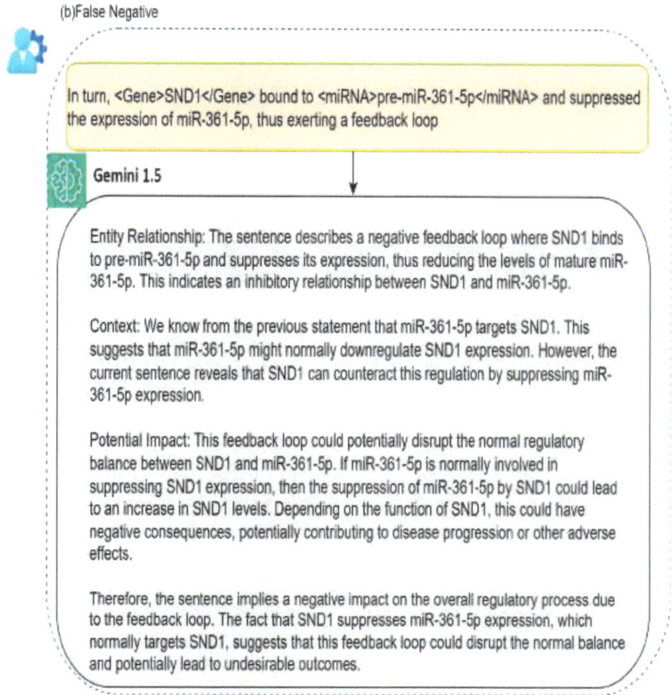

Fig. (6b). Snapshot of false negative prediction by Gemini on miRNA-mRNA interaction corpus.

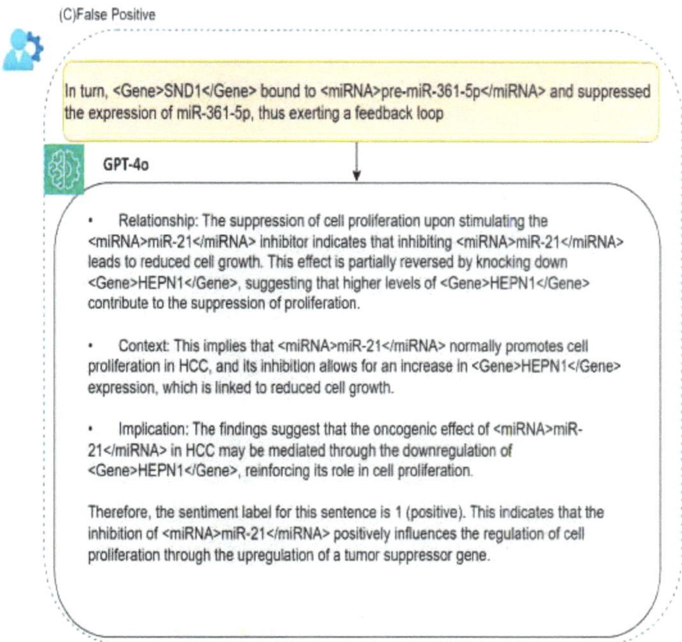

Fig. (6c). Snapshot of false positive prediction by GPT-4o on miRNA-mRNA interaction corpus.

Fig. **(6a-d)**. Illustrates the true positive, false negative, false positive, and accurate negative instances for both GPT-4o and Gemini LLMs. The interpretation of true predictions offers more profound insights into RNA interactions.

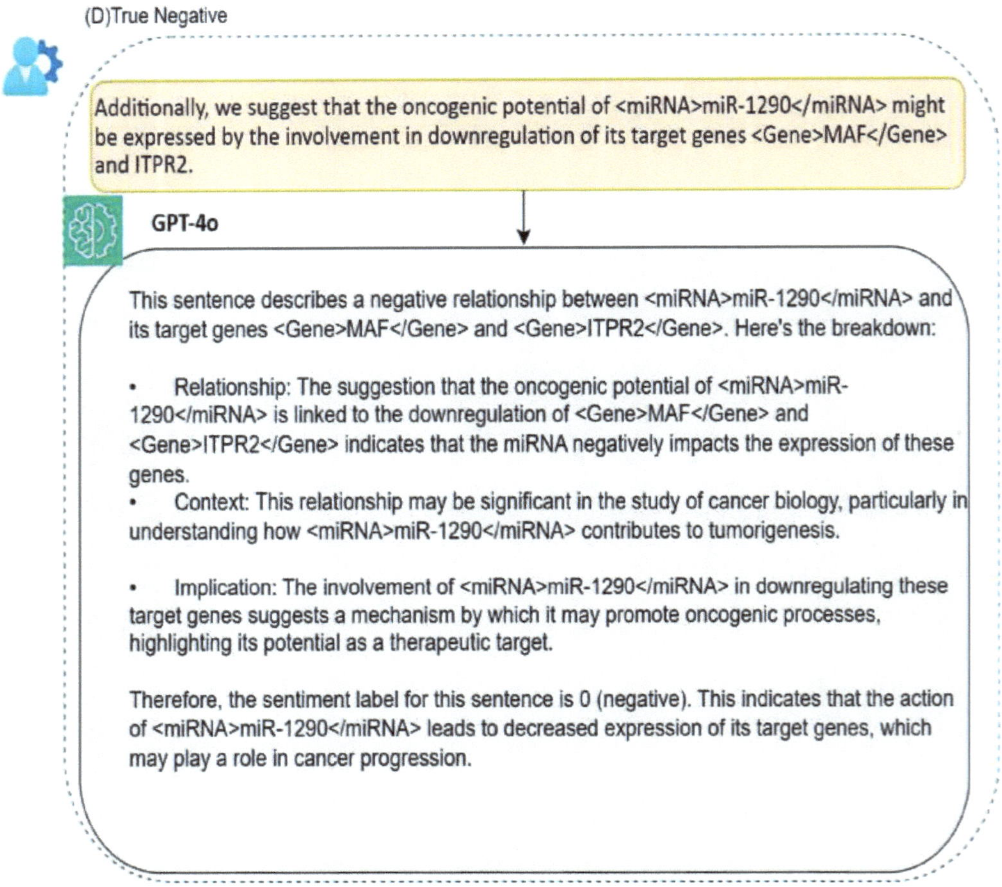

Fig. (6d). Snapshot of true negative prediction by GPT-4o on miRNA-mRNA interaction corpus.

DISCUSSION

The study's application of Large Language Models (LLMs) to extract miRNA-lncRNA interactions from the scientific literature offers valuable insights into the molecular mechanisms underlying cancer progression. The miRNA dataset highlights both oncogenic and tumor-suppressive roles. The models found a true positive association between miR-223 and the FBXW7 gene. miR-223 is critical in regulating apoptosis, proliferation, and invasion in gastric cancer by targeting FBXW7/hCdc4, a tumor suppressor gene, suggesting its potential as a therapeutic target. True positive interactions in the analysis reflect accurate predictions. These insights reinforce the dual roles of miRNAs, serving as oncogenic drivers and tumor suppressors depending on the molecular context.

Similarly, the lncRNA dataset emphasizes the nuanced roles of lncRNAs in cancer biology. The GPT-40 model correctly predicted the relation between lncRNA-ATB and the TGF-β1 protein. lncRNA-ATB promotes migration and invasion in Papillary Thyroid Carcinoma (PTC) under the regulation of TGF-beta1, suggesting its utility as a therapeutic target. On the other hand, lncRNA Evf2 inhibits BRG1's ATPase and chromatin remodeling activities, potentially impairing its tumor-suppressive function, while AK294004 downregulates CCND1, affecting cell cycle regulation. True positive findings accurately capture functional relationships, such as the role of lncRNA-ATB in enhancing cancer cell invasion.

The study's comparative analysis of GPT-4o and Gemini highlights the effectiveness of LLMs in extracting these RNA interactions. For miRNA-mRNA interactions, GPT-4o achieved higher precision and recall, showcasing its ability to capture relevant interactions while minimizing false negatives. In lncRNA-protein interactions, GPT-4o prioritized recall, capturing a broader set of interactions, while Gemini demonstrated superior precision, reducing false positives. These complementary strengths of the two models illustrate their suitability for different biomedical tasks—GPT-4o for comprehensive exploration and Gemini for minimizing erroneous predictions. Accurately identifying true positive and true negative interactions further emphasizes the models' potential to streamline RNA interaction research, enabling automated extraction from vast scientific literature and guiding targeted therapeutic strategies.

CONCLUSION

This study demonstrates the utility of Large Language Models (LLMs) in extracting RNA interactions from scientific literature, specifically focusing on miRNA–mRNA and lncRNA–protein interactions. By leveraging existing annotated corpora, the study highlights that advanced LLMs like GPT-4o and Gemini can extract complex RNA interactions without additional data preprocessing steps, such as entity recognition or manual annotation. GPT-4o consistently outperforms in terms of recall, capturing more relevant interactions, while Gemini shows higher precision, minimizing false positives. These complementary strengths suggest that LLMs can serve different purposes in biomedical research, enhancing either completeness or accuracy based on specific needs. Overall, this evaluation underscores the potential of LLMs in automating information extraction from biomedical texts, paving the way for streamlined RNA research and aiding in the identification of therapeutic targets. Future work should focus on refining model performance to achieve even higher precision and recall in diverse biomedical tasks.

CONSENT FOR PUBLICATION

All authors provide consent for publication.

CONFLICT OF INTEREST

The authors declare no conflict of interest.

ACKNOWLEDGEMENT

This research received no external funding.

REFERENCES

[1] A.M. Cohen, and W.R. Hersh, "A survey of current work in biomedical text mining", *Brief. Bioinform.,* vol. 6, no. 1, pp. 57-71, 2005. [http://dx.doi.org/10.1093/bib/6.1.57] [PMID: 15826357]

[2] PN Ahmad, AM Shah, and K Lee, "A review on electronic health record text-mining for biomedical name entity recognition in healthcare domain", *Healthcare,* vol. 11, no. 9, p. 1268, Apr 2023. [http://dx.doi.org/10.3390/healthcare11091268]

[3] D. Rebholz-Schuhmann, A. Oellrich, and R. Hoehndorf, "Text-mining solutions for biomedical research: enabling integrative biology", *Nat. Rev. Genet.,* vol. 13, no. 12, pp. 829-839, 2012. [http://dx.doi.org/10.1038/nrg3337] [PMID: 23150036]

[4] S. Zhao, C. Su, Z. Lu, and F. Wang, "Recent advances in biomedical literature mining", *Brief. Bioinform.,* vol. 22, no. 3, p. bbaa057, 2021. [http://dx.doi.org/10.1093/bib/bbaa057] [PMID: 32422651]

[5] B. Bhasuran, "Combining literature mining and machine learning for predicting biomedical discoveries", *Methods Mol. Biol.,* vol. 2496, pp. 123-140, 2022. [http://dx.doi.org/10.1007/978-1-0716-2305-3_7] [PMID: 35713862]

[6] J. Lee, W. Yoon, S. Kim, D. Kim, S. Kim, C.H. So, and J. Kang, "BioBERT: a pre-trained biomedical language representation model for biomedical text mining", *Bioinformatics,* vol. 36, no. 4, pp. 1234-1240, 2020. [http://dx.doi.org/10.1093/bioinformatics/btz682] [PMID: 31501885]

[7] Q. Chen, "An extensive benchmark study on biomedical text generation and mining with ChatGPT", *Bioinformatics,* vol. 39, no. 9, p. btad557, Sep 2023. [http://dx.doi.org/10.1093/bioinformatics/btad557]

[8] R. González-Márquez, L. Schmidt, B.M. Schmidt, P. Berens, and D. Kobak, "The landscape of biomedical research", *Patterns,* vol. 5, no. 6, p. 100968, Jun 2024. [http://dx.doi.org/10.1016/j.patter.2024.100968]

[9] B. Bhasuran, G. Murugesan, S. Abdulkadhar, and J. Natarajan, "Stacked ensemble combined with fuzzy matching for biomedical named entity recognition of diseases", *J. Biomed. Inform.,* vol. 64, pp. 1-9, 2016. [http://dx.doi.org/10.1016/j.jbi.2016.09.009] [PMID: 27634494]

[10] M. Lan, "Natural language processing and text mining", In: *Artificial Intelligence for Drug Design,* H. Li, M. Zheng, F. Zhu, F. Bai, Eds., Springer Nature Singapore: Singapore, 2026, pp. 189-215.

[http://dx.doi.org/10.1007/978-981-95-2525-6_18]

[11] J. Kim, S. So, H.J. Lee, J.C. Park, J.J. Kim, and H. Lee, "DigSee: Disease gene search engine with evidence sentences (version cancer)", *Nucleic Acids Research,* vol. 41, pp. W510-W517, Jul 2013. [http://dx.doi.org/10.1093/nar/gkt531]

[12] L. Luo, P.T. Lai, C.H. Wei, C.N. Arighi, and Z. Lu, "BioRED: A rich biomedical relation extraction dataset", *Briefings in Bioinformatics,* vol. 23, no. 5, p. bbac282, Sep 2022. [http://dx.doi.org/10.1093/bib/bbac282]

[13] R. Luo, "BioGPT: generative pre-trained transformer for biomedical text generation and mining", *Briefings in Bioinformatics,* vol. 23, no. 6, p. bbac409, Nov 2022. [http://dx.doi.org/10.1093/bib/bbac409]

[14] Z. Zhang, "Large-Scale biomedical relation extraction across diverse relation types: Model development and usability study on COVID-19", *Journal of Medical Internet Research,* vol. 25, p. e48115, Sep 2023. [http://dx.doi.org/10.2196/48115]

[15] N. Maroli, "Molecular mechanism of T-2 toxin-induced cerebral edema by aquaporin-4 blocking and permeation", *Journal of Chemical Information and Modeling,* vol. 59, no. 11, pp. 4942-4958, Nov 2019. [http://dx.doi.org/10.1021/acs.jcim.9b00711]

[16] M.T. Tahir, M. Ibrahim, N. Sarwar, A. Irshad, and G. Atteia, "Enhanced drug-drug interaction extraction from biomedical text using deep learning-based sentence representations", *Scientific Reports,* vol. 15, no. 1, p. 37842, Oct 2025. [http://dx.doi.org/10.1038/s41598-025-21782-0]

[17] K. Singhal, "Large language models encode clinical knowledge", *Nature,* vol. 620, no. 7972, pp. 172-180, 2023. [http://dx.doi.org/10.1038/s41586-023-06291-2] [PMID: 37438534]

[18] A.J. Thirunavukarasu, D.S.J. Ting, K. Elangovan, L. Gutierrez, T.F. Tan, and D.S.W. Ting, "Large language models in medicine", *Nat. Med.,* vol. 29, no. 8, pp. 1930-1940, 2023. [http://dx.doi.org/10.1038/s41591-023-02448-8] [PMID: 37460753]

[19] S. Tian, Q. Jin, L. Yeganova, P.T. Lai, Q. Zhu, X. Chen, Y. Yang, Q. Chen, W. Kim, D.C. Comeau, R. Islamaj, A. Kapoor, X. Gao, and Z. Lu, "Opportunities and challenges for ChatGPT and large language models in biomedicine and health", *Brief. Bioinform.,* vol. 25, no. 1, p. bbad493, 2023. [http://dx.doi.org/10.1093/bib/bbad493] [PMID: 38168838]

[20] OpenAI *et al*, "GPT-4 technical report", *arXiv,* 2023. [http://dx.doi.org/10.48550/arXiv.2303.08774]

[21] OpenAI *et al*, "The llama 3 herd of models", *arXiv,* 2024. [http://dx.doi.org/10.48550/arXiv.2407.21783]

[22] Gemini Team *et al*, "Gemini: A family of highly capable multimodal models", *arXiv,* 2023. [http://dx.doi.org/10.48550/arXiv.2312.11805]

[23] Q Jiang, "Mixtral of experts", *arXiv,* 2024. [http://dx.doi.org/10.48550/arXiv.2401.04088]

[24] B. Bhasuran, S. Manoharan, O.R. Iyyappan, G. Murugesan, A. Prabahar, and K. Raja, "Large language models and genomics for summarizing the role of microRNA in regulating mRNA expression", *Biomedicines,* vol. 12, no. 7, p. 1535, 2024. [http://dx.doi.org/10.3390/biomedicines12071535] [PMID: 39062108]

[25] Y. Li, L. Wei, C. Wang, J. Zhao, S. Han, Y. Zhang, and W. Du, "LPInsider: a webserver for lncRNA–protein interaction extraction from the literature", *BMC Bioinformatics,* vol. 23, no. 1, p. 135, 2022. [http://dx.doi.org/10.1186/s12859-022-04665-3] [PMID: 35428172]

[26] Poe: A Platform for AI-Powered Conversations," Poe.com. [Online]. Available: [Accessed: Sep. 6, 2024]
[http://dx.doi.org/10.48550/ARXIV.2407.21783]

CHAPTER 6

Futuristic Approach for Enhancing Healthcare Using Bi-LSTM and NLP

R. Deepalakshmi[1,*] and **S. Mary Praveena**[2]

[1] *Department of ECE, CARE College of Engineering, Tiruchirappalli, Tamil Nadu, India*

[2] *Department of ECE, Sri Ramakrishna Institute of Technology, Coimbatore, India*

Abstract: Healthcare informatics transforms modern medicine using advanced computational techniques to enhance patient care and clinical decision-making. Natural Language Processing (NLP) is a key innovation in this field, which extracts critical insights from unstructured clinical data, including Electronic Health Records (EHRs), medical notes, and research articles. The vast complexity of healthcare data demands sophisticated models capable of interpreting intricate medical language. One such model, the Bidirectional Long Short-Term Memory (Bi-LSTM) algorithm, a recurrent neural network, excels in this domain. By processing sequences in both forward and backward directions, Bi-LSTM effectively captures contextual dependencies, making it invaluable for tasks such as named entity recognition, medical text classification, and sentiment analysis. By integrating Bi-LSTM with NLP, healthcare informatics can improve diagnostic accuracy, detect adverse drug reactions, and streamline clinical workflows. Bi-LSTM's ability to handle sequential data and adapt to diverse NLP tasks enables intelligent systems that support informed decision-making in healthcare. This study highlights the effectiveness of Bi-LSTM in addressing real-world challenges like early disease detection and personalized treatment planning. Experiments show that Bi-LSTM outperforms conventional LSTM models, demonstrating superior handling of long-range dependencies and higher predictive accuracy. Integrating Bi-LSTM and NLP is revolutionizing healthcare delivery, offering opportunities for personalized medicine and improved patient outcomes. Future work will focus on optimizing model performance and broadening its application across various healthcare domains, further enhancing the efficiency and precision of data-driven healthcare solutions.

Keywords: AI-driven diagnostics, Bi-directional LSTM (Bi-LSTM), Healthcare efficiency, Healthcare informatics, Natural Language Processing (NLP).

INTRODUCTION

Healthcare informatics has become a cornerstone of modern medical practice, bridging the gap between clinical needs and computational advancements to

[*] **Corresponding author R. Deepalakshmi:** Department of ECE, CARE College of Engineering, Tiruchirappalli, Tamil Nadu, India; E-mail: rdeepalakshmi@care.ac.in

improve the quality, efficiency, and accessibility of patient care. As the medical field continues to generate vast amounts of data, innovative methods are required to manage, interpret, and utilize this information effectively.

Among these, Natural Language Processing (NLP) has drawn significant interest due to its ability to convert unstructured clinical data into valuable insights, including research papers, medical notes, and Electronic Health Records (EHRs). In healthcare informatics, Natural Language Processing (NLP) is an essential component that helps healthcare providers make better decisions and improve patient outcomes.

The rapid expansion of clinical data presents a unique challenge. Unlike structured data that is neatly organized in databases, clinical data is often unstructured, containing diverse information types and complex language. This complexity necessitates advanced computational models to understand the intricate terminologies and contexts unique to healthcare [1]. NLP meets these demands by allowing computers to process and analyze human language, making it possible to interpret medical records, flag potential adverse drug reactions, and assist with diagnostic support. These capabilities can provide clinicians with timely, relevant information, improving patient care in various ways [2].

The Bidirectional Long Short-Term Memory (Bi-LSTM) algorithm, a Recurrent Neural Network (RNN) designed specifically to process sequential input, is an emerging method in NLP for healthcare. Conventional LSTM networks process information in a single direction, usually from the past to the future. Despite its effectiveness, this method is limited for tasks requiring context comprehension across past and future data. By processing data forward and backward, Bi-LSTM improves this, enabling the model to identify dependencies across a sequence. In healthcare applications, where accurate analysis requires knowledge of a patient's full medical history or symptoms, this bidirectional processing is beneficial.

The Bi-LSTM architecture has demonstrated significant potential across various NLP tasks in healthcare, such as named entity recognition, medical text classification, and sentiment analysis. Named entity recognition involves identifying specific medical terms within a text, such as medications, symptoms, or diagnoses. This capability allows Bi-LSTM to automatically identify and categorize important information within patient records, aiding in developing structured databases and facilitating easier retrieval of relevant information. Medical text classification, another application, involves categorizing unstructured data into predefined categories, such as diagnoses or treatment plans. By accurately sorting information, Bi-LSTM can streamline workflows, assist in documentation, and provide healthcare providers with organized insights [3].

One specific application of Bi-LSTM in healthcare informatics is cancer prediction and diagnosis. Traditional diagnostic methods often rely on visual assessments of medical images, which can sometimes lack the precision needed for early detection of cancer cells. The Bi-LSTM algorithm offers a more nuanced approach by leveraging textual and contextual data, potentially revealing patterns or correlations that may go unnoticed through conventional analysis. By incorporating Bi-LSTM, the model can interpret the complex, nuanced language in clinical data, improving the model's ability to detect cancer cells with higher precision. For example, the model can process detailed descriptions from pathology reports or radiology notes, helping clinicians identify subtle cancer markers more accurately [4].

The bidirectional approach of Bi-LSTM also enhances the personalization of healthcare. Personalized medicine tailors treatment and care to the individual characteristics of each patient, often requiring an in-depth understanding of medical history, genetic profiles, and previous treatment responses. By processing data in both directions, Bi-LSTM can account for a patient's historical medical context and anticipate future needs, assisting clinicians in creating treatment plans that are both timely and specific to the individual. Furthermore, in pharmacovigilance, Bi-LSTM models can analyze patient records to detect potential adverse reactions, enhancing patient safety by providing early alerts to clinicians.

This study explores the integration of Bi-LSTM with NLP in healthcare informatics and underscores its transformative potential. Experimental results indicate that Bi-LSTM outperforms traditional LSTM models, particularly in handling long-range dependencies, which are common in medical data. This capability is critical in tasks such as analyzing a patient's medical history, where events are interconnected across multiple data points. The results further demonstrate Bi-LSTM's superior predictive accuracy, validating its effectiveness in real-world healthcare applications like early disease detection and personalized treatment planning [5].

As healthcare generates vast amounts of complex data, the demand for sophisticated tools like Bi-LSTM combined with NLP will only grow [6]. These tools are set to revolutionize healthcare informatics by enabling faster, more precise extraction of insights from unstructured data, improving patient care and clinical workflow. By streamlining data interpretation and enhancing diagnostic accuracy, Bi-LSTM and NLP have the potential to reshape clinical practices, making them more data-driven and patient-centered [7].

Future work will aim to enhance the performance of Bi-LSTM models by optimizing their architecture, minimizing computational overhead, and extending their capabilities to handle multimodal data. This includes integrating textual information with other data types, such as medical images or laboratory results, to provide more comprehensive and accurate analyses. Refining these models to understand specialized medical terminology better and implementing them across various healthcare domains can further unlock their potential [8]. Ultimately, the ongoing development of Bi-LSTM and NLP-based solutions will contribute to a new era of healthcare, where informed, timely decisions are made possible by intelligent, data-driven insights. This evolution in healthcare informatics promises to enhance operational efficiency and provide a higher standard of patient care across diverse medical settings [9].

LITERATURE REVIEW AND EXISTING MODEL

Bi-LSTM in Natural Language Processing (NLP)

Since the introduction of Bi-LSTM, NLP has seen extensive applications of this architecture due to its ability to capture bidirectional context in text sequences. A study by Huang *et al.* (2015) showed Bi-LSTM's effectiveness in Named Entity Recognition (NER) by leveraging both preceding and succeeding words in sentences, significantly improving accuracy over unidirectional LSTM and traditional NER models. Bi-LSTM was also used in sentiment analysis tasks [10], effectively capturing complex dependencies in sentiment phrases. These applications underscore Bi-LSTM's ability to enhance understanding of semantic relationships in text.

Subsequent studies advanced this use by combining Bi-LSTM with attention mechanisms. For instance [11], a study demonstrated that the attention-based Bi-LSTM model could improve document classification by focusing on informative words within a sequence, enhancing interpretability and precision. Similarly, it found that coupling Bi-LSTM with transformer architectures yielded further improvements in tasks that required fine-grained linguistic structure understanding [12].

Bi-LSTM in Time-Series Analysis

Bi-LSTM has also become prominent in time-series analysis, where bidirectional dependency capture is vital. Bi-LSTM was implemented for financial time-series forecasting, showing that bidirectional LSTM could more effectively capture complex temporal patterns, leading to better forecasting accuracy than traditional statistical methods such as ARIMA or conventional LSTM models [13].

Additionally, this approach was extended by integrating attention mechanisms with Bi-LSTM for time-series data, highlighting improved performance in capturing relevant trends over long sequences [14].

Bi-LSTM has been used in biomedical signal processing to predict events based on physiological signals. The study found that Bi-LSTM could accurately classify sequential health data, such as electrocardiograms (ECGs), outperforming unidirectional RNNs and demonstrating its potential for real-time monitoring in healthcare [15].

Speech Recognition and Audio Processing

Bi-LSTM has been shown to capture both forward and backward temporal dependencies in speech and audio processing, which are essential for understanding phonetic patterns. The study applied Bi-LSTM with Connectionist Temporal Classification (CTC) for end-to-end speech recognition [16]. Their work revealed that Bi-LSTM could process speech sequences bidirectionally, significantly reducing error rates compared to unidirectional LSTM approaches. Furthermore, recent advancements in integrating Bi-LSTM with deep convolutional layers have further improved recognition rates, especially in noisy environments [17].

Bi-LSTM in Machine Translation and Cross-Lingual Tasks

Bi-LSTM has also advanced machine translation tasks by enhancing the translation of both forward and backward sentence contexts [18]. Research on sequence-to-sequence learning laid the foundation for Bi-LSTM in translation by showing that encoding sentences bidirectionally could improve the quality of translations in both short and long text sequences [19]. Recent studies have also integrated attention mechanisms with Bi-LSTM for translation, allowing the model to focus on relevant parts of input sentences, thereby improving translation quality for complex languages.

While Bi-LSTM shows impressive results across various domains, several limitations persist. First, training Bi-LSTM models requires significant computational resources due to the dual processing layers, which can slow down real-time applications [20]. To address this, current research focuses on optimizing Bi-LSTM architectures through pruning, quantization, and other techniques to make them more efficient [21]. Additionally, integrating Bi-LSTM with transformer-based models and attention mechanisms shows promise in enhancing model interpretability and performance, suggesting a trend toward hybrid architectures.

Healthcare informatics has steadily evolved to improve the quality and efficiency of patient care by integrating advanced computational techniques into clinical workflows [22]. Recent research has focused on harnessing Artificial Intelligence (AI) and Machine Learning (ML) methods, especially in processing and analyzing large, unstructured datasets, such as those found in Electronic Health Records (EHRs), diagnostic imaging reports, and medical research literature [23].

One notable development in this domain is the application of Natural Language Processing (NLP) to make sense of vast amounts of clinical text data [24]. Traditional NLP approaches, like rule-based systems, initially provided structured insights from unstructured text. However, these systems often lacked flexibility and struggled with the complex language and variability in clinical documentation [25]. Over time, more robust techniques, such as neural network-based models, were introduced to address these limitations. For example, Convolutional Neural Networks (CNNs) and Recurrent Neural Networks (RNNs) have shown considerable promise in extracting relevant medical information [26]. However, they may still encounter limitations in capturing healthcare's nuanced and context-dependent language.

The Bidirectional Long Short-Term Memory (Bi-LSTM) model is one of the newer architectures applied to healthcare informatics, offering a unique advantage over traditional LSTM models by processing input sequences in both directions [27]. This bidirectional capability allows the model to understand context more effectively, which is particularly useful in domains where both past and future data points influence outcomes, such as cancer prediction from clinical notes or imaging descriptions [28]. Bi-LSTM-based approaches have demonstrated promising results in identifying clinical patterns, contributing to precision medicine by enhancing diagnostic accuracy and personalizing treatment recommendations [29].

PROPOSED MODEL

Bi-LSTM Algorithm and Approach

An improved Recurrent Neural Network (RNN) called Bidirectional Long Short-Term Memory (Bi-LSTM) is made to process sequential data both forward and backward. Bi-LSTM efficiently extracts contextual information from historical and prospective data inside the input sequence by fusing the powers of LSTM with bidirectional processing [30].

A more sophisticated form of Recurrent Neural Network (RNN) architecture created especially to process sequential input is called Bidirectional Long Short-Term Memory (Bi-LSTM) (Fig. **1**). Conventional LSTM models analyze data in a single direction, often forward, using the previous data points as a basis for processing each time step in a sequence. This method, however, occasionally restricts the model's comprehension of dependencies over lengthy sequences. By enabling information to flow forward and backward, Bi-LSTM overcomes this restriction and offers a deeper understanding of the sequence context. Because of this, Bi-LSTM models are particularly helpful in applications where knowledge of both past and future information is essential, and information order is important.

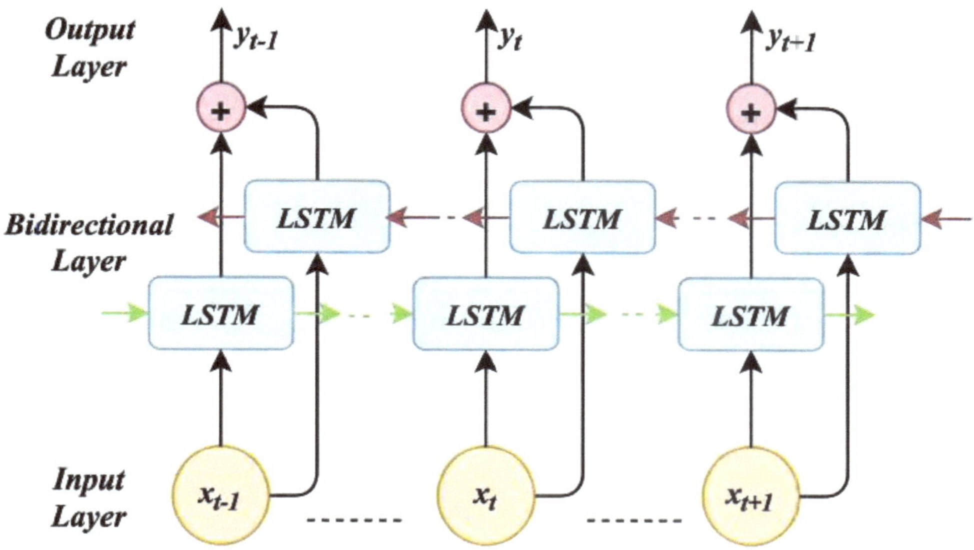

Fig. (1). Bi-LSTM model.

By adding two LSTM layers, Bi-LSTM expands on LSTM: One that processes the input sequence forward, from beginning to end, and another that processes the data in a reverse direction, from beginning to end [31]. At each time step, the outputs of these two layers, which operate concurrently and independently, are merged.

To determine the best model for deciphering navigational safety information, the study assesses six Bi-LSTM CRF-based deep learning models for the semantic classification of NAVTEX signals [32].

To improve prediction accuracy in drilling operations, the study presents an end-to-end ROP prediction model that combines bidirectional long short-term memory

(Bi-LSTM) with self-attention and an improved Dragonfly Algorithm. The ROP prediction method is based on an improved BiLSTM-SA-IDBO.

Workflow of the Bi-LSTM

Forward LSTM: This layer processes the input data sequence forward. For example, in a sequence of words, the forward LSTM starts with the first word and moves to the last word.

Backward LSTM: In parallel, the backward LSTM layer processes the input in reverse order, starting from the last word and moving toward the first word.

Combining the Outputs: At the time step, the outputs from the forward and backward LSTM layers are concatenated, summed, or otherwise combined to form the final output. This combination allows the network to use past and future information to predict its current state.

Data Preprocessing

- Normalization: Each input feature (Features 1–6) is normalized to fall within a standard range (e.g., 0 to 1) to aid in convergence during training.
- Sequencing: The input data is transformed into sequences compatible with the Bi-LSTM input structure. Sequences are padded to ensure uniformity in length, allowing for batch processing.

Model Architecture

- Combining Outputs: At each time step, the outputs from the forward and backward layers are concatenated, enabling the model to consider both preceding and succeeding contexts simultaneously.
- Dense Layer and Activation: After concatenation, the combined output is passed through a dense layer, often with a ReLU or softmax activation, to produce the final prediction.

Training the Model

- Loss Function: The model is trained to minimize a loss function appropriate to the task. For regression, Mean Squared Error (MSE) may be used, while categorical cross-entropy is typically used for classification.
- Optimization: An adaptive optimizer such as Adam is used for gradient descent to enhance learning efficiency.

- Regularization: Dropout layers are added between layers to reduce overfitting, especially given the complex nature of bidirectional networks.

Model Evaluation and Analysis

- Evaluation Metrics: Performance is evaluated using metrics appropriate to the problem domain, such as accuracy, F1-score for classification, or Mean Absolute Error (MAE) for regression.
- Scatter Plot Analysis of Features and Target Variable: A detailed examination of input feature-target variable relationships is conducted to identify potential predictive patterns. Scatter plots reveal that most data points cluster at lower target values, suggesting that the target variable is primarily influenced by low feature values.

Key Advantages of Bi-LSTM.

- ***Access to past and future contexts***: In traditional LSTM, the model can only learn dependencies from previous time steps, whereas Bi-LSTM captures information from both directions. For instance, in Natural Language Processing (NLP), the meaning of a word depends on the words before and after it.
- ***Improved Performance in Sequential Tasks***: Tasks such as machine translation, speech recognition, and time-series analysis often require knowledge of both past and future contexts. Bi-LSTM models outperform regular LSTM models in such tasks by having access to both sides of the sequence.
- ***Better Handling of Long Dependencies***: Bi-LSTM further enhances LSTM's ability of LSTM to capture long-range dependencies, making it more suitable for tasks with complex, long sequences.

The datasets for cancer cell prediction were collected from the following resources.

1. **Kaggle's Cancer Data**: This dataset includes patient characteristics and cancer diagnoses, useful for predictive modeling.
2. **Cancer Research Data Commons (CRDC)**: Provides access to a variety of datasets from NCI- and NIH-funded programs, including genomic, proteomic, and clinical data.
3. **Lung and Colon Cancer Histopathological Image Dataset (LC25000)**: Contains 25,000 histopathological images across five classes, aiding in image-based cancer cell prediction.

These datasets can serve as valuable resources for developing and testing models in cancer cell prediction research.

Algorithm and Coding using MATLAB:

```
% Load and read the dataset
data = xlsread('RESULTS_2.xlsx');
% Replace NaN with zeros
disp(data);
% Normalization of data
normalizedData = normalize(data);
data_nor = abs(normalizedData);
data_nor(isnan(data_nor)) = 0;
% Split the dataset into X and Y
X = data_nor(:, 1:end-2); % Input features (all columns except the last one)
Y = data_nor(:, end); % Output labels (last column)
% Shuffle the data
shuffle_indices = randperm(size(X, 1));
X = X(shuffle_indices,:);
Y = Y(shuffle_indices,:);
% Exploratory data analysis
% Histogram of the target variable
figure;
histogram(Y);
title('Histogram of Target Variable');
xlabel('Values');
ylabel('Frequency');
% Scatter plots of input features vs. target variable
```

```
numFeatures = size(X, 2);
figure;
for i = 1:numFeatures
subplot(1, numFeatures, i);
scatter(X(:, i), Y);
xlabel(['Feature ', num2str(i)]);
ylabel('Target Variable');
end
sgtitle('Scatter Plots: Input Features vs. Target Variable');
% Correlation matrix of input features
correlation_matrix = corr(X);
figure;
imagesc(correlation_matrix);
colorbar;
title('Correlation Matrix of Input Features for PTFE (Polytetrafluoroethylene) Lossy Material');
xlabel('Features');
ylabel('Features');
% Print the shape of predictors
disp(['Shape of predictors: ', num2str(size(X))]);
% Print the shape of target
disp(['Shape of target: ', num2str(size(Y))]);
% Split the data into training and testing sets
train_ratio = 0.8; % 90% for training, 10% for testing
```

```
train_samples = round(train_ratio * size(data_nor, 1));
X_train = X(1:train_samples,:);
X_test = X(train_samples+1:end,:);
Y_train = Y(1:train_samples,:);
Y_test = Y(train_samples+1:end,:);
% Print the shape of predictors
disp(['Shape of train data: ', num2str(size(X_train))]);
disp(['Shape of test data: ', num2str(size(X_test))]);
% Print the shape of target
disp(['Shape of train labels: ', num2str(size(Y_train))]);
disp(['Shape of test labels: ', num2str(size(Y_test))]);
% Define the BiLSTM architecture
numFeatures = size(X_train, 2); % Number of input features
numHiddenUnits = 100; % Number of hidden units in the LSTM layer
numClasses = 1; % Number of output classes (for regression, it is 1)
layers = [ ...
sequenceInputLayer(numFeatures)
lstmLayer(numHiddenUnits)
fullyConnectedLayer(numClasses)
regressionLayer];
% Set training options
options = trainingOptions('adam', ...
'MaxEpochs', 500, ...
'MiniBatchSize', 10, ...
```

```
'ValidationData', {X_test', Y_test'}, ...

'ValidationFrequency', 10, ...

'Shuffle', 'every-epoch', ...

'Plots', 'training-progress', ...

'Verbose', 1);

% Assuming you have already defined and compiled the LSTM architecture

net = trainNetwork(X_train', Y_train', layers, options);

% Predict using the trained LSTM on test data

Y_lstm_pred = predict(net, X_test')';

% Train the Random Forest

rf = fitrensemble(X_train, Y_train, 'Method', 'Bag', 'NumLearningCycles', 100,
'Learners', 'Tree');

% Assuming you want to view the first tree

view(rf.Trained{1}, 'Mode', 'graph');

% Predict using the Random Forest on test data

Y_rf_pred = predict(rf, X_test);

% Take the average of LSTM and Random Forest predictions

Y_combined_pred = (Y_lstm_pred + Y_rf_pred) / 2;

% Define metrics functions

mse = @(y_true, y_pred) mean((y_true - y_pred).^2);

rmse = @(y_true, y_pred) sqrt(mse(y_true, y_pred));

mae = @(y_true, y_pred) mean(abs(y_true - y_pred));

r_square = @(y_true, y_pred) 1 - sum((y_true - y_pred).^2) / sum((y_true -
mean(y_true)).^2);

% Calculate metrics
```

```
mse_combined = mse(Y_test, Y_combined_pred);
rmse_combined = rmse(Y_test, Y_combined_pred);
mae_combined = mae(Y_test, Y_combined_pred);
r_square_combined = r_square(Y_test, Y_combined_pred);
% Apply the threshold to convert to binary classes
Y_binary = Y > 0.5; % Values greater than 0.5 will be 1, and others will be 0
% Print the shape of binary target
disp(['Shape of binary target: ', num2str(size(Y_binary))]);
sum_zeros = sum(Y_binary == 0);
sum_ones = sum(Y_binary == 1);
disp("-
-
----------------------------------------------------------------------------------------------------------
----------------");
disp(['Number of 0s: ', num2str(sum_zeros)]);
disp("-
-
----------------------------------------------------------------------------------------------------------
----------------");
disp(['Number of 1s: ', num2str(sum_ones)]);
disp("-
-
----------------------------------------------------------------------------------------------------------
----------------");
X_train = X(1:train_samples,:);
X_test = X(train_samples+1:end,:);
Y_train = Y_binary(1:train_samples,:);
Y_test = Y_binary(train_samples+1:end,:);
```

```
% Print the shape of data splits
disp(['Shape of train data: ', num2str(size(X_train))]);
disp(['Shape of test data: ', num2str(size(X_test))]);
disp(['Shape of train labels: ', num2str(size(Y_train))]);
disp(['Shape of test labels: ', num2str(size(Y_test))]);
% Train the Random Forest for classification
numTrees = 100; % Number of trees in the forest
rf_classifier = TreeBagger(numTrees, X_train, Y_train, 'Method', 'classification');
% Plot ROC curve
figure;
plot(fpr_1, tpr_1);
xlabel('False Positive Rate');
ylabel('True Positive Rate');
```

Algorithm and Coding using Python:

```
train_dataset, test_dataset = dataset['train'], dataset['test']
batch_size = 32
train_dataset = train_dataset.shuffle(10000)
train_dataset = train_dataset.batch(batch_size)
test_dataset = test_dataset.batch(batch_size)
example, label = next(iter(train_dataset))
print('Text:\n', example.numpy()[0])
print('\nLabel: ', label.numpy()[0])
encoder = tf.keras.layers.TextVectorization(max_tokens=10000)
encoder.adapt(train_dataset.map(lambda text, _: text))
```

```
vocabulary = np.array(encoder.get_vocabulary())
original_text = example.numpy()[0]
encoded_text = encoder(original_text).numpy()
decoded_text = ' '.join(vocabulary[encoded_text])
print('original: ', original_text)
print('encoded: ', encoded_text)
print('decoded: ', decoded_text)
model = tf.keras.Sequential([
encoder,
tf.keras.layers.Embedding(
len(encoder.get_vocabulary()), 64, mask_zero=True),
tf.keras.layers.Bidirectional(
tf.keras.layers.LSTM(64, return_sequences=True)),
tf.keras.layers.Bidirectional(tf.keras.layers.LSTM(32)),
tf.keras.layers.Dense(64, activation='relu'),
tf.keras.layers.Dense(1)
])
model.summary()
# Compile the model
model.compile(
loss=tf.keras.losses.BinaryCrossentropy(from_logits=True),
optimizer=tf.keras.optimizers.Adam(),
metrics=['accuracy']
)
```

```
# Training the model and validating it on test set
history = model.fit(
train_dataset,
epochs=5,
validation_data=test_dataset,
)
# Plotting the accuracy and loss over time
# Training history
history_dict = history.history
# Seperating validation and training accuracy
acc = history_dict['accuracy']
val_acc = history_dict['val_accuracy']
# Seperating validation and training loss
loss = history_dict['loss']
val_loss = history_dict['val_loss']
# Plotting
plt.figure(figsize=(8, 4))
plt.subplot(1, 2, 1)
plt.plot(acc)
plt.plot(val_acc)
plt.title('Training and Validation Accuracy')
plt.xlabel('Epochs')
plt.ylabel('Accuracy')
plt.legend(['Accuracy', 'Validation Accuracy'])
```

```
plt.subplot(1, 2, 2)
plt.plot(loss)
plt.plot(val_loss)
plt.title('Training and Validation Loss')
plt.xlabel('Epochs')
plt.ylabel('Loss')
plt.legend(['Loss', 'Validation Loss'])
plt.show()
# Making predictions
predictions = model.predict(np.array([sample_text]))
print(*predictions[0])
# Print the label based on the prediction
if predictions[0] > 0:
print('The review is positive')
else:
print('The review is negative')
```

The image (Fig. **2**) represents scatter plots that compare six different input features (features 1–6) with a target variable.

Input Features (Features 1–6): Each plot shows one of the features on the x-axis, with values ranging between 0 and 5 for all features.

Target Variable (y-axis): The values of the target variable range between 1 and 6.

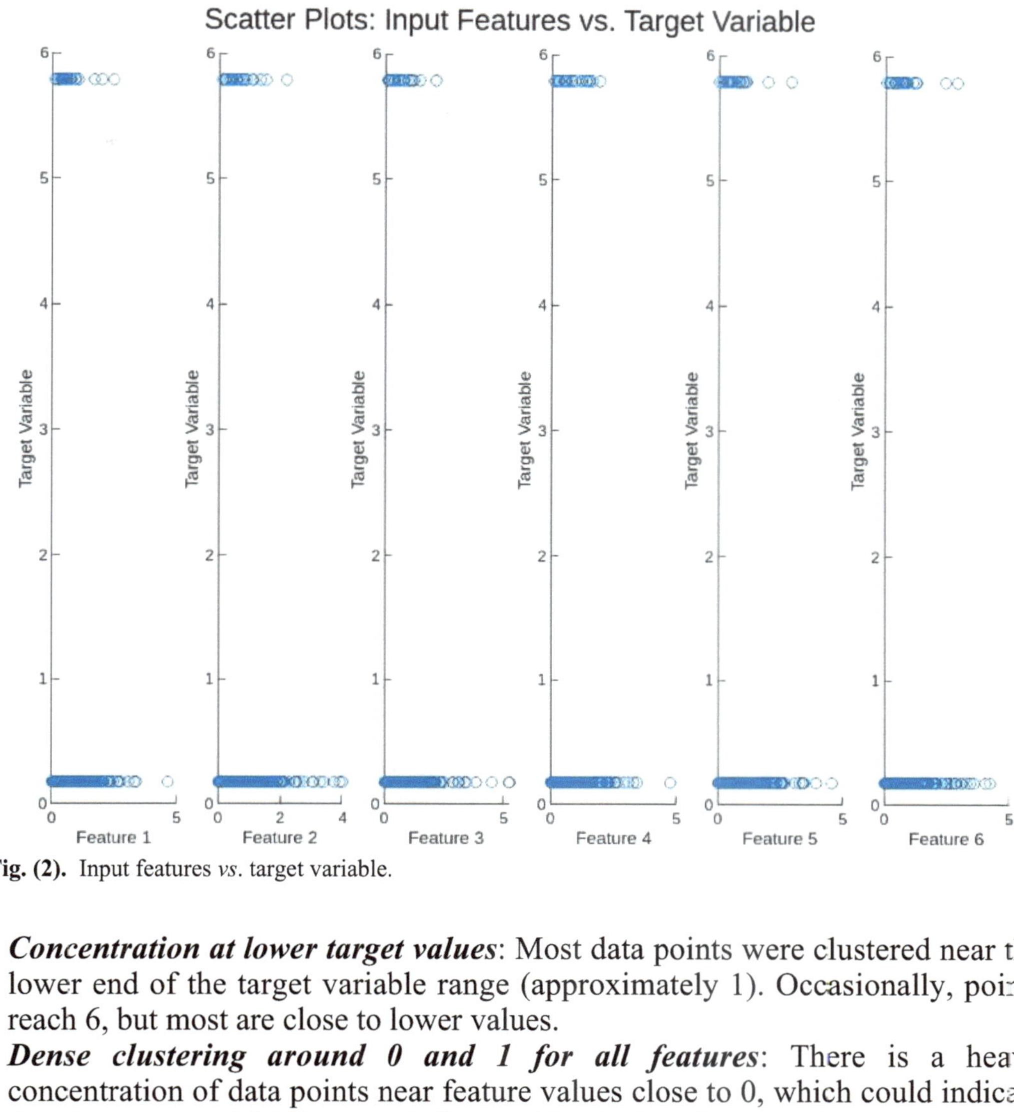

Fig. (2). Input features *vs*. target variable.

- ***Concentration at lower target values***: Most data points were clustered near the lower end of the target variable range (approximately 1). Occasionally, points reach 6, but most are close to lower values.
- ***Dense clustering around 0 and 1 for all features***: There is a heavy concentration of data points near feature values close to 0, which could indicate that the target variable is more influenced by the low feature values.
- ***No strong correlation***: Based on the scatter plots, there does not appear to be a clear, strong relationship between any of the features and the target variable. The points appear to be uniformly distributed along the y-axis across the entire range of feature values, suggesting that none of the features alone are strong predictors of the target variable.

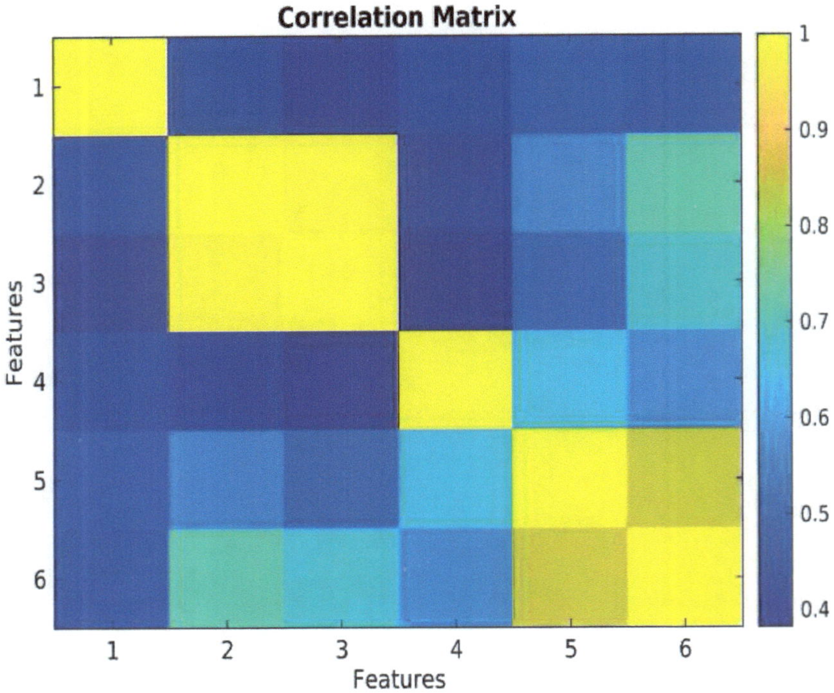

Fig. (3). Correlation matrix.

The image (Fig. **3**) represents a correlation matrix for the six features and is displayed as a heatmap. The matrix shows the pairwise correlation values between these features, with values ranging from -1 to 1.

Color Range: The color bar on the right represents the correlation scale, where yellow (1) indicates a strong positive correlation (features increase together), dark blue (0) indicates no correlation (features are independent), and intermediate colors (green to light blue) show moderate correlations.

Strong Positive Correlations: The bright yellow blocks in the matrix suggest strong positive correlations between certain features: Features 2 and 3 have the highest correlation (close to 1), indicating that they are strongly related; Features 3 and 6 also display a relatively high correlation; Features 2 and 4 exhibit another noticeable correlation.

Moderate/Weak Correlations: Feature 1 shows low to moderate correlations with most of the other features, as indicated by the dark blue and greenish colors. Features 5 and 6 have a moderate correlation, as depicted by the yellow-green block.

No Strong Negative Correlations: The matrix lacks deep red or darker shades, indicating no strong negative correlations among the features (negative correlations would appear as red hues).

The correlation matrix shows that features 2 and 3 are highly correlated, while the other feature pairs exhibit moderate to weak correlations. These insights can help in feature selection and engineering by potentially removing highly correlated features to avoid multicollinearity in the predictive models.

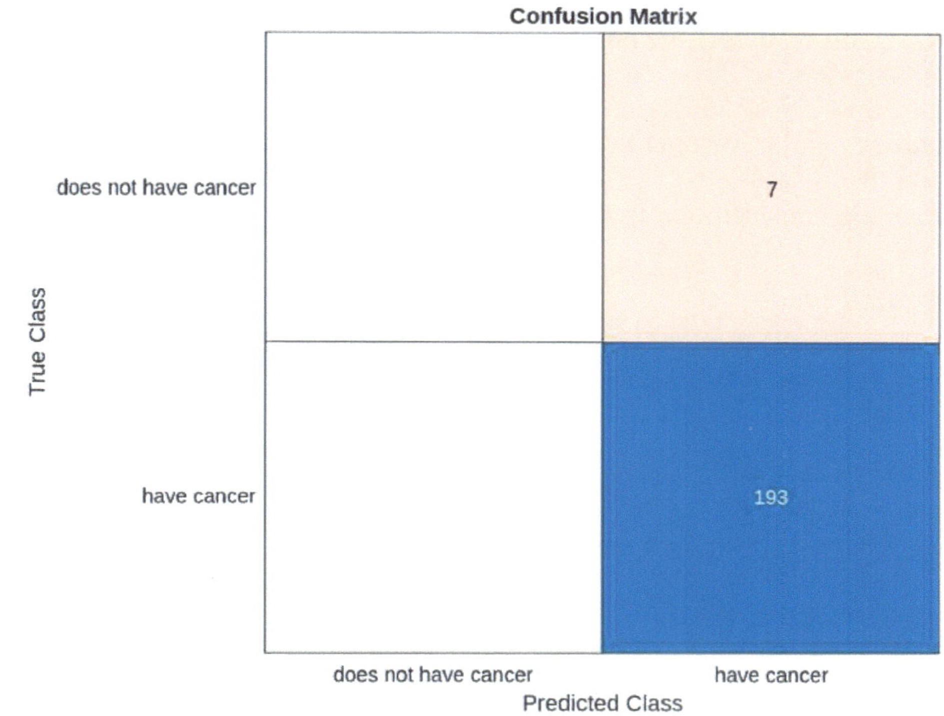

Fig. (4). Confusion matrix.

The image (Fig. **4**) represents a **Confusion Matrix** that summarizes the performance of a binary classification model that predicts whether patients have cancer. The matrix was divided into four quadrants, each showing the number of true positives, false positives, true negatives, and false negatives.

- ***True Positives (TP)***: The model correctly predicts "have cancer" (193 in this case).
- ***False Positives (FP)***: The model incorrectly predicts "have cancer" for patients who do not have cancer (7 in this case).

- ***True Negatives (TN)***: The model correctly predicts "does not have cancer" (This value is not provided in the matrix, but is assumed to be zero based on this representation).
- ***False Negatives (FN)***: The model incorrectly predicts "does not have cancer" for patients who actually have cancer (No cases in this quadrant indicate a high recall).

Observations

- ***High True Positive Rate***: The model correctly identified 193 cases of cancer, indicating strong predictive power for identifying positive cases.
- ***Low False Positive Rate***: The model made only seven false positive predictions, meaning it rarely misclassified non-cancer patients as having cancer.
- ***Imbalance***: No true-negative or false-negative data are shown, which may indicate that the dataset is heavily skewed toward cancer-positive cases. This is an important consideration in model evaluation.

The confusion matrix suggests that the classifier performed well in detecting cancer, with a high number of correct positive classifications (TP = 193) and very few false alarms (FP = 7). However, further details on the negative cases are necessary for a comprehensive evaluation of the model's overall accuracy and precision.

Precision: Precision is the ratio of True Positives (TP) to the sum of True Positives and False Positives (TP + FP). Higher precision means fewer false positives, that is, fewer incorrect predictions of cancer in non-cancer patients.

Precision=TPTP+FP= 193193+7= 0.965

This indicated that the model was highly precise, with 96.5% of its cancer predictions being correct.

Since no False Negatives (FN) were shown, we can assume perfect recall (1.0) in the given scenario, meaning the model has detected all cancer-positive patients.

The model demonstrated high accuracy in detecting cancer patients, with **high precision** (96.5%) and seemingly perfect recall. However, the absence of true-negative and false-negative data makes it difficult to fully evaluate the model's performance. Further analysis with a more balanced dataset is required for a comprehensive assessment.

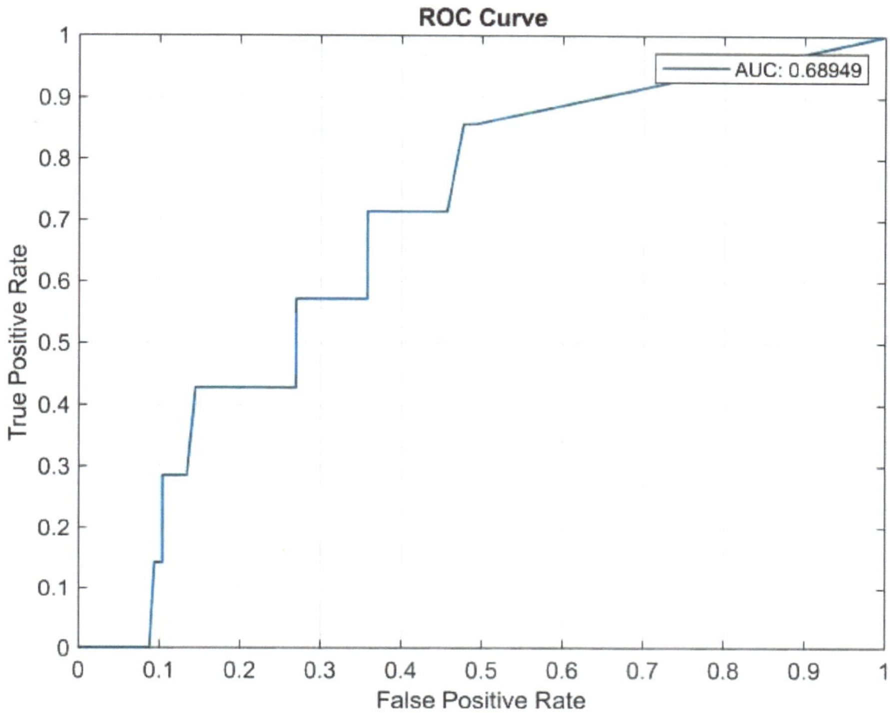

Fig. (5). ROC curve.

The ROC curve (Fig. **5**) illustrates the performance of a binary classifier that predicts the presence or absence of cancer cells. A curve is a tool used to measure the effectiveness of a model across various classification thresholds. The performance of this classifier is quantified by the Area Under the Curve (AUC), which helps us understand its discriminative power in distinguishing between cancerous and noncancerous cells.

1. **True Positive Rate (sensitivity)**: The Y-axis represents the True Positive Rate (TPR) or sensitivity, which measures the proportion of actual cancerous cells that are correctly predicted by the model. Higher values indicate a better detection of cancerous cells. The graph indicates that the model can achieve a sensitivity close to 0.9 in some threshold settings.
2. **False Positive Rate**: The X-axis represents the False Positive Rate (FPR), which shows the proportion of non-cancerous cells that are incorrectly classified as cancerous. Ideally, FPR should be low, indicating fewer incorrect positive predictions. In this curve, FPR ranged from 0 to 0.5.

3. **Area Under the Curve (AUC)**: The AUC value is approximately **0.68949**, which provides a good understanding of the overall performance of the classifier:
   - **0.5** represents random guessing.
   - **1.0** represents a perfect classification.

An AUC of 0.68949 suggests that the model performs better than random guessing, but is not highly accurate. It has moderate discriminatory power for distinguishing cancerous cells from non-cancerous cells.

Interpretation of Classifier Performance

Sensitivity and Specificity Trade-off: As shown in the ROC curve, the model maintains a reasonable balance between sensitivity (true positive rate) and specificity (low false positive rate). At certain points on the curve, the model achieved a TPR close to 0.9, while maintaining a manageable FPR, making it useful in scenarios where cancer detection is prioritized over the risk of false positives.

Model Utility in Cancer Detection: In cancer prediction models, high sensitivity is crucial to ensure that cancerous cells are not missed, even at the cost of an increased number of false positives. The ROC curve shows that the classifier achieves a high sensitivity. However, because the AUC is less than 0.7, the classifier's predictions are not very reliable, suggesting that further optimization is required to improve performance.

Threshold Adjustments: The varying slope of the ROC curve demonstrates how adjusting the decision threshold affects the balance between the true positive and false positive rates. For a practical cancer detection system, fine-tuning this threshold can help determine whether to prioritize minimizing false negatives (missing cancer cells) or false positives (misclassifying healthy cells as cancerous).

CONCLUSION

Enhancing the model's input features can improve its ability to distinguish between cancerous and non-cancerous cells. Feature selection techniques can help identify the most important predictors of cancer. It may be beneficial to tune the classifier's hyperparameters or explore more advanced models (such as ensemble methods or neural networks) to increase the AUC score. Given the consequences of false negatives (missed cancerous cells), cost-sensitive learning approaches can be applied to penalize the model more heavily for such errors and improve the detection of cancerous cells.

The ROC curve for this cancer cell prediction model showed moderate predictive power, with an AUC of approximately 0.68949. Although the model achieves a high true positive rate, its overall accuracy can be improved through feature optimization, hyperparameter tuning, and cost-sensitive approaches to better handle the trade-off between sensitivity and specificity.

CONSENT FOR PUBLICATION

None Declared

CONFLICT OF INTEREST

None Declared

ACKNOWLEDGEMENT

None Declared

REFERENCES

[1] Y. Wang, M. Zhang, and Y. Li, "A Bidirectional LSTM and Attention-based model for extracting medical events from clinical notes", *J. Biomed. Inform.*, vol. 138, 2023.104233

[2] A. Sharma, P. Gupta, and S. Verma, "Healthcare NLP: Transforming Clinical Data with Bidirectional LSTM", *IEEE Trans. Biomed. Eng.*, vol. 70, no. 4, pp. 1102-1115, 2023. [PMID: 36269902]

[3] R. Arora, and V. Singh, "Leveraging Bidirectional LSTM for Named Entity Recognition in Clinical Texts", *Health Informatics J.*, vol. 28, no. 2, pp. 194-208, 2022.

[4] V. Thanikachalam, and S. Shanthi, "Intelligent Deep Learning Based Disease Diagnosis Using Biomedical Tongue Images, Computers", *Materials & Continua,* vol. 70, no. 3, pp. 5667-5681, 2022. [http://dx.doi.org/10.32604/cmc.2022.020965]

[5] S. Liu, J. Yang, and X. Du, "Natural Language Processing for Healthcare using LSTM Networks: A Review", *IEEE Access,* vol. 10, pp. 35878-35891, 2022.

[6] A. Rajkomar, J. Dean, and I. Kohane, "Machine learning in medicine", *N. Engl. J. Med.*, vol. 380, no. 14, pp. 1347-1358, 2019. [http://dx.doi.org/10.1056/NEJMra1814259] [PMID: 30943338]

[7] L. Rokach, and O. Maimon, *Data mining with decision trees: theory and applications.* World Scientific, 2020.

[8] Y. Wang, L. Wang, M. Rastegar-Mojarad, S. Moon, F. Shen, N. Afzal, S. Liu, Y. Zeng, S. Mehrabi, S. Sohn, and H. Liu, "Clinical information extraction applications: A literature review", *J. Biomed. Inform.*, vol. 77, pp. 34-49, 2018. [http://dx.doi.org/10.1016/j.jbi.2017.11.011] [PMID: 29162496]

[9] R. Kumar, and P. Patel, "Enhancing Medical Information Retrieval with Bi-LSTM and Deep Learning Techniques", *J. Med. Syst.*, vol. 46, p. 127, 2022.

[10] K. Gupta, P. Reddy, and R. Chauhan, "BiLSTM-CRF Based Healthcare Named Entity Recognition Using Clinical Texts", *ACM Trans. Intell. Syst. Technol.*, vol. 13, no. 1, p. 20, 2022.

[11] M. Patil, and S. Swami, "AI-driven Healthcare: Natural Language Processing with LSTM Models for Disease Diagnosis", *J. Healthc. Inform. Res.*, vol. 5, no. 3, pp. 491-505, 2021.

[12] Y. Chen, and X. Huang, "Bidirectional Long Short-Term Memory Networks for Medical Text Classification in Electronic Health Records", *J. Med. Internet Res.,* vol. 23, no. 7, 2021.e23456

[13] H. Zhang, D. Xu, and W. Li, "A Bi-LSTM Approach for Medical Named Entity Recognition in Low-resource Settings", *BMC Med. Inform. Decis. Mak.,* vol. 21, p. 189, 2021.

[14] K. Rao, and N. Saxena, "An Efficient Medical Text Summarization Approach Using Bi-LSTM and Attention Mechanism", *IEEE J. Biomed. Health Inform.,* vol. 25, no. 9, pp. 3373-3384, 2021. [PMID: 33729962]

[15] Vanitha R, Deepalakshmi R, Shiva Shankari M. "COVID precaution system design using IoT and AI for facemask detection." In: Pandian AP, Palanisamy R, Narayanan M, Senjyu T, editors. Proceedings of the Third International Conference on Intelligent Computing, Information and Control Systems. Adv Intell Syst Comput. 2022;1415. Singapore: Springer. [http://dx.doi.org/10.1007/978-981-16-7330-6_55]

[16] D. Lee, and H. Kang, "Healthcare Dialogue Systems: An Application of Bidirectional LSTM and NLP Techniques", *Artif. Intell. Med.,* vol. 104, 2020.102168

[17] Z. Hu, and Y. Wu, "Improving Disease Detection with Bi-Directional LSTM Models", *Comput. Methods Programs Biomed.,* vol. 187, 2020.105063

[18] C. Xiao, E. Choi, and J. Sun, "Opportunities and challenges in developing deep learning models using electronic health records data: a systematic review", *J. Am. Med. Inform. Assoc.,* vol. 25, no. 10, pp. 1419-1428, 2018. [http://dx.doi.org/10.1093/jamia/ocy068] [PMID: 29893864]

[19] T. Nguyen, and J. Lee, "Bi-LSTM and Clinical Concept Extraction: A Study on Healthcare Informatics", *BMC Med. Inform. Decis. Mak.,* vol. 20, no. 1, p. 245, 2020. [PMID: 32993640]

[20] K. Jha, and S. Prasad, "A Survey on NLP in Healthcare: Leveraging Bi-LSTM for Efficient Data Processing", *Health Inf. Sci. Syst.,* vol. 8, no. 1, p. 3, 2020. [PMID: 31915522]

[21] M. Li, and Q. Zhao, "Medical Text Mining Using Bidirectional LSTM and Neural Network Approaches", *J. Biomed. Inform.,* vol. 94, 2019.103206

[22] J. Lee, W. Yoon, S. Kim, D. Kim, S. Kim, C.H. So, and J. Kang, "BioBERT: a pre-trained biomedical language representation model for biomedical text mining", *Bioinformatics,* vol. 36, no. 4, pp. 1234-1240, 2020. [http://dx.doi.org/10.1093/bioinformatics/btz682] [PMID: 31501885]

[23] K. Srinivasan, and R. Prasad, "Advancements in Healthcare Diagnostics Using NLP and Bi-LSTM Techniques", *Healthc. Technol. Lett.,* vol. 6, no. 3, pp. 96-104, 2019.

[24] M. Xiong, S. Zheng, W. Liu, *et al.*, "A Rate of Penetration (ROP) prediction method based on improved dung beetle optimization algorithm and BiLSTM-SA," Scientific Reports, vol. 14, p. 25856, 2024. [http://dx.doi.org/10.1038/s41598-024-75703-8]

[25] H. Sun, and T. Zhang, "Deep Learning in Medical Information Processing: A Review of Bi-LSTM Applications", *IEEE Access,* vol. 7, pp. 123-135, 2019.

[26] Y. Luo, and Q. Wu, "Bidirectional Long Short-Term Memory for Disease Prediction from Clinical Text", *J. Healthc. Eng.,* vol. 2018, 2018.4123459

[27] Q. Xie, and W. Yu, "Utilizing Bidirectional LSTM Networks for Clinical Text Classification", *J. Med. Syst.,* vol. 42, no. 5, p. 87, 2018. [PMID: 29611142]

[28] C. Lee, H. Cho, and S. Lee, "Analysis of Bi-LSTM CRF Series Models for Semantic Classification of NAVTEX Navigational Safety Messages", *J. Mar. Sci. Eng.,* vol. 12, no. 9, p. 1518, 2024.

[http://dx.doi.org/10.3390/jmse12091518]

[29] Z. Huang, W. Xu, and K. Yu, "Bidirectional LSTM-CRF Models for Sequence Tagging",

[30] P.B. Jensen, L.J. Jensen, and S. Brunak, "Mining electronic health records: towards better research applications and clinical care", *Nat. Rev. Genet.,* vol. 13, no. 6, pp. 395-405, 2012. [http://dx.doi.org/10.1038/nrg3208] [PMID: 22549152]

[31] F. Liu, Y. Wang, and W.J. Zheng, "Medical named entity recognition using Bi-LSTM-CRF with neuromorphic features", *BMC Bioinformatics,* vol. 19, no. 1, pp. 1-9, 2018. [PMID: 29291722]

[32] Y. Peng, S. Yan, and Z. Lu, "Transfer learning in biomedical natural language processing: A survey", *J. Biomed. Inform.,* vol. 115, 2021.103686

CHAPTER 7

Role of Knowledge Graph in Rare Disease Prediction

Sabenabanu Abdulkadhar[1,3,*], **Gurusamy Murugesan**[1] and **Yasmin Abdulkadhar**[2]

[1] *Department of Computer Science and Engineering, Koneru Lakshmaiah Education Foundation, Vaddeswaram, Guntur, Andhra Pradesh-522302, India*

[2] *Department of Artificial Intelligence and Data Science, Excel Engineering College (Autonomous), Pallakapalayam, Namakkal, Tamil Nadu-637303, India*

[3] *Department of Computer Applications, Faculty of Science and Humanities, SRM Institute of Science and Technology, Kattankulathur, Chennai-603203, Tamil Nadu, India*

Abstract: Rare Diseases (RD), or orphan diseases, affect a small portion of the population. It is considered rare to affect less than 1 in 2,000 people. Although RDs are rare, their numbers are high: between 6,000 and 8,000 RDs are known to exist. In addition, this disease is often long and lethal. RD is characterized by phenotypic diversity that varies from one disease to another and between patients with the same disease. It became difficult to predict despite the low prediction rate and several problems, such as limited access to accurate diagnosis, a lack of knowledge about the disease, and a lack of scientific understanding of the condition. Biomedical text mining has become an essential tool in recent years to extract information from structured and unstructured text and provide valuable insights for drug discovery, disease prediction, and disease-disease interaction prediction. This chapter introduces rare diseases and the techniques and tools used to predict rare diseases.

Keywords: Biomedical text mining, Knowledge graphs, Phenotypic diversity, Rare diseases.

INTRODUCTION

Rare diseases, often known as orphan diseases, typically afflict tiny groups of people, with an estimated 1 in 2000 persons affected, in contrast to diseases like cancer and Alzheimer's [1 - 3]. As the World Health Organization (WHO) indicates, RDs are those where the number of people infected is 0.65 % to 1 % of the total population. Even though they are uncommon, some RDs have a sizable

* **Corresponding author Sabenabanu Abdulkadhar, Current affiliation:** Department of Computer Applications, Faculty of Science and Humanities, SRM Institute of Science and Technology, Kattankulathur, Chennai-603203, Tamil Nadu, India; E-mail: sabenabanu.a@hotmail.com

A. Shankar, Saranya Jayapalan, & Basant. K. Tiwary (Eds.)

population afflicted by specific illnesses [4, 5]. RDs are characterized by a wide range of phenotypes that vary from one infection to the next and from one patient to another who has a similar sickness [6, 7]. *Alkaptonuria, Cystic fibrosis, Muscular dystrophy, Angelman syndrome, Haemophilia, Achalasia, etc.,* are some of the examples of rare diseases [8].

Alkaptonuria is a rare inherited genetic disease that is brought about by a change in the HGD gene for the chemical homogentisate 1,2-dioxygenase; if an individual receives a strange duplicate from the two guardians, the body collects a moderate substance called homogentisic acid in the blood and tissues [9, 10]. *Cystic fibrosis* (otherwise called "mucoviscidosis" is liable for respiratory and gastrointestinal issues, affecting around 1 in 5,000. A group of illnesses known as *muscular dystrophy* results in progressive weakness and muscle mass loss. Children with muscular dystrophy, a primary immune deficiency, have symptoms that include aberrant gene mutations that prevent the body from producing the proteins necessary to form healthy muscle [11, 12].

Angelman syndrome is a complex hereditary problem that essentially influences the sensory system. Trademark elements of this condition include delayed development, intellectual disability, severe communication disability, and issues with motor development and coordination. Most impacted kids likewise have intermittent seizures (epilepsy) and a small head size [13, 14]. One fascinating disorder that affects the blood's ability to clot is *hemophilia*. Males are affected by the vast majority of *hemophilia* [15, 16]. *Achalasia* is a swallowing disorder that affects the esophagus, the tube that connects the mouth and stomach. When nerves are damaged, it is difficult for the throat muscles to move food and liquids into the stomach [17, 18].

Since it provides a detailed picture of infections, the data extraction regarding RD phenotypes is critical and could be used to guide clinical judgment and clinical consideration [19]. In addition, this disease is often long and lethal. The prediction rate of RDs is low [20 - 22]. A large volume of information about rare diseases is encoded in organized sources like databases and ontologies, yet in addition in composed texts, for example, research articles, clinical cases, clinical trials, drug safety reports, health agency newsletters, as well as information from social media, websites, and health forums [23, 24].

Recently, biomedical text mining has become one of the most critical areas to process and dissect enormous volumes of unstructured data accessible in any space or field of information, and it gives valuable knowledge in disease predictions, disease-disease interaction predictions, drug discovery, and so on [25 - 27]. A few shared tasks, such as BioCreative [28], i2b2 [29], BioNLP shared tasks [30], and DDI Extraction [31], have contributed to the development of examination in NLP strategies as applied to the areas of science and biomedicine. Subsequently, numerous frameworks and instruments (MetaMap [32], cTakings [33], and MedLEE [34]) have been produced to acknowledge the substances and extract connections between these domains.

This chapter briefly introduces rare diseases and symptoms, biomedical resources, architecture, and state-of-the-art approaches to extract knowledge about RDs from biomedical literature. (Fig. **1**) illustrates the architecture of the rare disease knowledge graph.

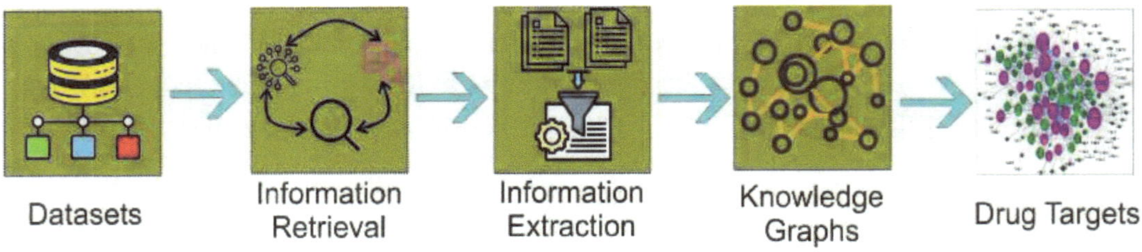

Fig. (1). The architecture of rare disease knowledge graph.

Biomedical Resources/Corpora and Databases

Selecting the appropriate corpus and biomedical resources is crucial for assessing the effectiveness of any text-based knowledge discovery process [35 - 37]. Different types of corpora and databases are available as open-source [37].

ICD: As a medical services order system, the ICD offers a set of demonstrative codes for classifying illnesses, including a broad range of symptoms, adverse effects, unexpected findings, demonstrations, social circumstances, and external causes of illness or injury [ICD07]. It is utilized for factual purposes and as a coding framework in clinical data sets [38]. The ICD's inability to resist perceiving the outcome of the treatment course is one of its limitations [KPM+08]. Similarly, the final ICD-coded finding may need several patient visits and is rarely clarified during the initial visit [39].

DO: Human Disease Ontology (DO) DO is an ontology for portraying the characterization of human diseases coordinated according to a clinical viewpoint of disease etiology and area [KAF+15]. DO was created to make a solitary structure for the arrangement of diseases to combine the portrayal of diseases into an ontology from the numerous and different existing phrasings and vocabularies [40]. The target of DO gives an unmistakable definition to every disease. It empowers the predictable use and application for explaining biomedical information and is incorporated with other phrase-based ontologies like MeSH [41], ICD [38], NCI's thesaurus [42], SNOMED [43], and OMIM [44].

KEGG Disease Database: The KEGG DISEASE database is an assortment of disease entries, each containing a list of human disease genes and microorganisms. The subtleties of how atomic organizations are bothered by such perturbants are addressed as organization variety maps in the KEGG Organization data set. KEGG DISEASE is used to contain ecological variables. However, they are included exclusively in the KEGG Organization when atomic-level data is free. The H number recognizes every disease section and may contain the connection to organize variety maps (see, for instance, the disease passage of spinal muscular decay H00455) [45, 46]. Remedial drugs are displayed in the drug field; those demonstrated on the FDA drug labels are in the English variant, and those on the Japanese drug labels are in the Japanese rendition [46].

OMIM (Online Mendelian Inheritance in Man): It is an exhaustive, definitive outline of human genes and hereditary conditions that is unreservedly accessible and updated daily. The full text, called outlines in OMIM, contains data on undeniably known Mendelian problems and more than 16,000 qualities. OMIM centers around the connection between aggregate and genotype [44]. It is refreshed daily, and the passages contain extensive connections to other hereditary qualities assets [47].

NORD Rare Disease Database: The NORD Rare Disease Database has over 1,300 reports on rare issues. These reports give point-by-point data about side effects, causes, diagnosis, medicines, clinical studies, and supporting assets, including patient support associations. Each report incorporates references from course readings, articles, sites, and government offices (https://rarediseases.org/rare-diseases/) [48].

Orphanet: Orphanet is a novel resource that assembles and develops information on rare diseases, organized to work on finding, caring for, and treating patients with uncommon illnesses. Orphanet expects to give significant data on intriguing diseases and guarantee equal access to information for all partners. Orphanet additionally keeps up with the Orphanet uncommon illness terminology (ORPHAcode), which is fundamental in working on the permeability of intriguing diseases in well-being and exploration data frameworks(https://www.orpha.net/) [49].

Orphanet Rare Disease Ontology (ORDO): It is a structured vocabulary for RDs, catching connections between RDs, qualities, and other pertinent highlights [50]. ORDO is created from the Orphanet data set [Orp15b] [3]. It features an order of RDs, information (*e.g.*, quality illness connections), and connections with different phrasings (MeSH [41], SNOMED [43], UMLS [51], MedDRA [52],

ICD [38]) and databases (OMIM [44], UniProtKB [53], HGNC [54], Ensembl [55], Reactome [56], IUPHAR [57]).

NCBI Disease Corpus: As a research tool for the biomedical natural language processing community, the NCBI disease corpus is thoroughly annotated at the mention and concept level [58]. 91% of the 6,892 disease mentions, which are split into training, developing, and testing sets, correspond to a single disease concept, according to Medical Subject Headings (MeSH) [41], Online Mendelian Inheritance in Man (OMIM) [44], and 790 distinct disease concepts. 91% of the mentions map to a single disease concept, divided into training, developing, and testing sets [41, 44].

BioCreative V CDR Disease Corpus: The 1500 PubMed publications in the BC5CDR corpus include 5818 diseases, 3116 chemical-disease interactions, and 4409 annotated chemicals. Each entity annotation contains both the mentioned text spans and normalized concept identifiers [59].

Rare Disease Corpus (RareDis): It is a choice of 1,041 texts included in the corpus, the explanation interaction, and the comment rules. The substances (disease, rare disease, side effect, sign, and anaphor) and the connections (produces, is a, is a cron, is synon, expands the chance of, anaphora) were commented on. This corpus contains over 5,000 rare diseases, and about 6,000 clinical manifestations are annotated [60, 61].

According to the exact match criteria, this corpus yields an F-score of 83.5 for the entities and 81.3% for the relations. Given the evaluation results, this corpus is of excellent quality. It represents a significant advancement for the field, as there is a dearth of easily accessible corpora that explain rare diseases [60].

A wide range of databases and biomedical corpora are available as open source, from which Orphanet, ORDO, NORD, and the RareDis corpus played an essential role in the rare disease knowledge discovery process. (Table **1**) depicts the number of entities and annotation relations in each dataset.

Table 1. Number of entities and annotations in datasets.

Dataset	Task	Entity	Number of Relation Annotations
BC5CDR (disease) (Li, *et al.*, 2016) [59]	NER	Disease	12864
NCBI (disease) (Gerner *et al.*, 2010) [58]	NER	Disease	6892
BC5CDR (chemical) (Li, *et al.*, 2016) [59]	NER	Chemical	15933
CHEMDNER (Krallinger, *et al.*, 2015) [62]	NER	Chemical	84355

(Table 1) cont.....

Dataset	Task	Entity	Number of Relation Annotations
BC2GM (Ando, 2007) [63]	NER	Gene	24583
GAD (Bravo, *et al.*, 2015) [64]	RE	Gene-disease	5330
EU-ADR (Van Mulligen, *et al.*, 2012) [65]	RE	Gene-disease	355
ChemDisGene (Zhang, *et al.*, 2022) [66]	RE	Chemical-Gene	3911
Rare disease Corpus [60]	NER, RE	Disease, Symptoms	11,000

Architecture of Rare Disease Knowledge Discovery Process

The rare disease knowledge discovery process architecture includes the following components [3, 36]. The first component is preprocessing, which provides for sentence segmentation, tokenization, POS tagging, lemmatization, chunking, and dependency parsing. The information extraction component includes Named Entity Recognition (NER) and biological event extraction. Next, different methodologies are used in the knowledge discovery process [36].

Pre-processing: In preprocessing, the following common pre-processing steps are involved, such as i) sentence segmentation, ii) tokenization, iii) POS tagging, iv) lemmatization, v) chunking, vi) stop word removal, and vii) dependency parsing. (Fig. **2**) illustrates the pre-processing steps of the disease knowledge process [3, 36].

Sentence Segmentation: Sentence Segmentation divides the sentence into meaningful units [67]. For example, if we have taken an abstract or an article to extract the disease knowledge, the abstract is divided into meaningful sentences using delimiters such as a full-stop (.).

Tokenization: Tokenization is the first step in biomedical natural language processing, and it is used to segment text into primary blocks called tokens [68, 69]. For example, if we take the sentence "Mutations of the CFTR gene cause cystic fibrosis.".

Original sentence (PMID: 25046381): Cystic fibrosis is caused by mutations of the CFTR gene.

After Tokenization: Cystic/ fibrosis/ is/caused/by/mutations/of/CFTR/gene

POS tagging: Part of speech (POS) tagging detects the word's grammatical role in a given sentence [70].

Lemmatization: Lemmatization converts the token into the word's basic form [3, 71, 72]. For example, in the above sentence PMID: 25046381, the word “activated ” is converted into ”activate ” to preprocess the text for the particular task.

Chunking: Chunking is a natural language processing technique that attempts to provide some machine understanding of the structure of a sentence [36, 73]. The process of chunking splits the text into grammatical units, namely a Noun Phrase (NP), a Verb Phrase (VP), or a Preposition Phrase (PP).

Stop Word Removal: Stop word removal is the process of taking out meaningless words (“and,” “or,” “this,” *etc.*) in a given sentence [74].

Dependency Parsing: It is formalized as a directional grammatical relationship that includes two words (headword and dependent word), and a sentence is represented as a graph of dependency relations [75]. The advantage of using dependency parsing is to find the grammatical relationships between two words from the syntactic representation of a given sentence [72]. (Fig. **3**) represents the dependency graph of a given sentence. Stanford parser [76] and GDep parser [77] are the two commonly available parsers for the dependency parsing of biomedical text.

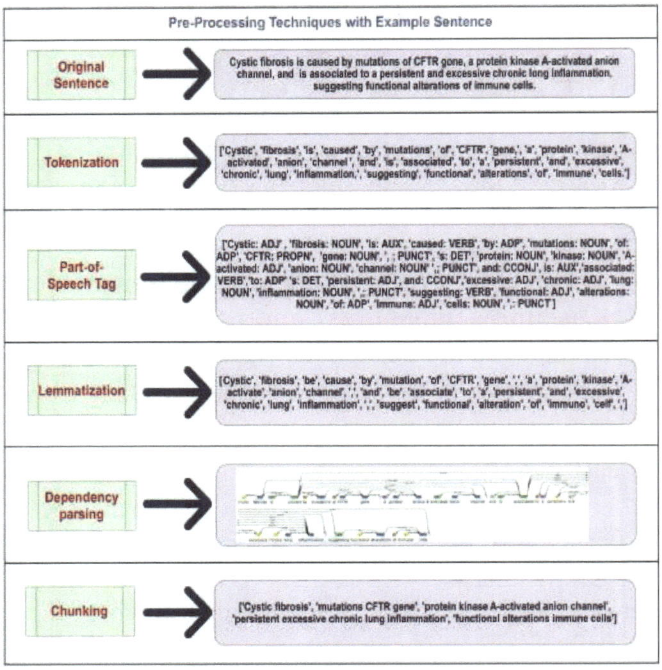

Fig. (2). Preprocessing techniques with example sentence.

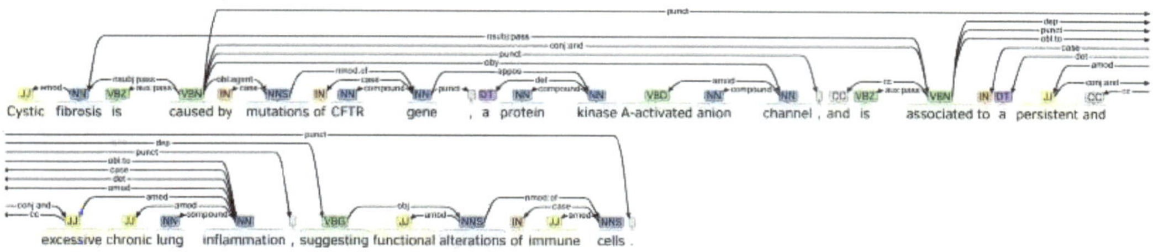

Fig. (3). Dependency graph of a given sentence.

Information Extraction

Named Entity Recognition

It is the first step and foundation of information extraction in NLP [78 - 82]. It is the process of finding names, organization, and location in general text, detecting the biological entities such as genes, proteins, diseases, species, RNA, cell, cell line, and chemical names from the biomedical text [79]. Different methodologies, such as rule-based, dictionary-based, machine learning based, and hybrid approaches, are utilized to extract the biomedical entities. After implementing the preliminary preprocessing steps, we next employed a named entity recognition process. Recently, hybrid named entity recognition methodologies have achieved better accuracy [78]. For example, Cousyn *et al.* proposed automatically extracting rare disease symptoms from the PubMed Central (PMC) database. In this study, they implemented numerical statistics, Term Frequency - Inverse Document Frequency, and a dictionary-based approach to extract the rare disease entities [83].

Bio-Relation or Event Extraction

The next step is extracting biomedical relations/events from the text [70]. The event extraction process consists of two common steps: trigger detection and argument detection. Identifying trigger words comprises the detection of event triggers and their types, as quantified by the selected ontology [84, 85]. The process of identifying arguments for the events is called argument detection, edge detection, or event theme construction. These arguments could be identified as biological entities represented by trigger words [85].

Knowledge Discovery Process by Network and Pathway Curation

Biological pathways and regulatory networks are essential components of the biomedical knowledge discovery process that contribute to understanding complex illnesses, the hierarchical relationships between transcription factors and diseases, and the development of new therapeutics [86]. A biological pathway, also known as a regulatory network, is a group of molecular regulators that can activate modifications in cell processes and cause new molecules to form through a sequence of interactions between the molecules [36]. Recently, there has been a lot of focus on automatically extracting and building biological pathways and regulatory networks from biomedical literature [87, 88]. The advancement of Natural Language Processing (NLP) and integration of biomedical semantics and knowledge discovery support the development of a large number of biomedical text mining systems to extract the biological pathways and networks from text [89, 90].

Drug Targets Extraction

A drug target is a particular molecule, frequently a protein, in the body that is firmly connected to a specific disease process and can be impacted by a drug to create an ideal therapeutic result [91]. Recently, text-mining applications incorporate an expansive range of heterogeneous information sources, giving methodologies and tools to investigate, extract, and visualize data, which helps researchers transform available data into usable information to extract the drug targets [92]. Pharmacogenomic facts and therapeutic innovations are pertinent to the automated curation of drug targets from the biomedical literature [93, 94].

Postprocessing

The post-processing phase is used to remove errors from the model, and it helps to improve the accuracy of the system [95]. Various post-processing approaches, such as rule-based, dictionary-based, and hybrid approaches, were implemented to remove the errors in the knowledge discovery process [78, 79]. Some important post-processing techniques were used in biomedical knowledge discovery, such as surrounding text features, an abbreviation resolution algorithm, contextual patterns, and semantic role labelling [79].

Visualization of Rare Disease Knowledge Graph

Many tools were developed and are available for biological networks and pathway visualization, such as Gephi [36, 96], VisANT [97], Pathway Studio [98], PATIKA [99], *etc*., *Gephi* (https://github.com/gephi/gephi) [96] that runs as a simple Java-based desktop program on Windows, Mac, or Linux to visualize the pathways. It is a flexible and multi-task architecture with complex data sets and produces valuable visual results. Several key features of Gephi, such as filtering, navigating, manipulating, and clustering, provide easy and broad access to our network visualization. VisANT(https://bio.tools/visant) is an integrative visual analysis tool for biological networks and pathways that contains modules for querying and integrating KEGG pathways with expression data.

VisANT [97] is Java-based and can be run as a Java applet, as a Java web application, or downloaded and run locally. New functions allow determination of over-representation and expression enrichment, integrated search and navigation of disease and drug hierarchies, drug/disease annotation, *etc.*

Pathway Studio is developed as a software application for the purpose of navigating and analyzing gene regulation networks, protein interaction maps, and biological pathways [98]. On the other hand, Patika is an integrated, multi-user environment for visualizing and modifying a network of cellular events. It is made up of client-side editors and a server-side, scalable, object-oriented database. Advanced querying, functional calculation support, automatic pathway creation, and an intuitive graphical user interface are all aspects of this application.

Evaluation Metrics

Different types of metrics were used to explore the performance of the rare disease knowledge discovery process approaches [36, 100]. These are accuracy, precision, recall, and F-score. F-score is measured by four metrics- True Positive (TP), True Negative (TN), False Positive (FP), and False Negative (FN). Where TP refers to the number of proportion of rare disease entities correctly identified by the system, FN refers to the number of proportion of biological entities that the approach failed to identify, and FP refers to the number of proportion of disease entities that were incorrectly identified by the system. The F-score, Precision, and Recall are designed by following the procedure; these are

$$\text{F-Score} = \frac{2*P*R}{P+R} \quad \textbf{(1)}$$

$$\text{Precision (P)} = \frac{TP}{(TP+FP)} \quad \textbf{(2)}$$

$$\text{Recall (R)} = \frac{TP}{(TP+FN)} \quad \textbf{(3)}$$

Rare Disease Knowledge Discovery Process Approaches

Different types of approaches were used to extract the knowledge of rare diseases, these are rule-based approaches, dictionary-based approaches, machine learning based approaches, and hybrid approaches [78]. A set of rules is used to extract the entities in rule-based approaches, in dictionary-based approaches, a rare disease dictionary was created, and we employ some rules to match the lexicons [78, 79]. Rule and dictionary-based approaches are time-consuming and expensive. Machine learning methods were introduced to overcome the limitations of baseline approaches and obtained better results than the dictionary and rule-based methods. Machine learning based approaches need more training sets. In recent years, hybrid approaches have gained popularity and achieved state-of-the-art results in various tasks such as NER, relation extraction, and knowledge discovery of rare diseases [83].

NER Approaches

Li *et al.* employed soft margin SVM to identify disease entities [101], Bhasuran *et al.* proposed a general disease named entity tagger, which consists of Bidirectional-Conditional Random Fields (bidirectional CRF), fuzzy logic approaches to detect the disease entities [79], Xu *et al.* proposed a hybrid approach combined with bidirectional Long Short Term Memory (LSTM) and CRF to identify disease mentions [102].

Shyr *et al.* proposed a prompt learning ChatGPT, a large language model, to extract rare disease entities. In this study, they identified rare diseases and their phenotypes (disease, symptoms, and signs) [103]. Davis *et al.* proposed a NER for multiple sclerosis from Electronic Health Records (EHR). The authors used manually curated relevant keywords and rule-based algorithms to determine disease progression and type [104].

Lo *et al.* [23] extracted phenotypes related to *Dravet syndrome* from UML Metathesaurus with the subset of 20,000 phenotypic words and expressions [105]. Deisseroth *et al.* [106] developed ClinPhen, a rule-based phenotype extractor for genetic diseases. Nigwekar *et al.* [107] used an unnamed NLP software to identify "calciphylaxis" or "calcific uremic arteriolopathy" from medical records. Fabregat *et al.* [108] used a BiLSTM model with a recurrent neural network to identify rare diseases. Segura Bedmaret *et al.* implemented Conditional Random Fields (CRF) as the output layer and domain-specific BERT models for the NER task.

Wei *et al.* proposed a DNER (Disease NER) and Normalization. The authors proposed two models, one consisting of CRF and post-processing rules, and another one containing bi-directional recurrent neural networks. Finally, both models combined with SVM can recognize diseases [109]. Holat *et al.* implemented a pattern mining and Conditional Random Field (CRF) to get rare disease symptoms. In that work, they used 100 diseases and then 100 publications per disease [110]. Martin *et al.* proposed a tagger with pattern matching, a tree tagger, and NLP. In this, they only considered 25 rare diseases [111]. Harsh Patel introduced BioNerFlair, a methodology combined with Bidirectional LSTM-CRF and Flair plus GloVe word embeddings to detect disease entities [112].

Relation Extraction and Knowledge Discovery Approaches

Béchet *et al.* proposed a sequential pattern mining approach to extract the relation between genes and rare diseases [113]. Lang Cao *et al.* proposed AutoRD, a rare disease relation extraction system to find the disease entities, relations, and knowledge graphs from the text. In this study, the author employed Large Language Models (LLMs) [114]. Fabregat *et al.* implemented Convolutional Neural Networks (CNN) and Bi-directional LSTM to identify the relationships between disease and disabilities [115]. Shashank Gupta proposed an End-To-End Relation Extraction (E2ERE) approach to extract the chemical-protein and disease-protein relations. In this study, the author used the GPT model and the sequence-to-sequence model [116].

Fabregat *et al.* proposed CRF and Bi-LSTM to extract the relations and entities in the rare diseases [108]. Bhasuran and Natarajan proposed supervised machine learning, rich features covering conceptual, syntactic, and semantic features, and domain-specific word embedding, ensemble learning to extract the relations between genes and diseases [117]. Alam *et al.* [118] proposed a chemical-disease relation extraction approach. In this study, they employed Support Vector Machines and domain-specific knowledge resources on PubMed abstracts and achieved better performance.

Hassan *et al.* [3] constructed a rare disease-symptom knowledge graph with lexico-syntactic patterns and a dependency graph. Bhasuran and Natarajan [119] proposed the DisGeReExT knowledge graph of gene-disease associations. In this study, they employed ABC principal and joint ensemble learning for prioritizing and rationalizing potential informative discoveries of the genetic role in diseases. Xing *et al.* [120] proposed RDBridge, a text-mining framework, which offers search functions for genes, potential drugs, pathways, literature, and medical imaging data that will support mechanistic research, drug development, diagnosis, and treatment for rare diseases. Lee *et al.* [121] employed Bio-BERT (a domain-specific model based on BERT architecture) for Named Entity Recognition (NER) and Relation Extraction (RE) tasks and knowledge discovery.

Frisoni *et al.* [122] proposed knowledge-graph learning coupled with text mining and semantic web techniques on social posts of patients. Lang Cao *et al.* [114] proposed that AutoRD is a pipeline system that involves data preprocessing, entity extraction, relation extraction, entity calibration, and knowledge graph construction. In this context, the authors implemented LLMs and medical knowledge graphs developed from open-source medical ontologies on the RareDis Corpus. Zhu *et al.* [123] proposed a meta-ontology-based integrative knowledge graph for rare diseases. This integrative knowledge graph includes a total of 3,819,623 nodes and 84,223,681 relations from 34 different biomedical data resources, including curated drug and rare disease associations. Chen *et al.* [124] proposed a dynamic few-shot prompt methodology on LLMs to leverage a comprehensive rare disease knowledge graph synthesized from multiple knowledge bases.

CONCLUSION

The primary source of knowledge for finding new information is scientific literature, which is also a resource for interpreting experimental results across different domains. Researchers utilize this literature data to find relevant information for research purposes and also to construct primary and secondary databases by extracting structured information in the biomedical domain. According to NORD, a Rare Disease is a disease, illness, or condition that affects a small group of people. Regardless of whether RDs are uncommon, their number is enormous in some cases. In addition, this disease is often long and lethal. RD is characterized by phenotypic diversity that varies not only from one disease to another but also between patients with the same disease. Several factors are making research on RDs difficult, these are i) correct diagnosis, ii) lack of information, and iii) poor knowledge about the diseases. The implementation of biomedical text mining procedures on unstructured and structured rare disease text shows that it is feasible to improve symptomatic accuracy and competence, addressing the critical difficulties presented by the unique case and intricacy of these circumstances. State-of-the-art rare disease knowledge discovery methodologies and gold standard corpora played a vital role. In conclusion, this study helps researchers to generate reliable, innovative hypotheses and knowledge about rare diseases.

REFERENCES

[1] S. Arora, and S. Arora, *Rare diseases and orphan drugs: challenges, regulatory movements and market strategy.* Information Booklet, 2014, pp. 1-22.

[2] C. Chen, R. Dubin, and M.C. Kim, "Orphan drugs and rare diseases: a scientometric review (2000 – 2014)", *Expert Opin. Orphan Drugs,* vol. 2, no. 7, pp. 709-724, 2014. [http://dx.doi.org/10.1517/21678707.2014.920251]

[3] M. Hassan, Knowledge discovery considering domain literature and ontologies: Application to rare diseases, 2017.

[4] C.C.Y. Chung, A.T.W. Chu, and B.H.Y. Chung, "Rare disease emerging as a global public health priority", *Front. Public Health,* vol. 10, 2022.1028545 [http://dx.doi.org/10.3389/fpubh.2022.1028545] [PMID: 36339196]

[5] L. Jaya, P. Rutuja, A. Korbu, and S. Barage, *Rare disease diagnosis as information retrieval task.* Semantic Web for Effective Healthcare, 2021, pp. 269-292. [http://dx.doi.org/10.1002/9781119764175.ch12]

[6] L.R. Prince, N.C. Maxwell, S.K. Gill, D.H. Dockrell, I. Sabroe, E.P. McGreal, S. Kotecha, and M.K. Whyte, "Macrophage phenotype is associated with disease severity in preterm infants with chronic

lung disease", *PLoS One,* vol. 9, no. 8, 2014.e103059
[http://dx.doi.org/10.1371/journal.pone.0103059] [PMID: 25115925]

[7] J.E. Magnani, and S.M. Donn, "Persistent respiratory distress in the term neonate: Genetic surfactant deficiency diseases", *Curr. Pediatr. Rev.,* vol. 16, no. 1, pp. 17-25, 2020.
[http://dx.doi.org/10.2174/1573396315666190723112916] [PMID: 31544695]

[8] A. Schieppati, J.I. Henter, E. Daina, and A. Aperia, "Why rare diseases are an important medical and social issue", *Lancet,* vol. 371, no. 9629, pp. 2039-2041, 2008.
[http://dx.doi.org/10.1016/S0140-6736(08)60872-7] [PMID: 18555915]

[9] J.A. Gallagher, J.P. Dillon, N. Sireau, O. Timmis, and L.R. Ranganath, "Alkaptonuria: An example of a "fundamental disease"—A rare disease with important lessons for more common disorders", *Semin. Cell Dev. Biol.,* vol. 52, pp. 53-57, 2016.
[http://dx.doi.org/10.1016/j.semcdb.2016.02.020] [PMID: 26891864]

[10] A. Zatkova, L. Ranganath, and L. Kadasi, "Alkaptonuria: current perspectives", *Appl. Clin. Genet.,* vol. 13, pp. 37-47, 2020.
[http://dx.doi.org/10.2147/TACG.S186773] [PMID: 32158253]

[11] S.A. Hussain, E. Sezgin, K. Krivchenia, J. Luna, S. Rust, and Y. Huang, "A natural language processing pipeline to synthesize patient-generated notes toward improving remote care and chronic disease management: a cystic fibrosis case study", *JAMIA Open,* vol. 4, no. 3, 2021.ooab084
[http://dx.doi.org/10.1093/jamiaopen/ooab084] [PMID: 34604710]

[12] C. Martin, E. Burnet, A. Ronayette-Preira, P. de Carli, J. Martin, L. Delmas, B. Prieur, and P.R. Burgel, "Patient perspectives following initiation of elexacaftor-tezacaftor-ivacaftor in people with cystic fibrosis and advanced lung disease", *Respir. Med. Res.,* vol. 80, 2021.100829
[http://dx.doi.org/10.1016/j.resmer.2021.100829] [PMID: 34091202]

[13] E. Pearson, L. Wilde, M. Heald, R. Royston, and C. Oliver, "Communication in Angelman syndrome: a scoping review", *Dev. Med. Child Neurol.,* vol. 61, no. 11, pp. 1266-1274, 2019.
[http://dx.doi.org/10.1111/dmcn.14257] [PMID: 31074506]

[14] M. Fujimoto, "Genotype-phenotype correlation over time in Angelman syndrome: Researching 134 patients", *Hum. Genet. Genomics Adv.,* vol. 5, no. 4, 2024.
[http://dx.doi.org/10.1016/j.xhgg.2024.100342]

[15] T.J.S. Lopes, R. Rios, and T. Nogueira, "Computational analyses reveal fundamental properties of the hemophilia literature in the last 6 decades", *Bioinform. Biol. Insights,* vol. 16, 2022.11779322221125604
[http://dx.doi.org/10.1177/11779322221125604] [PMID: 36172338]

[16] M.W. Skinner, G. Hanson, T. Xu, R. Ofori-Asenso, R.H. Ko, E. Cibelli, F. Nissen, M. Witkop, F. Sanabria, and A.D. Shapiro, "A novel methodology for building longitudinal, patient-centric real world datasets in hemophilia A", *Blood,* vol. 138, suppl. Suppl. 1, p. 594, 2021.
[http://dx.doi.org/10.1182/blood-2021-146160]

[17] M. Kalantari, A. Hollywood, R. Lim, and M. Hashemi, "Mapping the experiences of people with achalasia from initial symptoms to long□term management", *Health Expect.,* vol. 24, no. 1, pp. 131-139, 2021.
[http://dx.doi.org/10.1111/hex.13160] [PMID: 33210821]

[18] S.K. Chuah, C.S. Lim, C.M. Liang, H.I. Lu, K.L. Wu, C.S. Changchien, and W.C. Tai, "Bridging the gap between advancements in the evolution of diagnosis and treatment towards better outcomes in achalasia", *BioMed Res. Int.,* vol. 2019, pp. 1-10, 2019.
[http://dx.doi.org/10.1155/2019/8549187] [PMID: 30881999]

[19] P. Buphamalai, T. Kokotovic, V. Nagy, and J. Menche, "Network analysis reveals rare disease signatures across multiple levels of biological organization", *Nat. Commun.,* vol. 12, no. 1, p. 6306, 2021.
[http://dx.doi.org/10.1038/s41467-021-26674-1] [PMID: 34753928]

[20] V.M. Alves, D. Korn, V. Pervitsky, A. Thieme, S.J. Capuzzi, N. Baker, R. Chirkova, S. Ekins, E.N. Muratov, A. Hickey, and A. Tropsha, "Knowledge-based approaches to drug discovery for rare diseases", *Drug Discov. Today,* vol. 27, no. 2, pp. 490-502, 2022.
[http://dx.doi.org/10.1016/j.drudis.2021.10.014] [PMID: 34718207]

[21] F. Shen, Y. Zhao, L. Wang, M.R. Mojarad, Y. Wang, S. Liu, and H. Liu, "Rare disease knowledge enrichment through a data-driven approach", *BMC Med. Inform. Decis. Mak.,* vol. 19, no. 1, p. 32, 2019.
[http://dx.doi.org/10.1186/s12911-019-0752-9] [PMID: 30764825]

[22] Q. Zhu, D.T. Nguyen, I. Grishagin, N. Southall, E. Sid, and A. Pariser, "An integrative knowledge graph for rare diseases, derived from the Genetic and Rare Diseases Information Center (GARD)", *J. Biomed. Semantics,* vol. 11, no. 1, p. 13, 2020.
[http://dx.doi.org/10.1186/s13326-020-00232-y] [PMID: 33183351]

[23] J. Sanjak, J. Binder, A.S. Yadaw, Q. Zhu, and E.A. Mathé, "Clustering rare diseases within an ontology-enriched knowledge graph", *J. Am. Med. Inform. Assoc.,* vol. 31, no. 1, pp. 154-164, 2023.
[http://dx.doi.org/10.1093/jamia/ocad186] [PMID: 37759342]

[24] W.Z. Kariampuzha, G. Alyea, S. Qu, J. Sanjak, E. Mathé, E. Sid, H. Chatelaine, A. Yadaw, Y. Xu, and Q. Zhu, "Precision information extraction for rare disease epidemiology at scale", *J. Transl. Med.,* vol. 21, no. 1, p. 157, 2023.
[http://dx.doi.org/10.1186/s12967-023-04011-y] [PMID: 36855134]

[25] N. Hallowell, M. Parker, and C. Nellåker, "Big data phenotyping in rare diseases: some ethical issues", *Genet. Med.,* vol. 21, no. 2, pp. 272-274, 2019.
[http://dx.doi.org/10.1038/s41436-018-0067-8] [PMID: 29907800]

[26] S. Decherchi, E. Pedrini, M. Mordenti, A. Cavalli, and L. Sangiorgi, "Opportunities and challenges for machine learning in rare diseases", *Front. Med. (Lausanne),* vol. 8, 2021.747612
[http://dx.doi.org/10.3389/fmed.2021.747612] [PMID: 34676229]

[27] M. Abulaish, M.A. Parwez, and Jahiruddin, "DiseaSE: A biomedical text analytics system for disease symptom extraction and characterization", *J. Biomed. Inform.,* vol. 100, 2019.103324
[http://dx.doi.org/10.1016/j.jbi.2019.103324] [PMID: 31678590]

[28] M. Rastegar-Mojarad, S. Liu, Y. Wang, N. Afzal, L. Wang, F. Shen, S. Fu, and H. Liu, "BioCreative/OHNLP Challenge 2018," in Proc. BioCreative/OHNLP Challenge, New York, NY, USA: ACM, 2018.
[http://dx.doi.org/10.1145/3233547.3233672]

[29] W. Sun, A. Rumshisky, and O. Uzuner, "Evaluating temporal relations in clinical text: 2012 i2b2 Challenge", *J. Am. Med. Inform. Assoc.,* vol. 20, no. 5, pp. 806-813, 2013.
[http://dx.doi.org/10.1136/amiajnl-2013-001628] [PMID: 23564629]

[30] C. Nédellec, "Overview of BioNLP shared task 2013", *Proc. BioNLP Shared Task 2013 Workshop,* 2013 pp. 1-7

[31] A. Miranda-Escalada, F. Mehryary, J. Luoma, D. Estrada-Zavala, L. Gasco, S. Pyysalo, A. Valencia, and M. Krallinger, "Overview of DrugProt task at BioCreative VII: data and methods for large-scale text mining and knowledge graph generation of heterogenous chemical–protein relations", *Database (Oxford),* vol. 2023, 2023.baad080
[http://dx.doi.org/10.1093/database/baad080] [PMID: 38015956]

[32] A.R. Aronson, and F.M. Lang, "An overview of MetaMap: historical perspective and recent advances", *J. Am. Med. Inform. Assoc.,* vol. 17, no. 3, pp. 229-236, 2010.
[http://dx.doi.org/10.1136/jamia.2009.002733] [PMID: 20442139]

[33] R. Reátegui, and S. Ratté, "Comparison of MetaMap and cTAKES for entity extraction in clinical notes", *BMC Med. Inform. Decis. Mak.,* vol. 18, no. S3, suppl. Suppl. 3, p. 74, 2018.
[http://dx.doi.org/10.1186/s12911-018-0654-2] [PMID: 30255810]

[34] C. Friedman, L. Shagina, S. A. Socratous, and X. Zeng, "A web-based version of MedLEE: A medical language extraction and encoding system," in Proceedings of the AMIA Annual Fall Symposium, American Medical Informatics Association, 1996, p. 938.

[35] S. Abdulkadhar, G. Murugesan, and J. Natarajan, "Classifying protein-protein interaction articles from biomedical literature using many relevant features and context-free grammar, J. King Saud Univ", *Comput. Inf. Sci.,* vol. 32, no. 5, pp. 553-560, 2020.

[36] S. Abdulkadhar and J. Natarajan, "A text mining protocol for mining biological pathways and regulatory networks from biomedical literature," in Biomedical Text Mining, K. Raja, Ed. New York, NY, USA: Humana Press, 2022, pp. 149–168, Methods in Molecular Biology, vol. 2496. [http://dx.doi.org/10.1007/978-1-0716-2305-3_8]

[37] G. Murugesan, S. Abdulkadhar, and J. Natarajan, "Distributed smoothed tree kernel for protein-protein interaction extraction from the biomedical literature", *PLoS One,* vol. 12, no. 11, 2017.e0187379 [http://dx.doi.org/10.1371/journal.pone.0187379] [PMID: 29099838]

[38] D.S. Lee, A.D. Krahn, J.S. Healey, D. Birnie, E. Crystal, P. Dorian, C.S. Simpson, Y. Khaykin, D. Cameron, A. Janmohamed, R. Yee, P.C. Austin, Z. Chen, J. Hardy, and J.V. Tu, "Evaluation of early complications related to *De Novo* cardioverter defibrillator implantation insights from the Ontario ICD database", *J. Am. Coll. Cardiol.,* vol. 55, no. 8, pp. 774-782, 2010. [http://dx.doi.org/10.1016/j.jacc.2009.11.029] [PMID: 20170816]

[39] J.W. Chae, C.S. Song, H. Kim, K.B. Lee, B.S. Seo, and D.I. Kim, "Prediction of mortality in patients undergoing maintenance hemodialysis by Charlson Comorbidity Index using ICD-10 database", *Nephron Clin. Pract.,* vol. 117, no. 4, pp. 379-384, 2011. [http://dx.doi.org/10.1159/000321525] [PMID: 21071962]

[40] L.M. Schriml, J.B. Munro, M. Schor, D. Olley, C. McCracken, V. Felix, J.A. Baron, R. Jackson, S.M. Bello, C. Bearer, R. Lichenstein, K. Bisordi, N.C. Dialo, M. Giglio, and C. Greene, "The human disease ontology 2022 update", *Nucleic Acids Res.,* vol. 50, no. D1, pp. D1255-D1261, 2022. [http://dx.doi.org/10.1093/nar/gkab1063] [PMID: 34755882]

[41] A. Hliaoutakis, Semantic similarity measures in MeSH ontology and their application to information retrieval on Medline, Master's thesis, Technical University of Crete, Greece, 2005. [Online]. Available: http://www.intelligence.tuc.gr/publications/Hliautakis.pdf

[42] G. Fragoso, S. de Coronado, M. Haber, F. Hartel, and L. Wright, "Overview and utilization of the NCI Thesaurus", *Comp. Funct. Genomics,* vol. 5, no. 8, pp. 648-654, 2004. [http://dx.doi.org/10.1002/cfg.445] [PMID: 18629178]

[43] S. El-Sappagh, F. Franda, F. Ali, and K.S. Kwak, "SNOMED CT standard ontology based on the ontology for general medical science", *BMC Med. Inform. Decis. Mak.,* vol. 18, no. 1, p. 76, 2018. [http://dx.doi.org/10.1186/s12911-018-0651-5] [PMID: 30170591]

[44] A. Hamosh, A.F. Scott, J. Amberger, D. Valle, and V.A. McKusick, "Online Mendelian Inheritance In Man (OMIM)", *Hum. Mutat.,* vol. 15, no. 1, pp. 57-61, 2000. [http://dx.doi.org/10.1002/(SICI)1098-1004(200001)15:1<57::AID-HUMU12>3.0.CO;2-G] [PMID: 10612823]

[45] M. Kanehisa, "The KEGG database", *in In Silico Simulation of Biological Processes: Novartis Foundation Symposium 247, Chichester, UK: John Wiley & Sons, Ltd.,* vol. 247, pp. 91-103, 2002. [http://dx.doi.org/10.1002/0470857897.ch8]

[46] M. Kanehisa, Y. Sato, M. Furumichi, K. Morishima, and M. Tanabe, "New approach for understanding genome variations in KEGG", *Nucleic Acids Res.,* vol. 47, no. D1, pp. D590-D595, 2019. [http://dx.doi.org/10.1093/nar/gky962] [PMID: 30321428]

[47] J.S. Amberger, C.A. Bocchini, F. Schiettecatte, A.F. Scott, and A. Hamosh, "OMIM.org: Online Mendelian Inheritance in Man (OMIM®), an online catalog of human genes and genetic disorders",

Nucleic Acids Res., vol. 43, no. D1, pp. D789-D798, 2015. [http://dx.doi.org/10.1093/nar/gku1205] [PMID: 25428349]

[48] K. Hogan Smith, "Review of Rare Diseases Resources: National Organization for Rare Disorders (NORD) Rare Disease Database, NIH Genetic and Rare Diseases Information Center, and Orphanet", *J. Consum. Health Internet,* vol. 21, no. 2, pp. 216-225, 2017. [http://dx.doi.org/10.1080/15398285.2017.1311613]

[49] S.S. Weinreich, R. Mangon, J.J. Sikkens, M.E. Teeuw, and M.C. Cornel, "[Orphanet: a European database for rare diseases]", *Ned. Tijdschr. Geneeskd.,* vol. 152, no. 9, pp. 518-519, 2008. [PMID: 18389888]

[50] M. Mohtashamian, R. Abeysinghe, X. Hao, and L. Cui, "Identifying missing IS-A relations in Orphanet rare disease ontology", *in Proc. IEEE Int. Conf. Bioinformatics Biomed. (BIBM),* pp. 3274-3279, Dec. 2022. [http://dx.doi.org/10.1109/BIBM55620.2022.9995614]

[51] O. Bodenreider, "The unified medical language system (UMLS): Integrating biomedical terminology", *Nucleic Acids Res.,* vol. 32, no. suppl_1, pp. D267-D270, 2004. [http://dx.doi.org/10.1093/nar/gkh061]

[52] P. Mozzicato, "MedDRA", *Pharmaceut. Med.,* vol. 23, no. 2, pp. 65-75, 2009. [http://dx.doi.org/10.1007/BF03256752]

[53] L. Breuza, S. Poux, A. Estreicher, M.L. Famiglietti, M. Magrane, M. Tognolli, A. Bridge, D. Baratin, and N. Redaschi, "The UniProtKB guide to the human proteome", *Database (Oxford),* vol. 2016, 2016.bav120 [http://dx.doi.org/10.1093/database/bav120] [PMID: 26896845]

[54] S. Povey, R. Lovering, E. Bruford, M. Wright, M. Lush, and H. Wain, "The HUGO Gene Nomenclature Committee (HGNC)", *Hum. Genet.,* vol. 109, no. 6, pp. 678-680, 2001. [http://dx.doi.org/10.1007/s00439-001-0615-0] [PMID: 11810281]

[55] A. Yates, W. Akanni, M.R. Amode, D. Barrell, K. Billis, D. Carvalho-Silva, C. Cummins, P. Clapham, S. Fitzgerald, L. Gil, C.G. Girón, L. Gordon, T. Hourlier, S.E. Hunt, S.H. Janacek, N. Johnson, T. Juettemann, S. Keenan, I. Lavidas, F.J. Martin, T. Maurel, W. McLaren, D.N. Murphy, R. Nag, M. Nuhn, A. Parker, M. Patricio, M. Pignatelli, M. Rahtz, H.S. Riat, D. Sheppard, K. Taylor, A. Thormann, A. Vullo, S.P. Wilder, A. Zadissa, E. Birney, J. Harrow, M. Muffato, E. Perry, M. Ruffier, G. Spudich, S.J. Trevanion, F. Cunningham, B.L. Aken, D.R. Zerbino, and P. Flicek, "Ensembl 2016", *Nucleic Acids Res.,* vol. 44, no. D1, pp. D710-D716, 2016. [http://dx.doi.org/10.1093/nar/gkv1157] [PMID: 26687719]

[56] G. Joshi-Tope, M. Gillespie, I. Vastrik, P. D'Eustachio, E. Schmidt, B. de Bono, B. Jassal, G. R. Gopinath, G. R. Wu, L. Matthews, S. Lewis, E. Birney, and L. Stein, "Reactome: a knowledgebase of biological pathways," *Nucleic Acids Research,* vol. 33, suppl. 1, pp. D428–D432, Jan. 2005. [Online]. Available: https://doi.org/10.1093/nar/gki072

[57] A. J. Harmar, "IUPHAR-DB: The IUPHAR database of G protein-coupled receptors and ion channels", *Nucleic Acids Res.,* vol. 37, no. suppl_1, pp. D680-D685, 2009. [http://dx.doi.org/10.1093/nar/gkn728]

[58] R.I. Doğan, R. Leaman, and Z. Lu, "NCBI disease corpus: A resource for disease name recognition and concept normalization", *J. Biomed. Inform.,* vol. 47, pp. 1-10, 2014. [http://dx.doi.org/10.1016/j.jbi.2013.12.006] [PMID: 24393765]

[59] J. Li, Y. Sun, R. J. Johnson, D. Sciaky, C. H. Wei, R. Leaman, A. P. Davis, C. J. Mattingly, T. C. Wiegers, and Z. Lu, "BioCreative V CDR task corpus: A resource for chemical disease relation extraction," Database (Oxford), vol. 2016, May 9 2016, p. baw068. [http://dx.doi.org/10.1093/database/baw068]

[60] C. Martínez-deMiguel, I. Segura-Bedmar, E. Chacón-Solano, and S. Guerrero-Aspizua, "The RareDis corpus: A corpus annotated with rare diseases, their signs and symptoms", *J. Biomed. Inform.,* vol.

125, 2022.103961
[http://dx.doi.org/10.1016/j.jbi.2021.103961] [PMID: 34879250]

[61] H. Fabregat, L. Araujo, and J. Martinez-Romo, "Deep neural models for extracting entities and relationships in the new RDD corpus relating disabilities and rare diseases", *Comput. Methods Programs Biomed.*, vol. 164, pp. 121-129, 2018.
[http://dx.doi.org/10.1016/j.cmpb.2018.07.007] [PMID: 30195420]

[62] M. Krallinger, O. Rabal, F. Leitner, M. Vazquez, D. Salgado, Z. Lu, R. Leaman, Y. Lu, D. Ji, D.M. Lowe, R.A. Sayle, R.T. Batista-Navarro, R. Rak, T. Huber, T. Rocktäschel, S. Matos, D. Campos, B. Tang, H. Xu, T. Munkhdalai, K.H. Ryu, S.V. Ramanan, S. Nathan, S. Žitnik, M. Bajec, L. Weber, M. Irmer, S.A. Akhondi, J.A. Kors, S. Xu, X. An, U.K. Sikdar, A. Ekbal, M. Yoshioka, T.M. Dieb, M. Choi, K. Verspoor, M. Khabsa, C.L. Giles, H. Liu, K.E. Ravikumar, A. Lamurias, F.M. Couto, H.J. Dai, R.T.H. Tsai, C. Ata, T. Can, A. Usié, R. Alves, I. Segura-Bedmar, P. Martínez, J. Oyarzabal, and A. Valencia, "The CHEMDNER corpus of chemicals and drugs and its annotation principles", *J. Cheminform.*, vol. 7, no. S1, suppl. Suppl 1 Text mining for chemistry and the CHEMDNER track, p. S2, 2015.
[http://dx.doi.org/10.1186/1758-2946-7-S1-S2] [PMID: 25810773]

[63] L. Smith, L.K. Tanabe, R.J. Ando, C.J. Kuo, I.F. Chung, C.N. Hsu, Y.S. Lin, R. Klinger, C.M. Friedrich, K. Ganchev, M. Torii, H. Liu, B. Haddow, C.A. Struble, R.J. Povinelli, A. Vlachos, W.A. Baumgartner Jr, L. Hunter, B. Carpenter, R.T.H. Tsai, H.J. Dai, F. Liu, Y. Chen, C. Sun, S. Katrenko, P. Adriaans, C. Blaschke, R. Torres, M. Neves, P. Nakov, A. Divoli, M. Maña-López, J. Mata, and W.J. Wilbur, "Overview of BioCreative II gene mention recognition", *Genome Biol.*, vol. 9, no. S2, suppl. Suppl. 2, p. S2, 2008.
[http://dx.doi.org/10.1186/gb-2008-9-s2-s2] [PMID: 18834493]

[64] À. Bravo, J. Piñero, N. Queralt-Rosinach, M. Rautschka, and L.I. Furlong, "Extraction of relations between genes and diseases from text and large-scale data analysis: implications for translational research", *BMC Bioinformatics,* vol. 16, no. 1, p. 55, 2015.
[http://dx.doi.org/10.1186/s12859-015-0472-9] [PMID: 25886734]

[65] E.M. van Mulligen, A. Fourrier-Reglat, D. Gurwitz, M. Molokhia, A. Nieto, G. Trifiro, J.A. Kors, and L.I. Furlong, "The EU-ADR corpus: Annotated drugs, diseases, targets, and their relationships", *J. Biomed. Inform.*, vol. 45, no. 5, pp. 879-884, 2012.
[http://dx.doi.org/10.1016/j.jbi.2012.04.004] [PMID: 22554700]

[66] Li J, Sun Y, Johnson RJ, Sciaky D, Wei CH, Leaman R, Davis AP, Mattingly CJ, Wiegers TC, Lu Z. BioCreative V CDR task corpus: a resource for chemical disease relation extraction. Database (Oxford). 2016 May 9;2016:baw068. doi: 10.1093/database/baw068. PMID: 27161011; PMCID: PMC4860626.

[67] D.D. Palmer, "Tokenisation and sentence segmentation", *in Handbook of Natural Language Processing, R. Dale, H. Moisl, and H. Somers, Eds.,* 2000.

[68] S. Vijayarani, M.J. Ilamathi, and M. Nithya, "Preprocessing techniques for text mining—An overview", *Int. J. Comput. Sci. Commun. Netw.,* vol. 5, no. 1, pp. 7-16, 2015.

[69] S. Kannan, V. Gurusamy, S. Vijayarani, J. Ilamathi, and M. Nithya, "Preprocessing techniques for text mining", *Int. J. Comput. Sci. Commun. Netw.,* vol. 5, no. 1, pp. 7-16, 2014.

[70] S. Abdulkadhar, B. Bhasuran, and J. Natarajan, "Multiscale Laplacian graph kernel combined with lexico-syntactic patterns for biomedical event extraction from literature", *Knowl. Inf. Syst.,* vol. 63, no. 1, pp. 143-173, 2021.
[http://dx.doi.org/10.1007/s10115-020-01514-8]

[71] M. Gross, "Lemmatization of compound tenses in English", *Lingvist. Investiga.,* vol. 22, no. 1–2, pp. 71-122, 1998.

[72] H. Liu, T. Christiansen, W.A. Baumgartner Jr, and K. Verspoor, "BioLemmatizer: a lemmatization tool for morphological processing of biomedical text", *J. Biomed. Semantics,* vol. 3, no. 1, p. 3, 2012.

[http://dx.doi.org/10.1186/2041-1480-3-3] [PMID: 22464129]

[73] R. Collobert, J. Weston, L. Bottou, M. Karlen, K. Kavukcuoglu, and P. Kuksa, "Natural Language Processing (almost) from Scratch, arXiv preprint arXiv:1103.0398, 2011. [Online]. Available: https://doi.org/10.48550/arXiv.1103.0398

[74] S. Ferilli, F. Esposito, and D. Grieco, "Automatic learning of linguistic resources for stopword removal and stemming from text", *Procedia Comput. Sci.,* vol. 38, pp. 116-123, 2014. [http://dx.doi.org/10.1016/j.procs.2014.10.019]

[75] S. Kübler, R. McDonald, and J. Nivre, "Dependency parsing", *Synthesis Lectures on Human Language Technologies,* vol. 1, no. 1, pp. 1-127, 2009. [http://dx.doi.org/10.1007/978-3-031-02131-2]

[76] M.C. De Marneffe, and C.D. Manning, "The Stanford typed dependencies representation", *Workshop on Cross-Framework and Cross-Domain Parser Evaluation,* pp. 1-8, 2008. [Online]. Available: https://aclanthology.org/W08-1301/

[77] K. Sagae, and J.I. Tsujii, "Dependency parsing and domain adaptation with data-driven LR models and parser ensembles", *Trends in Parsing Technology,* pp. 57-68, 2010. [http://dx.doi.org/10.1007/978-90-481-9352-3_4]

[78] G. Murugesan, S. Abdulkadhar, B. Bhasuran, and J. Natarajan, "BCC-NER: bidirectional, contextual clues named entity tagger for gene/protein mention recognition", *EURASIP J. Bioinform. Syst. Biol.,* vol. 2017, no. 1, p. 7, 2017. [http://dx.doi.org/10.1186/s13637-017-0060-6] [PMID: 28477208]

[79] B. Bhasuran, G. Murugesan, S. Abdulkadhar, and J. Natarajan, "Stacked ensemble combined with fuzzy matching for biomedical named entity recognition of diseases", *J. Biomed. Inform.,* vol. 64, pp. 1-9, 2016. [http://dx.doi.org/10.1016/j.jbi.2016.09.009] [PMID: 27634494]

[80] R. Leaman, and G. Gonzalez, "BANNER: An executable survey of advances in biomedical named entity recognition", *in Biocomputing 2008,* pp. 652-663, 2008. PMID: 18229723.

[81] B. Settles, "ABNER: an open source tool for automatically tagging genes, proteins and other entity names in text", *Bioinformatics,* vol. 21, no. 14, pp. 3191-3192, 2005. [http://dx.doi.org/10.1093/bioinformatics/bti475] [PMID: 15860559]

[82] Q. Wei, T. Chen, R. Xu, Y. He, and L. Gui, "Disease named entity recognition by combining conditional random fields and bidirectional recurrent neural networks", *Database (Oxford),* vol. 2016, 2016.baw140 [http://dx.doi.org/10.1093/database/baw140] [PMID: 27777244]

[83] C. Cousyn, K. Bouchard, S. Gaboury, and B. Bouchard, "Towards using scientific publications to automatically extract information on rare diseases", *Mob. Netw. Appl.,* vol. 25, no. 3, pp. 953-960, 2020. [http://dx.doi.org/10.1007/s11036-019-01237-3]

[84] J.A. Vanegas, S. Matos, F. González, and J.L. Oliveira, "An overview of biomolecular event extraction from scientific documents", *Comput. Math. Methods Med.,* vol. 2015, pp. 1-19, 2015. [http://dx.doi.org/10.1155/2015/571381] [PMID: 26587051]

[85] S. Ananiadou, P. Thompson, R. Nawaz, J. McNaught, and D.B. Kell, "Event-based text mining for biology and functional genomics", *Brief. Funct. Genomics,* vol. 14, no. 3, pp. 213-230, 2015. [http://dx.doi.org/10.1093/bfgp/elu015] [PMID: 24907365]

[86] X. Chen, D. Xie, Q. Zhao, and Z.H. You, "MicroRNAs and complex diseases: from experimental results to computational models", *Brief. Bioinform.,* vol. 20, no. 2, pp. 515-539, 2019. [http://dx.doi.org/10.1093/bib/bbx130] [PMID: 29045685]

[87] S. Ananiadou, S. Pyysalo, J. Tsujii, and D.B. Kell, "Event extraction for systems biology by text mining the literature", *Trends Biotechnol.,* vol. 28, no. 7, pp. 381-390, 2010.

[http://dx.doi.org/10.1016/j.tibtech.2010.04.005] [PMID: 20570001]

[88] M. Krallinger, F. Leitner, and A. Valencia, "Analysis of biological processes and diseases using text mining approaches", *Bioinformatics Methods Clin. Res,* pp. 341-382, 2010. [http://dx.doi.org/10.1007/978-1-60327-194-3_16]

[89] O. Bodenreider, "Biomedical ontologies in action: role in knowledge management, data integration and decision support", *Yearb. Med. Inform.,* vol. 17, no. 1, pp. 67-79, 2008. [http://dx.doi.org/10.1055/s-0038-1638585] [PMID: 18660879]

[90] C. Friedman, T.C. Rindflesch, and M. Corn, "Natural language processing: State of the art and prospects for significant progress, a workshop sponsored by the National Library of Medicine", *J. Biomed. Inform.,* vol. 46, no. 5, pp. 765-773, 2013. [http://dx.doi.org/10.1016/j.jbi.2013.06.004] [PMID: 23810857]

[91] J.A. Malik, and J.N. Agrewala, "Future perspectives of emerging novel drug targets and immunotherapies to control drug addiction", *Int. Immunopharmacol.,* vol. 119, 2023.110210 [http://dx.doi.org/10.1016/j.intimp.2023.110210] [PMID: 37099943]

[92] Y. Garten, A. Coulet, and R.B. Altman, "Recent progress in automatically extracting information from the pharmacogenomic literature", *Pharmacogenomics,* vol. 11, no. 10, pp. 1467-1489, 2010. [http://dx.doi.org/10.2217/pgs.10.136] [PMID: 21047206]

[93] A.A. Kalinin, G.A. Higgins, N. Reamaroon, S. Soroushmehr, A. Allyn-Feuer, I.D. Dinov, K. Najarian, and B.D. Athey, "Deep learning in pharmacogenomics: from gene regulation to patient stratification", *Pharmacogenomics,* vol. 19, no. 7, pp. 629-650, 2018. [http://dx.doi.org/10.2217/pgs-2018-0008] [PMID: 29697304]

[94] G. Potamias, K. Lakiotaki, T. Katsila, M.T.M. Lee, S. Topouzis, D.N. Cooper, and G.P. Patrinos, "Deciphering next-generation pharmacogenomics: an information technology perspective", *Open Biol.,* vol. 4, no. 7, 2014.140071 [http://dx.doi.org/10.1098/rsob.140071] [PMID: 25030607]

[95] A. Kumar, P. Kumar, R.K. Mittal, and H. Singh, "Preprocessing and postprocessing in additive manufacturing," in Advances in Additive Manufacturing", *in Advances in Additive Manufacturing, Elsevier,* pp. 141-165, 2023.

[96] M. Bastian, S. Heymann, and M. Jacomy, "Gephi: An open source software for exploring and manipulating networks", *in Proc. Int. AAAI Conf. Web Soc. Media,* vol. 3, no. 1, pp. 361-362s, Mar. 2009. [http://dx.doi.org/10.1609/icwsm.v3i1.13937]

[97] Z. Hu, J. Mellor, J. Wu, T. Yamada, D. Holloway, and C. DeLisi, "VisANT: data-integrating visual framework for biological networks and modules", *Nucleic Acids Res.,* vol. 33, no. Web Server, suppl. Suppl. 2, pp. W352-W357, 2005. [http://dx.doi.org/10.1093/nar/gki431] [PMID: 15980487]

[98] A. Nikitin, S. Egorov, N. Daraselia, and I. Mazo, "Pathway studio—the analysis and navigation of molecular networks", *Bioinformatics,* vol. 19, no. 16, pp. 2155-2157, 2003. [http://dx.doi.org/10.1093/bioinformatics/btg290] [PMID: 14594725]

[99] E. Demir, O. Babur, U. Dogrusoz, A. Gursoy, G. Nisanci, R. Cetin-Atalay, and M. Ozturk, "P atika : an integrated visual environment for collaborative construction and analysis of cellular pathways", *Bioinformatics,* vol. 18, no. 7, pp. 996-1003, 2002. [http://dx.doi.org/10.1093/bioinformatics/18.7.996] [PMID: 12117798]

[100] J. Makhoul, F. Kubala, R. Schwartz, and R. Weischedel, "Performance measures for information extraction", *Proc. DARPA Broadcast News Workshop,* pp. 249-252, 1999.

[101] X. Li, K. Chen, J. Yang, C. Wang, T. Yang, C. Luo, N. Li, and Z. Liu, "TLDA: A transfer learning based dual-augmentation strategy for traditional Chinese Medicine syndrome differentiation in rare disease", *Comput. Biol. Med.,* vol. 169, p. 107808, 2024.

[http://dx.doi.org/10.1016/j.compbiomed.2023.107808] [PMID: 38101119]

[102] K. Xu, Z. Zhou, T. Gong, T. Hao, and W. Liu, "SBLC: a hybrid model for disease named entity recognition based on semantic bidirectional LSTMs and conditional random fields", *BMC Med. Inform. Decis. Mak.,* vol. 18, no. S5, suppl. Suppl. 5, p. 114, 2018. [http://dx.doi.org/10.1186/s12911-018-0690-y] [PMID: 30526592]

[103] C. Shyr, Y. Hu, P.A. Harris, and H. Xu, "Identifying and extracting rare disease phenotypes with large language models", *arXiv preprint arXiv:2306.12656,* 2023.

[104] M.F. Davis, S. Sriram, W.S. Bush, J.C. Denny, and J.L. Haines, "Automated extraction of clinical traits of multiple sclerosis in electronic medical records", *J. Am. Med. Inform. Assoc.,* vol. 20, no. e2, pp. e334-e340, 2013. [http://dx.doi.org/10.1136/amiajnl-2013-001999] [PMID: 24148554]

[105] T. Lo Barco, M. Kuchenbuch, N. Garcelon, A. Neuraz, and R. Nabbout, "Improving early diagnosis of rare diseases using Natural Language Processing in unstructured medical records: an illustration from Dravet syndrome", *Orphanet J. Rare Dis.,* vol. 16, no. 1, p. 309, 2021. [http://dx.doi.org/10.1186/s13023-021-01936-9] [PMID: 34256808]

[106] C.A. Deisseroth, J. Birgmeier, E.E. Bodle, J.N. Kohler, D.R. Matalon, Y. Nazarenko, C.A. Genetti, C.A. Brownstein, K. Schmitz-Abe, K. Schoch, H. Cope, R. Signer, J.A. Martinez-Agosto, V. Shashi, A.H. Beggs, M.T. Wheeler, J.A. Bernstein, and G. Bejerano, "ClinPhen extracts and prioritizes patient phenotypes directly from medical records to expedite genetic disease diagnosis", *Genet. Med.,* vol. 21, no. 7, pp. 1585-1593, 2019. [http://dx.doi.org/10.1038/s41436-018-0381-1] [PMID: 30514889]

[107] S.U. Nigwekar, C.A. Solid, E. Ankers, R. Malhotra, W. Eggert, A. Turchin, R.I. Thadhani, and C.A. Herzog, "Quantifying a rare disease in administrative data: the example of calciphylaxis", *J. Gen. Intern. Med.,* vol. 29, no. S3, suppl. Suppl. 3, pp. 724-731, 2014. [http://dx.doi.org/10.1007/s11606-014-2910-1] [PMID: 25029979]

[108] M. Jiang, M. Li, W. Cao, M. Yang, and L. Zhou, "Multi-task convolutional deep neural network for recommendation based on knowledge graphs", *Neurocomputing,* vol. 619, pp. 129-136, 2025. [http://dx.doi.org/10.1016/j.neucom.2024.129136]

[109] S. Raj, V. Namdeo, P. Singh, and A. Srivastava, "Identification and prioritization of disease candidate genes using biomedical named entity recognition and random forest classification", *Computers in Biology and Medicine,* vol. 192, p. 110320, 2025. [http://dx.doi.org/10.1016/j.compbiomed.2025.110320]

[110] P. Holat, "Weakly-supervised symptom recognition for rare diseases in biomedical text", *15th Int. Symp. IDA 2016,* pp. 192-203, Oct. 13–15, 2016.Stockholm, Sweden [http://dx.doi.org/10.1007/978-3-319-46349-0_17]

[111] L. Martin, D. Battistelli, and T. Charnois, in 13th Workshop Biomed. Nat. Lang. Process. (BioNLP 2014), 2014.

[112] H. Patel, “BioNerFlair: Biomedical named entity recognition using flair embedding and sequence tagger,” arXiv, Nov. 2020, arXiv:2011.01504. doi: 10.48550/arXiv.2011.01504.

[113] N. Béchet, P. Cellier, T. Charnois, B. Crémilleux, and M.C. Jaulent, "Sequential pattern mining to discover relations between genes and rare diseases", *in 2012 25th IEEE Int. Symp. Comput.-Based Med. Syst. (CBMS), IEEE,* pp. 1-6, 2012. [http://dx.doi.org/10.1109/CBMS.2012.6266367]

[114] L. Cao, J. Sun, and A. Cross, "AutoRD: An automatic and end-to-end system for rare disease knowledge graph construction based on ontologies-enhanced large language models", *arXiv preprint arXiv:2403.00953,* 2024. [http://dx.doi.org/10.2196/preprints.60665]

[115] J. Du, G. Liu, J. Gao, X. Liao, J. Hu, and L. Wu, "Graph neural network-based entity extraction and

relationship reasoning in complex knowledge graphs", In: *2024 International Conference on Image Processing, Computer Vision and Machine Learning (ICICML)*, 2024, pp. 679-683.IEEE [http://dx.doi.org/10.48550/arXiv.2411.15195]

[116] S. Gupta, X. Ai, and R. Kavuluru, "Comparison of pipeline, sequence-to-sequence, and GPT models for end-to-end relation extraction: Experiments with the rare disease use-case", *arXiv preprint arXiv:2311.13729,* 2023.

[117] B. Bhasuran, and J. Natarajan, "Automatic extraction of gene-disease associations from literature using joint ensemble learning", *PLoS One,* vol. 13, no. 7, p. e0200699, 2018. [http://dx.doi.org/10.1371/journal.pone.0200699] [PMID: 30048465]

[118] F. Alam, A. Corazza, A. Lavelli, and R. Zanoli, "A knowledge-poor approach to chemical-disease relation extraction", *Database (Oxford),* vol. 2016, p. baw071, 2016. [http://dx.doi.org/10.1093/database/baw071] [PMID: 27189609]

[119] B. Bhasuran, and J. Natarajan, "DisGeReExT: a knowledge discovery system for exploration of disease–gene associations through large-scale literature-wide analysis study", *Knowl. Inf. Syst.,* vol. 65, no. 8, pp. 3463-3487, 2023. [http://dx.doi.org/10.1007/s10115-023-01862-1]

[120] H. Xing, D. Zhang, P. Cai, R. Zhang, and Q.N. Hu, "RDBridge: a knowledge graph of rare diseases based on large-scale text mining", *Bioinformatics,* vol. 39, no. 7, p. btad440, 2023. [http://dx.doi.org/10.1093/bioinformatics/btad440] [PMID: 37458501]

[121] J. Lee, W. Yoon, S. Kim, D. Kim, S. Kim, C.H. So, and J. Kang, "BioBERT: a pre-trained biomedical language representation model for biomedical text mining", *Bioinformatics,* vol. 36, no. 4, pp. 1234-1240, 2020. [http://dx.doi.org/10.1093/bioinformatics/btz682] [PMID: 31501885]

[122] G. Frisoni, G. Moro, and A. Carbonaro, "Unsupervised descriptive text mining for knowledge graph learning", *in Proc. 12th Int. Joint Conf. Knowl. Discov., Knowl. Eng., Knowl. Manag. (IC3K 2020),* vol. 1, pp. 316-324, 2020.

[123] X. Chen, X. Mao, Q. Guo, L. Wang, S. Zhang, and T. Chen, "RareBench: can LLMs serve as rare diseases specialists?", *Proceedings of the 30th ACM SIGKDD Conference on Knowledge Discovery and Data Mining,* pp. 4850-4861, 2024.ACM [http://dx.doi.org/10.48550/arXiv.2402.06341]

[124] X. Chen, "RareBench: can LLMs serve as rare diseases specialists?", *in Proc. 30th ACM SIGKDD Conf. Knowl. Discov. Data Min.,* pp. 4850-4861, Aug. 2024. [http://dx.doi.org/10.1145/3637528.3671576]

CHAPTER 8

Leveraging AI and ML to Enhance Focused Ultrasound Treatments for Essential Tremors

Tamilalagan S.[1], **R. K. Pongiannan**[1,*], **R. Brindha**[1], **Jishnu K. S.**[1], **Shijukumar K.**[1], **K. P. Naveen**[2] and **Telugu Maddileti**[3]

[1] *Department of Computing Technologies, School of Computing, CET, SRM Institute of Science and Technology, Kattankulathur Campus, Chennai, Tamil Nadu, India*

[2] *Pondicherry Institute of Medical Sciences, Puducherry, India*

[3] *Department of Electronics and Communication Engineering, Guru Nanak Institutions Technical Campus, Ibrahimpatnam, Ranga Reddy District, Telangana-501506, India*

Abstract: In today's world, technological advancements in the medical field have revolutionized healthcare, dramatically enhancing diagnosis, treatment, and patient care. For example, AI and ML algorithms can now precisely analyze and observe medical images. The quality of life of individuals with Essential Tremors (ET) is significantly affected, and Focused Ultrasound (FUS) has become a viable non-invasive therapeutic option. However, precision targeting and customized therapy regimens are necessary for maximizing FUS treatment for ET. To improve the effectiveness of FUS in ET therapy, this work investigates the integration of Artificial Intelligence (AI) and Machine Learning (ML). In order to assess patient data, enhance imaging precision, and customize therapy parameters, we implemented cutting-edge AI algorithms. According to research, utilizing AI and ML in FUS can transform ET management and provide a more efficient and personalized treatment choice. The creation of real-time AI tools and additional validation will be the main goals of future research. For instance, imaging processes can be performed using computer-assisted interpretation without human intervention and in a more accurate way. The quality of life of people affected by Essential Tremors (ET) is significantly low, and thus, Focused Ultrasound (FUS) has emerged as a promising non-invasive treatment. However, precision targeting and bespoke therapeutic approaches must be employed to bridge any resultant gaps in FUS treatment for ET. This work investigates ways in which Artificial Intelligence (AI) and Machine Learning (ML) can be employed to enhance the efficacy of FUS treatment in ET therapy.

Keywords: Artificial Intelligence (AI), Essential Tremors (ET), Focused Ultrasound (FUS), Machine Learning (ML), Precision targeting.

* **Corresponding author R. K. Pongiannan:** Department of Computing Technologies, School of Computing, CET, SRM Institute of Science and Technology, Kattankulathur Campus, Chennai, Tamilnadu, India;
E-mail: pongiank@srmist.edu.in

A. Shankar, Saranya Jayapalan, & Basant. K. Tiwary (Eds.)

INTRODUCTION

Essential tremor [1] is one of the most common movement disorders worldwide. This condition is mainly characterized by involuntary shaking of hands, head, or voice. According to an article in PubMed Central [2], the global prevalence of ET was estimated to be 0.32% (24.91 million people) in 2020. This prevalence rises with age, from 0.04% in people younger than 20 to 2.87% in those 80 or older. ET is also more prevalent in men as opposed to women, with a male prevalence of 0.36% and a female prevalence of 0.28%. Some patients derive relief from medication and lifestyle changes; however, in many cases, this fails to improve the condition, and therefore, attention has been drawn to seeking alternative treatments. On this basis, breakthroughs in Focused Ultrasound (FUS) provide promising non-invasive therapy options. Because FUS does not require surgical incisions, clinicians can target the brain areas where tremor generation occurs.

FUS works by overlaying high-frequency sound waves to create tight, focused thermal or mechanical impacts in specific brain tissues. The effectiveness of FUS therapy [3] lies in the extent to which remors decrease, making the patient's lifestyle simpler and more comfortable. The optimality of the treatment parameters, coupled with the proper selection of patients, will determine the success of the therapy. In real-time monitoring of responses to the procedure, responses from the patient are required to make alterations for better outcomes.

The introduction of AI combined with ML [4, 5] into FUS protocols can be a transformative opportunity to enhance efficiency and efficacy in treatment. These technologies will analyze large volumes of patient data to identify those likely to benefit from FUS, considering disease severity and comorbidities. AI and ML might further help in planning treatment by predicting optimal parameters involved in ultrasound application, such as frequency and intensity, tailored to the profile of each patient.

AI-driven real-time monitoring enables online adjustment of treatment parameters during treatment, efficiently and precisely targeting areas of the brain that cause tremors. It also uses AI in post-treatment analysis to predict long-term results so that the clinician can adjust follow-up care accordingly. Integrating AI and ML can significantly enhance the approach taken to treat essential tremors with FUS, ultimately improving patient outcomes and increasing personalization of the process [6].

RELATED WORKS

In one of the earliest studies conducted by Lynn *et al.* [7] in 1942, an efficient focused ultrasound generator was developed and successfully tested, which demonstrated the possibility of producing focal heating in paraffin blocks and the targeted destruction of fresh liver tissue with minimal surface effects. Local cerebral changes induced by high-intensity focused ultrasound were observed in animals and were evidenced by behavioral disabilities that resolved within 2 to 16 hours after exposure, despite passing through the scalp, skull, and meninges. However, previous attempts have resulted in severe injuries to the skin and subcutaneous tissues. The above article suggests ways to optimize focused ultrasound application to increase focal effects in the brain while reducing or removing surface injuries.

The study by Haar G. *et al.* [8] shows that High-Intensity Focused Ultrasound (HIFU) is quickly becoming accepted as a treatment modality, allowing non-invasive tissue heating and ablation for many applications. HIFU treatments are most commonly performed as a single session, often with the patient fully conscious, lightly sedated, or under light general anesthesia. The primary benefit of HIFU over any other thermal ablation technique is that there is no need to place probes into the target tissue. Such highly focused beams are created from sources that are either external to the body, used for the treatment of tumors in the liver, kidney, breast, uterus, pancreas, and bone, or located in the rectum, which is used for the treatment of the prostate, and intended for rapid heating of a target tissue volume with minimal effects on tissue in the ultrasound propagation path. However, because of the broad applicability of HIFU, many devices have been developed for extracorporeal, transrectal, and interstitial treatments to optimize application-specific delivery. Their principles of operation will be described, along with an overview of the physical mechanisms governing HIFU propagation and HIFU-induced heating. Current methods of characterizing HIFU fields and quantifying HIFU exposure and its associated effects are given much focus in the present article.

The paper by Bystritsky *et al.* [9] presents an approach to several neuromodulation techniques, such as DBS and VNS; there is increasing interest in these methods in clinical research. However, the currently available techniques suffer from problems associated with a lack of specificity and invasion. The present article looks into LIFUP, a noninvasive method of brain stimulation that can be delivered precisely through the skull and even integrated with another imaging technique like fMRI. LIFUP is in preclinical testing. There is, however, promise for future clinical applications in more than 50 years of focused ultrasound research on neuronal tissue.

A recent study by Gail R *et al.* [10] describes the noninvasive application of tightly focused ultrasound beams to selectively kill cells within a focal volume while sparing surrounding tissues. This makes it applicable in fields like urology, ophthalmology, and oncology. The primary mechanism is thermal, and renewed interest in HIFU is driven by progress in medical imaging that makes this high level of precision possible in targeting and monitoring the effects of the treatment. This article reviews this rapidly expanding area of HIFU-focused ultrasound surgery.

The study by Hynynen *et al.* [11] employs a historical and contemporary overview of focused ultrasound as a treatment for brain disorders, highlighting its evolution and current applications in neuromodulation and therapeutic interventions.

An article by Izadifar *et al.* [12] presents a treatment principle for the High-Intensity Focused Ultrasound (HIFU) technique for solid tumors, including the pancreas, liver, prostate, uterine fibroids, and soft-tissue sarcomas. It is a non-invasive thermal ablation technique that is augmented by visualization techniques such as MRI and ultrasound in real time, thus heralding an end to open craniocephal surgery for brain diseases. The article discusses the outcomes, side effects, and recent advancements in HIFU technology for treating various conditions—such as tumors, targeted drug delivery, vascular blockages, and movement disorders—along with the current challenges and future prospects of the field. Jolesz *et al.* [13] introduced a Magnetic Resonance imaging-guided Focused Ultrasound (MRgFUS) surgery, which is a noninvasive thermal surgical procedure. In MRgFUS, MRI identifies treatment sites, conceives treatment strategies, and monitors the energy delivered. Because of the ability of ultrasound to focus therapy by combining it with magnetic resonance, sonography with magnetic resonance imaging dramatically enhances the ability to focus energy onto a specific area and destroy soft tissues while ensuring that the surrounding typical structures are unaffected. All these factors contribute to making MRgFUS a viable replacement for surgery or radiation therapy for soft tissue tumors. Already in the market for the management of uterine fibroids, MRgFUS is being studied for breast cancer, liver cancer, and prostate and brain tumors, as well as for pain relief in cancerous bone lesions. There are also nonthermal ablation-related applications, including FUS with or without microbubbles, to transiently increase the permeability of blood vessels or cell membranes and deliver or uncage drugs for drug delivery or gene transfection. MRgFUS is a revolutionary tool in plate tectonics as it opens new therapeutic options and is bound to bring about drastic changes in the management of patients and many fields of medicine.

The study done by Clement *et al.* [14] deals with Focused ultrasound, which is gaining traction as a potential therapeutic tool, especially in light of the development of high-power phased arrays and noninvasive imaging that allow targeting in regions where the brain would otherwise be located beyond reach.

New developments, such as microbubble-assisted heating, are geared towards shortening treatment times efficiently. This paper examines the scientific and engineering developments that are making it possible to use focused ultrasound in the clinic, especially in treating brain disorders and improving drug delivery.

The paper presented by Nir Lipsman *et al.* [15] shows that Focused Ultrasound (FUS) is a revolutionary area of medicine that combines physics and engineering, imaging, biology, and neurosurgery, all of which make it possible to perform non-invasive procedures on brain circuits connected with various pathologies. Its uses include temporary blood-brain barrier opening, neuromodulation with high-intensity focused ultrasound, and permanent tissue thermoablation. Over the last five years, the clinical uses of focused ultrasound have grown dramatically, raising both academic and societal engagement. This review aims to systematically assess FUS's current uses and future possibilities regarding its use in treating various neurologic and psychiatric diseases, its capability to revolutionize brain treatments, and the obstacles to better utilization.

The researchers David P *et al.* [16] used Noninvasive neuromodulation using focused ultrasound, which has been used for more than 70 years. Much like therapeutic ultrasound, which is determined as one of the primary methods in imaging, focused ultrasound has also undergone a remarkable evolution. This has allowed for many transcranial-focused ultrasounds in the nervous system, wherein high-intensity focused ultrasounds can make irreversible deep-brain lesions. In contrast, low-intensity focused ultrasound temporarily alters brain functioning. The first focuses on the most recent developments within. Several studies add to the body of knowledge and explain something about the effects, although the reasons and mechanisms for these effects are still not fully understood. The transformative features of the technology, such as but not limited to multimodal compatibility, submillimeter focusing, and real-time monitoring, will support how it might be utilized as a potent clinical neuromodulatory platform in the future. However, various technical issues exist currently.

BACKGROUND

One of the benefits of Ultrasound is that it is a cutting-edge treatment option for many patients, and it is a non-invasive procedure. Compared to usual surgical methods, which require cuts in the body that would take longer healing time, FUS allows a non-invasive treatment with no need for anesthesia and hospital stay for an extended period. Patients go home following the procedure and often find immediate symptom relief with little, if any, downtime. The benefits are ideal for people who may be reluctant to go in for invasive surgeries, which may involve risks and long recovery processes.

Its precision directly correlates to how well the focused ultrasound works. Surgeons can see the area of interest in real-time throughout the procedure using sophisticated imaging modalities such as MRI. It allows for remarkably accurate targeting of the sound waves so that only a small portion of surrounding healthy tissues is damaged or destroyed, thus maximizing therapeutic benefits while minimizing collateral damage. Also, modifying the treatment enhances its safety and effectiveness, making it an excellent option for patients who have failed pharmacotherapy or are looking for an alternative to other noninvasive interventions.

This approach's ability to target different neurological disorders, such as epilepsy, some brain tumors, *etc*., is an example of its versatility. As technology matures and large trials find a home for focused ultrasound in neurology and beyond, many patients may ultimately experience improved quality of life with a new treatment arsenal that is more effective than current options and safer than traditional surgery.

Moreover, since focused ultrasound therapy does not require any cuts, it eliminates surgical dangers associated with postoperative wounds, allergic reactions to general anesthesia, or excessive blood loss. Compared to conventional surgery, FUS surgery is shorter and less intrusive towards the patient, allowing them to carry on with their everyday activities much faster. This outpatient treatment, coupled with the fact that the patient does not have to remain bedridden for ages after the procedure, is preferable for elderly or chronically ill patients who cannot be operated on using the conventional method. Moreover, since no cuts are made, there is no resultant scarring, an advantage for people looking for less invasive options. The precision in treatment reduces collateral tissue damage. It extends the safety margin of the procedures, giving the patients confidence that the treatment is effective and safe compared to the older treatment methods.

The rapid improvements in imaging and computer modeling techniques further enhance the efficacy of focused ultrasound. Focused ultrasound surgery that is MRI-guided in real-time has increased the accuracy of the surgeon's targeting, enabling the surgeon to find and destroy the relevant tissue with precision. This is especially the case in treating diseases such as essential tremors, where there is a need to treat the specific zone of aberrant brain activity. In the future, treatment planning *vis-à-vis* intervention will also be rational due to AI and ML algorithms and real-time imaging for the intervention in conjunction with treating the deep-seated brain areas. This integration of imaging-guided therapy, with precision targeting and flexible treatment manipulations, will likely lead to a paradigm shift in treating the paper's survey issue.

As a therapeutic technique, it has many applications and can be extended to several other disorders. It is not only applied to the treatment of essential tremors or movement disorders, but FUS is under study for more benefits in psychiatric treatment [17], such as for depression that targets the specific regions of the brain in charge of mood. It is being looked upon for the ability to help in using ultrasound for curing other conditions like Alzheimer's [18], where sound waves can help in either clearing out the conjectures from the brain or improving the blood flow in the brain. This potential in FUS for neurological applications is only scratching the surface; as more future analysis continues, more of such technology will apply to many diseases that are not currently being treated, thus giving more therapeutic options to patients with less harmful treatments as compared to the existing ones and in a shorter time frame than the current methods.

Role of ML and AI in the Treatment of Essential Tremor

For instance, Artificial Intelligence (AI) and Machine Learning (ML) are remodeling the healthcare sector with individualized care and improved treatments. These technologies use data to analyze big data sets, uncover complex patterns, predict patient outcomes, or provide optimized treatment protocols to healthcare providers. This move to a data-centric approach improves the quality of medical care and boosts operational efficiency in healthcare institutions.

AI and ML can be utilized in focused ultrasound treatments. Such technologies can map out a tumor's whole genome and predict what mutations are likely to be driving it, providing super-powerful personalized treatment regimes that target the mutations present in the patient. Key data points include demographics like age, gender, and medical history, all of which may affect the patient's response to the treatment. Understanding such factors in these conditions makes it possible for clinicians to make decisions that reflect each patient's unique profile.

Besides, clinical presentations, particularly the tremors' character and time trend, are essential information for AI and ML algorithms. These can be used to determine which therapies can be given priority as a function of the patient's specific signs, such as in the case of more complex or persistent situations. Imaging is essential, as in a focused ultrasound procedure. It may be an MRI or CT scan of the brain. AI shall analyze images and provide the proper diagnosis of the area in the brain to be treated. In this case, the degree of precision lessens the chances of damaging healthy tissue but raises the procedure's success rate. Integrating information from demographics, clinical symptoms, and image data, AI and ML allow healthcare providers to deliver treatments tailored to the patient's needs that, while with focused ultrasound and other similar medical interventions, effectively significantly enhance patient outcomes.

In addition, the assistance of machine learning together with artificial intelligence in the focused ultrasound surgery enables health care providers to have an extensive management of real-time patient monitoring, which improves the accuracy of treatment. In the course of FUS, AI assists in rendering the information obtained from the devices, MRI, ultrasound, or infrared monitoring systems, *i.e.*, the latter enables clinicians to modify the ultrasound parameters in real time in correspondence to the behavior of a patient. As such, the treatment becomes more progressive as the parameters, including ultrasound intensity, frequency, and duration, are adjusted on a feedback basis and used optimally with the least side effects. Such therapy has implications in rendering FUS techniques more effective in therapeutic interventions, as they would even minimize the possibility of damaging healthy tissues. For instance, due to such technologies, advanced artificial intelligence not only targets the success of the treatment but also the complications preventing the success of the processes in the long run.

AI and ML also play crucial roles in the evaluation and prediction of treatment outcomes. After treatment finishes, such technologies are applied in the analysis of data collected after treatment, such as follow-up scans and symptom monitoring, which help evaluate how the patient is responding and forecast the chances of recovery over time. AI models, for instance, using pre- and post-treatment datasets, can determine functional improvements in the brain or a decrease in symptoms that may be insignificant to the naked eye or standard approaches. This assists in rehabilitation and follow-up care management, including determining the necessity for further treatment options. Such a capacity provides a probability of complications of recurrence and allows protection of patients' recovery and quality of life. As AI evolves, its predictive functions will become the foundations of personalized care plan formulations, thus making sure that future treatments are even more focused and effective.

Embracing AI and ML in the clinical terrain encourages a more cooperative approach towards healthcare. Because it analyzes big data, intelligence systems generate an information quotient that helps multiple care providers when making decisions. For instance, a treatment system that has its various specialist inputs – neurologists, radiologists, and AI in imaging for complex global FUS neurosurgery. Also, the responsibility of the AI component in the healthcare predictive analytics model is to allow various providers to understand the patient before they arrive, thus preventing under- and over-supply of health care services, improving the average time to treatment. The more such technologies penetrate the healthcare system, the more specialists work together with fewer conflicts and overcome barriers to patients receiving care. It is through this path that AI not only improves the accuracy of treatment but also causes a shift in the paradigm of healthcare delivery to a system that is interwoven and revolves around the patient.

PATIENT SELECTION AND STRATIFICATION

The application of AI algorithms is indeed very important in selecting the right set of patients for focused ultrasound treatment. Upon reviewing the overall data from those previously analyzed patients, the algorithm will indicate to the user who most likely will benefit from the treatment procedure. Symptom severity, comorbidities, and even other previous treatments have been evaluated to create a profile about each patient. Such an approach not only ensures optimization of patients' outcomes but also conserves healthcare resources since efforts are made towards producing maximal benefit.

In this manner, patient selection and stratification guided by AI may help enhance the accuracy of focused ultrasound delivery. As an added benefit, machine learning algorithms can also sift through and draw predictive correlations within a big data set to establish treatment responders based on predictor variables, including age, disease stage, and comorbidities. Indeed, this approach to treatment provides evidence-based guidelines for health practitioners on who is a candidate for FUS so that those patients who will not have remarkable changes are not put through unnecessary procedures. Also, those systems may encode additional data and, consequently, change selection criteria and become even more exact with predictions. This improves the quality of care rendered to patients, reduces the chances of complications occurring, and focuses resources efficiently.

Fueled by AI and machine learning systems for patient selection, focused ultrasound treatment is a data-driven treatment with precise candidate identification processes. The algorithms are able to make sense of a lot of data and track the patterns to identify even the smallest of the factors that may be difficult to differentiate during the normal clinical assessments. For instance, AI can visualize how those factors, such as gender and its related genetic markers or even lifestyle, determine the development of the disease and the effectiveness of treatment in women. Therefore, it facilitates the understanding of perceived risks and advantages for each patient, theoretically telling the clinicians who is more likely to benefit from the FUS treatment. Moreover, by virtue of the fact that AI prediction structures can revise their forecasts when new data arrives, there will be further improvement of patients' profiles, making sure that at all times patient referral is correct and flexible with the incorporation of new knowledge.

One more positive characteristic of an AI-based patient selection system is its ability to aid clinical decision-making in difficult cases that could not be addressed by conventional evaluation techniques. For instance, consider patients with a multiplicity of co-morbid conditions, the AI systems are able to factor in the weight of success of FUS against all these potential co-morbid factors. Taking into account aspects like the health status of the individual, their history of treatment and its effectiveness, as well as the type of disease, AI-driven models can recommend the best intervention for a particular patient. This means that clinicians are unlikely to use treatment regimes that cut across all patients, given the fact that different patients present with different ailments. Therefore, complications are less, and the outcomes of treatment are more favorable to the patients.

Treatment Plans

This data-driven approach allows physicians to make decisions about eligibility so that those who will benefit most from the treatment are served first.

With ML-based predictions of the suitability of ultrasound parameters for a given patient, the treatment of FUS could be made significantly more effective. Some ultrasound parameters may involve frequency, intensity, and even duration of treatment with ultrasound waves. Beyond predictions, the ML model also simulates scenarios of varied treatments on given patients using patient data, which allows clinicians to identify active strategies that favor maximizing effectiveness while minimizing adverse effects. This personalized course of treatment has the added benefit of an increased chance of achieving a successful outcome and enhances patient safety because of decreased adverse effect profiles associated with inappropriate settings of treatment.

In addition to enhancing the accuracy of delivering ultrasound in treatment protocols, the incorporation of machine learning into treatment protocol development enables the establishment of real-time protocols that are flexible and can be changed. The system is capable of adjusting the ultrasound parameters, depending on the evaluation of the treatment effect, optimizing the therapeutic effect with reduced side effects or discomfort. For example, when a patient has a negative response to ultrasound at a certain frequency or intensity, the system will impose a limit that will set that frequency or intensity for the remaining sessions. This also reduces chances to undertreat the patient or over treat the patient, allowing for tailored treatment to each of the sessions. In addition, machine learning models forecast the treatment outcomes, understand the nature of its risks, and identify the risks during the course of treatment so that the clinician can prevent the event before it occurs. These treatment strategies will prove to be more effective and precise with the advancement of more sophisticated algorithms, which will limit adverse effects, consequently leading to better patient experience with focused ultrasound therapy.

Telemedicine is becoming a progressively popular treatment modality for managing essential tremors, which are an uncontrollable movement disorder of shaking. Tremor characteristic evaluation systems involve a mobile instrument that communicates *via* the internet, thereby permitting home-based patient evaluation, enabling recommendations to be sent directly from healthcare providers to the patients. It has diagnostic and follow-up care implications, as well as improves access to specialist care in underserved populations. Studies have indicated that telemedicine can effectively monitor tremors and assist in treatment changes, hence improving patient outcomes and saving healthcare costs.

Real-time Monitoring

Real-time monitoring of the responses of patients is especially important in FUS procedures. AI algorithms can process this information in real time and shed light on the effectiveness of the treatment as it progresses. This functionality allows for real-time alteration of ultrasound parameters during a session so that the therapy effects can be targeted optimally throughout the treatment session. For example, in a case where a patient is diagnosed as under-responding to the treatment, the settings could be modified in real-time to enhance outcomes. The dynamic of this adaptability enhances the specificity of the treatment and achieves a more personalized experience in dealing with the patient.

In addition, real-time monitoring allows the clinician performing the procedure to also monitor the patient's dynamics and understand how effectively ultrasound waves are delivered to the tissue of interest at any given moment. A synergistic combination of advanced imaging modalities, such as MRI or ultrasound imaging, and artificial intelligence-enabled monitoring of tissue changes offers the possibility of a real-time picture, which makes even small changes in a particular area visible, and sometimes even invisible to the eye. This enables ultrasound parameters—for example, frequency, intensity, and focal point—to be altered instantaneously so that the treatment remains appropriate to that person's physiological reaction at all times. Furthermore, the AI system is capable of predicting undesirable events, *e.g.*, excessive heating or unwanted damage to surrounding structures, and will warn the clinician in advance. Such persistent and accurate feedback not only improves treatment outcomes but also minimizes the risks of occurrence, which contributes to improved safety of the procedures and greater uniformity in results achievement. With the progression of technologies utilized, the real-time monitoring will likely prove imperative during all focused ultrasound treatments, transcending the confines of precision medicine.

Post-Treatment Analysis

The needs to predict outcomes after treatments with FUS further make them important for an overall assessment. AI and ML can analyze the pre-and post-treatment data in order to foresee long-term results, providing clinicians with significant information about the chances of success or complications. Indeed, early signs of either success or failure allow clinicians to make informed decisions about follow-up care and adapt treatment plans appropriately so that recovery is as good as possible, and patients improve their quality of life. This can be helpful in post-treatment assessments and hence helps to determine future treatment approaches.

The analysis and evaluation of treatment outcomes that have been achieved is where AI and ML have multifaceted applications, insofar as ultrasound intervention is concerned. This is done through the assessment of treatment effect, where the post-treatment data is compared and contrasted with the pre-treatment data in order to measure the degree of improvement in symptom severity. Such analyses can identify in which sites of the brain, or tissues rather, the intervention has achieved its purpose and whether regions devoid of abnormalities can benefit from intervention as well. Every time there is a change in the patient's state, machine-learning models can demonstrate the degree of the recovery process; in particular, subtle specifics that are not shown with the help of evaluation methods used in traditional medicine. It enables clinicians to fine-tune their recommendations with respect to, for example, medication or rehabilitative procedures, as the care system replicates a digital feedback system.

In addition, because of the use of AI, where the results of many patients are pooled together, it would assist in perfecting treatment protocols for various ailments, thus facilitating a more tailored approach in both intervention and control. Finally, with the assistance of AI insights, outcome analyses become treatment-oriented; that is, the patients undergoing therapy are assured of the highest quality, patient-centered treatment available, which improves their recovery curve and lessens the chances of any further therapeutic interventions, more so, invasive ones.

Improving with Feedback from Patients

Feedback from patients can refine the treatment protocols related to focused ultrasound. AI systems can scrutinize the patient-reported outcome to lead to further refinement of FUS strategies. Such systems form a feedback loop that incorporates patient experiences to help improve treatment efficacy with time. This framework of continuous learning enables clinicians to adapt and update the protocols for treatment based on real-world patient data, ensuring that FUS maintains its advanced character as a responsive therapeutic approach. In the long run, it assists with a more personalized and effective treatment experience both in the present and the future for patients.

Patient opinions can help improve the focused ultrasound treatment protocols. The systems of artificial intelligence can help scrutinize the outcome reported by the patient to call for a more advanced FUS strategy. Such systems make a circle of enhancement where the treatment is improved over time as per the interventions done by the patients. Such a Continuous Practice Learning framework allows clinicians to modify and upgrade treatment strategies based on patients' data after the introduction of the FUS system, considering its cutting-edge nature as a treatment modality. It helps in the long run for a better degree of care for the patient now and in the future.

CONCLUSION

The growth of focused ultrasound for the treatment of essential tremors will seek to foster greater integration between AI researchers, neurologists, and ultrasound technologists. Neuroimaging advancement and real-time stats analytics will enable the induction of more accurate and successful therapies. Besides, the additional studies regarding the modes of action of essential tremors will be supportive in building specifically customized artificial intelligence models. The advancement of the technology that employs artificial intelligence and ultrasound for the treatment of essential tremors is one of the greatest developments in modern medicine, specifically neurology. Data and technology will allow us to improve the results of patients, make treatment more accurate, and fundamentally change the approach to this disorder. The ongoing improvement of these methods and their combination will allow the fullest utilization of these innovations so that patients are provided with the best and most appropriate treatment.

REFERENCES

[1] R.J. Elble, "What is essential tremor?", *Curr. Neurol. Neurosci. Rep.,* vol. 13, no. 6, p. 353, 2013. [http://dx.doi.org/10.1007/s11910-013-0353-4] [PMID: 23591755]

[2] P. Song, Y. Zhang, M. Zha, Q. Yang, X. Ye, Q. Yi, and I. Rudan, "The global prevalence of essential tremor, with emphasis on age and sex: A meta-analysis", *J. Glob. Health,* vol. 11, p. 04028, 2021. [http://dx.doi.org/10.7189/jogh.11.04028] [PMID: 33880180]

[3] Lazzaro di Biase, "Focused ultrasound (FUS) for chronic pain management: approved and potential applications", *Neurology Research International,* 2021. 1 (2021): 8438498. [http://dx.doi.org/10.1155/2021/8438498]

[4] E. Tjoa, and C. Guan, "A survey on explainable artificial intelligence (xai): Toward medical xai", *IEEE Trans. Neural Netw. Learn. Syst.,* vol. 32, no. 11, pp. 4793-4813, 2021. [http://dx.doi.org/10.1109/TNNLS.2020.3027314] [PMID: 33079674]

[5] X. Xing, N. Luo, S. Li, L. Zhou, C. Song, and J. Liu, "Identification and classification of Parkinsonian and essential tremors for diagnosis using machine learning algorithms", *Front. Neurosci.,* vol. 16, 2022.701632 [http://dx.doi.org/10.3389/fnins.2022.701632] [PMID: 35386595]

[6] Q. Bi, K.E. Goodman, J. Kaminsky, and J. Lessler, "What is machine learning? A primer for the epidemiologist", *Am. J. Epidemiol.,* vol. 188, no. 12, 2019.kwz189

[http://dx.doi.org/10.1093/aje/kwz189] [PMID: 31509183]

[7] John G. Lynn, "A new method for the generation and use of focused ultrasound in experimental biology", *The Journal of general physiology,* vol. 26, no. 2, p. 179, 1942. [http://dx.doi.org/10.1085/jgp.26.2.179]

[8] G. ter Haar, and C. Coussios, "High intensity focused ultrasound: Physical principles and devices", *Int. J. Hyperthermia,* vol. 23, no. 2, pp. 89-104, 2007. [http://dx.doi.org/10.1080/02656730601186138] [PMID: 17578335]

[9] A. Bystritsky, A.S. Korb, P.K. Douglas, M.S. Cohen, W.P. Melega, A.P. Mulgaonkar, A. DeSalles, B.K. Min, and S.S. Yoo, "A review of low-intensity focused ultrasound pulsation", *Brain Stimul.,* vol. 4, no. 3, pp. 125-136, 2011. [http://dx.doi.org/10.1016/j.brs.2011.03.007] [PMID: 21777872]

[10] G.R. Ter Haar, "High intensity focused ultrasound for the treatment of tumors", *Echocardiography,* vol. 18, no. 4, pp. 317-322, 2001. [http://dx.doi.org/10.1046/j.1540-8175.2001.00317.x] [PMID: 11415504]

[11] K. Hynynen, and G. Clement, "Clinical applications of focused ultrasound—The brain", *Int. J. Hyperthermia,* vol. 23, no. 2, pp. 193-202, 2007. [http://dx.doi.org/10.1080/02656730701200094] [PMID: 17578343]

[12] Zahra Izadifar, "An introduction to high intensity focused ultrasound: systematic review on principles, devices, and clinical applications", *Journal of clinical medicine ,* vol. 9, no. 2, p. 460, 2020. [http://dx.doi.org/10.3390/jcm9020460]

[13] F.A. Jolesz, "MRI-guided focused ultrasound surgery", *Annu. Rev. Med.,* vol. 60, no. 1, pp. 417-430, 2009. [http://dx.doi.org/10.1146/annurev.med.60.041707.170303] [PMID: 19630579]

[14] G.T. Clement, "Perspectives in clinical uses of high-intensity focused ultrasound", *Ultrasonics,* vol. 42, no. 10, pp. 1087-1093, 2004. [http://dx.doi.org/10.1016/j.ultras.2004.04.003] [PMID: 15234170]

[15] Y. Meng, K. Hynynen, and N. Lipsman, "Applications of focused ultrasound in the brain: from thermoablation to drug delivery", *Nat. Rev. Neurol.,* vol. 17, no. 1, pp. 7-22, 2021. [http://dx.doi.org/10.1038/s41582-020-00418-z] [PMID: 33106619]

[16] D.P. Darrow, "Focused ultrasound for neuromodulation", *Neurotherapeutics,* vol. 16, no. 1, pp. 88-99, 2019. [http://dx.doi.org/10.1007/s13311-018-00691-3] [PMID: 30488340]

[17] A.R. Arulpragasam, M. van 't Wout-Frank, J. Barredo, C.R. Faucher, B.D. Greenberg, and N.S. Philip, "Low intensity focused ultrasound for non-invasive and reversible deep brain neuromodulation—a paradigm shift in psychiatric research", *Front. Psychiatry,* vol. 13, 2022.825802 [http://dx.doi.org/10.3389/fpsyt.2022.825802] [PMID: 35280168]

[18] Xiaodan Liu, "The applications of Focused Ultrasound (FUS) in Alzheimer's disease treatment: A systematic review on both animal and human studies", *Aging and disease,* vol. 12, no. 8, p. 1977, 2021. [http://dx.doi.org/10.14336/AD.2021.0510]

CHAPTER 9

A Mathematical Model for Future Trends and Directions in Healthcare NLP Using Ranking of Tetradecagonal Fuzzy Numbers

A. Britto Manoj[1] and **P. M. Benson Mansingh**[1,*]

[1] *Advanced Computer Science and Engineering, Vignan's Foundation for Science, Technology, and Research, Vadlamudi (Post), Guntur (Dist.), India*

Abstract: In this exploration, we adopted a ranking approach based on tetradecagonal fuzzy numbers, which are 14-sided polygons through which transit patterns such as demand, supply, and transportation value are represented. Vogel's Approximation Method (VAM), a traditional method in fuzzy studies, is used to solve fuzzy transportation problems to obtain fuzzy nominal results. Tetradecagonal fuzzy values suggest an excellent nutrient rate for a fruit diet at a low cost. The fruit diet will provide high-energy and nutritionally essential food for healthcare. This chapter indicates compelling growth in the use of fuzzy logic in healthcare NLP. The nominal result offers a constructive explanation that focuses on the data's imprecision while providing an initial solution. Our path is constructive in amending fruit diets. By assimilating tetradecagonal fuzzy numbers, which are 14-sided polygons, we can accurately model the costs and nutritional values of various fruits, ensuring that the diet remains within budget and provides high energy and essential nutrients. The ranking schema in fuzzy transportation for healthcare in NLP is adequately commensurate with cost moderation and health supplement requirements, making it feasible to map a well-balanced fruit that increases health benefits for healthcare NLP. Ranking tetradecagonal fuzzy numbers allows us to exhibit compelling upgrades in the application of fuzzy logic to transportation and dietary optimization, offering both practical and nutritional advantages.

Keywords: Fuzzy transportation problem, Fuzzy ranking approach, Healthcare data NLP, Macronutrients, Micronutrients, Nutritionally balanced diet, Tetradecagonal fuzzy number.

* **Corresponding author P. M. Benson Mansingh:** Advanced Computer Science and Engineering, Vignan's Foundation for Science, Technology, and Research, Vadlamudi (Post), Guntur(Dist.), India;
E-mail: benyuva@gmail.com

A. Shankar, Saranya Jayapalan, & Basant. K. Tiwary (Eds.)

INTRODUCTION

When discussing the nutrients and the strength of cuisine, it should complement the food. Most of the foods people eat depend on their interests. Gastronomy etiquette can diverge from one locality to another in society and from one home to another. Fruits are built in periodically to upgrade fitness conditions. Fruits are vital and are packed with iron, minerals, potassium, zinc, and trace metals [1] [2]. Fruits encompass an immense source of vitality that is important for our bodies. Fruits provide enough iron absorption and contain several vitamins and fibres that boost people's energy levels and help them sustain their health.

In health care, fruits are broadly excellent in the origin of macronutrients, and they also contain pectin, which contributes a considerable volume to a well-balanced diet and helps abdominal development. Everyone must take botanical fruits in their daily routine. As a result, it increases efficiency and intensity. It generates fresh vitality for all climatic conditions. The essence of a fair, well-balanced diet will be modified according to fiscal status, and the anatomical state, and fair health supplements of fruits can be appropriated into triple stipulations of massive amounts, reasonable amounts, and small amounts. Even nutritional theory constantly lifts the community's health and wealth care and pacts with fruit absorption, utilization, and management. The individual who takes fruit health supplements as part of a routine to measure their well-balanced diet will have long-term health benefits and avoid inflammation. It grants health care perquisites and protects us from sickness [3]. Blackberry, litchi, strawberry, sapota, and pomegranate are fruits regularly used by people all over the country because they are all upscale sources of macronutrients in health care supplements. It casts divergence for a well-balanced dietary element, giving macronutrients and micronutrients. Frequently passed down, Blackberries are the finest source of cellulose, and cellulose is a rich energy source for accomplishing work. Blackberries consist of manure, which is indeed a macronutrient for the body. Blackberries help us to epitome comfortably and contain a lot of vitamin C. Litchis are high in macronutrients. It aids in preventing many disorders and presents fair and fresh skin. Litchis consist of depressed calories. Litchis have inhibited oxidation, which protects health and indicates the avoidance of tumors. Health supplements make Litchi a tumor-vigilant fresh produce. Strawberries are typically termed a dietary element that contains carotene-beta and macronutrients that contain A. Strawberries contain enzymes that are very needed for digestion. Strawberries are rich in fiber, and they have developed a healthcare system. The accessible way to boost fiber absorption is to eat sapota, which is rich in health benefits and macronutrients. Sapota involves cuprum and calcium, a good source of evolving immunity within the body. Sapota guides curtail density, which will boost our metabolism. Sapota involves iron components, which are a significant part of plasma. Pomegranate deals like a cloak of oxygen, and it battles heart inflammation. Pomegranates contain many health supplements that protect us from many syndromes, and they are a rich source of macronutrients in healthcare.

In this exploration, we spotlight fruitage, which contains a fantastic amount of macronutrients that we require daily. For our well-balanced diet, blackberries, Litchis, Strawberries, Sapota, and Pomegranates are taken appropriately. Scaling the tetra-decagonal of uncertain sets mapped by the penalty method has been exceptional in acquiring the macronutrients and micronutrients for healthy supplements. The grit of the analysis contributes to illustrating the choice for fitness by adopting a fitting dietary element that has a minimal amount.

Methodology

- A fuzzy set $\tilde{C}$ X is characterized by a membership function. $\mu_{\tilde{c}}(x)$ Which associates each point in X with an actual number in the interval [0, 1]. The value of $\mu_{\tilde{c}}(x)$

Represents the grade of membership of $x \in \mu_{\tilde{c}}(x)$.

- The α-cut of the fuzzy set $\tilde{C}$ The universe of discourse X is defined as

$\widetilde{C_\alpha} = \{x \in x/\mu_{\tilde{c}}(x) \geq \alpha$, where $\in (0,1)$.

- A fuzzy set $\tilde{C}$ It is defined on the set of real numbers. R is a fuzzy number if it is a membership function. $\tilde{C}: R \to [\,0,1\,]$ has the following characteristics
  a. $\tilde{C}$ It is piecewise continuous.
  b. $\tilde{C}$ It is expected that if there is an $x \in R$ such that $\mu_{\tilde{c}}(x) = 1$

Tetradecagonal Fuzzy Number (a 14-sided fuzzy number)

An uncertain set of $\tilde{C}_T$ is a tetradecagonal uncertain set denoted by

$$\tilde{C}_T = (c_1, c_2, c_3, c_4, c_5, c_6, c_{7,} c_8, c_9, c_{10,} c_{11}, c_{12}, c_{13}, c_{14})$$

and $c_1, c_2, c_3, c_4, c_5, c_6, c_{7,} c_8, c_9, c_{10,} c_{11}, c_{12}, c_{13}, c_{14}$ The numbers are accurate, and the group function is given below,

$$
\mu_{\tilde{C}_T}(\theta)=\begin{cases}
\mu_1\dfrac{(\theta-c_1)}{(c_2-c_1)}, & c_1\le\theta\le c_2\\
\mu_1+(1-\mu_1)\dfrac{(\theta-c_2)}{(c_3-c_2)}, & c_2\le\theta\le c_3\\
\mu_2\dfrac{(\theta-c_3)}{(c_4-c_3)}, & c_3\le\theta\le c_4\\
\mu_2+(1-\mu_2)\dfrac{(\theta-c_4)}{(c_5-c_4)}, & c_4\le\theta\le c_5\\
\mu_3\dfrac{(\theta-c_5)}{(c_6-c_5)}, & c_5\le\theta\le c_6\\
\mu_3+(1-\mu_3)\dfrac{(\theta-c_6)}{(c_7-c_6)}, & c_6\le\theta\le c_7\\
1, & c_7\le\theta\le c_8\\
\mu_3+(1-\mu_3)\dfrac{(c_9-\theta)}{(c_9-c_8)}, & c_8\le\theta\le c_9\\
\mu_3\dfrac{(c_{10}-\theta)}{(c_{10}-c_9)}, & c_9\le\theta\le c_{10}\\
\mu_2+(1-\mu_2)\dfrac{(c_{11}-\theta)}{(c_{11}-c_{10})}, & c_{10}\le\theta\le c_{11}\\
\mu_2\dfrac{(c_{12}-\theta)}{(c_{12}-c_{11})}, & c_{11}\le\theta\le c_{12}\\
\mu_1+(1-\mu_1)\dfrac{(c_{13}-\theta)}{(c_{13}-c_{12})}, & c_{12}\le\theta\le c_{13}\\
\mu_1\dfrac{(c_{14}-\theta)}{(c_{14}-c_{13})}, & c_{13}\le\theta\le c_{14}\\
0, & \theta\ge c_{14}
\end{cases}
$$

Tetradecagonal Fuzzy Number of Ranking

Tetradecagonal Fuzzy numbers are accurately brought into the absolute line by ranking uncertain sets. Let $\tilde{C}_T$ be an epitomized tetradecagonal number of uncertain sets [7]. The standard and ranking of $\tilde{C}_T$ is stands followsR ($\tilde{C}_T$) are determined as follows:

$$
R(\tilde{C}_T)=\left[\frac{c_1+c_2+c_3+c_4+c_5+c_6+c_7+c_8+c_9+c_{10}+c_{11}+c_{12}+c_{13}+c_{14}}{14}\right]
$$

Application and Results

From exploration, we transmit the dietary value of fruits such as blackberries, litchis, strawberries, sapota, and pomegranates, giving an upscale authority to macronutrients and micronutrients. Evident input was consumed, and a measure of nutritious food in the fruits was recorded from the Nutritive value of Indian foods given by the National Institute of Nutrition [4], Indian Food Composition tables [5]. The lowest, natural, and highest contents of macronutrients and micronutrients in each fruit item are treated as 14-sided polygons of uncertain sets. The cost of nutrients such as macronutrients and micronutrients for each fruit component is appropriated as stock [6]. The edible segment supplement contents for every fruit dietary element are ordered.

The uncertain set of transportation problems considering the given fruit item is perhaps established in the subsequent mathematical statement [7].

Min Z = R (1.35, 1.39, 1.43, 1.47, 1.51, 1.55, 1.59, 1.63, 1.67, 1.71, 1.75, 1.79, 1.83, 1.91) a_{11} +R (0.49, 0.50, 0.51, 0.52, 0.53, 0.54, 0.55, 0.56, 0.57, 0.58, 0.59, 0.60, 0.61, 0.69) a_{12} +R (2.08, 2.10, 2.12, 2.14, 2.16, 2.18, 2.20, 2.22, 2.24, 2.26, 2.28, 2.30, 2.32, 2.40) a_{13} +R (11.64, 11.69, 11.74, 11.79, 11.84, 11.89, 11.94, 11.99, 12.04, 12.09, 12.14, 12.19, 12.24, 12.32) a_{14} +R (0.71, 0.73, 0.75, 0.77, 0.79, 0.81, 0.83, 0.85, 0.87, 0.89, 0.91, 0.93, 0.95, 1.03) a_{21}+R (0.38, 0.38, 0.38, 0.38, 0.38, 0.38, 0.38, 0.38, 0.38, 0.38, 0.38, 0.38, 0.38, 0.46) a_{22} +R (1.29, 1.31, 1.33, 1.35, 1.37, 1.39, 1.41, 1.43, 1.45, 1.47, 1.49, 1.51, 1.53, 1.61) a_{23} +R (12.71, 12.81, 12.91, 13.01, 13.11, 13.21, 13.31, 13.41, 13.51, 13.61, 13.71, 13.81, 13.91, 13.99) a_{24}+R (1.43, 1.45, 147, 1.49, 1.51, 1.53, 1.55, 1.57, 1.59, 1.61, 1.63, 1.65, 1.67, 1.75) a_{31}+R (0.37, 0.38, 0.39, 0.40, 0.41, 0.42, 0.43, 0.44, 0.45, 0.46, 0.47, 0.48, 0.49, 0.57) a_{32} +R (4.88, 4.94, 5.00, 5.06, 5.12, 5.18, 5.24, 5.30, 5.36, 5.42, 5.48, 5.54, 5.60, 5.68) a_{33}+R (8.62, 8.63, 8.64, 8.65, 8.66, 8.67, 8.68, 8.69, 8.70, 8.71, 8.72, 8.73, 8.74, 8.82) a_{34} +R (0.51, 0.53, 0.55, 0.57, 0.59, 0.61, 0.63, 0.65, 0.67, 0.69, 0.71, 0.73, 0.75, 0.83) a_{41} +R (0.22, 0.22, 0.22, 0.22, 0.22, 0.22, 0.22, 0.22, 0.22, 0.22, 0.22, 0.22, 0.22, 0.30) a_{42} + R (3.42, 3.44, 3.46, 3.48, 3.50, 3.52, 3.54, 3.56, 3.58, 3.60, 3.62, 3.64, 3.66, 3.74) a_{43}+R (8.35, 8.54, 8.73, 8.92, 9.11, 9.30, 9.49, 9.68, 9.87, 10.06, 10.25, 10.44, 10.63, 10.71) a_{44} + R (0.59, 0.61, 0.63, 0.65, 0.67, 0.69, 0.71, 0.73, 0.75, 0.77, 0.79, 0.81, 0.83, 0.91) a_{51}+R (0.32, 0.35, 0.38, 0.41, 0.44, 0.47, 0.50, 0.53, 0.56, 0.59, 0.62, 0.65, 0.68, 0.76) a_{52}+R (1.79, 1.85, 1.91, 1.97, 2.03, 2.09, 2.15, 2.21, 2.27, 2.33, 2.39, 2.45,2.51, 2.59) a_{53}+R (10.71, 10.96, 11.21, 11.46, 11.71, 11.96, 12.21, 12.46, 12.71, 12.96, 13.21, 13.46, 13.71, 13.79) a_{54}

Table (**1**) provides a comprehensive overview of the nutritional composition of fruits like Blackberry, Litchi, Strawberry, Sapota, and Pomegranate, along with their supply and demand data, providing insights into their dietary value and market availability, crucial for health promotion and healthcare recommendations [8].

Table 1. Nutrient content of fruit dietary elements.

Fruits	Protein	Fat	Total Fibre	Carbohydrates	Supply
Blackberry	1.35, 1.39, 1.43, 1.47, 1.51, 1.55, 1.59, 1.63, 1.67, 1.71, 1.75, 1.79, 1.83, 1.91	0.49, 0.50, 0.51, 0.52, 0.53, 0.54, 0.55, 0.56, 0.57, 0.58, 0.59, 0.60, 0.61, 0.69	2.08, 2.10, 2.12, 2.14, 2.16, 2.18, 2.20, 2.22, 2.24, 2.26, 2.28, 2.30, 2.32, 2.40	11.64, 11.69, 11.74, 11.79, 11.84, 11.89, 11.94, 11.99, 12.04, 12.09, 12.14, 12.19, 12.24, 12.32	1.30, 1.31, 1.32, 1.33, 1.34, 1.35, 1.36, 1.37, 1.38, 1.39, 1.40, 1.41, 1.42, 1.50
Litchi	0.71, 0.73, 0.75, 0.77, 0.79, 0.81, 0.83, 0.85, 0.87, 0.89, 0.91, 0.93, 0.95, 1.03	0.38, 0.38, 0.38, 0.38, 0.38, 0.38, 0.38, 0.38, 0.38, 0.38, 0.38, 0.38, 0.38, 0.46	1.29, 1.31, 1.33, 1.35, 1.37, 1.39, 1.41, 1.43, 1.45, 1.47, 1.49, 1.51, 1.53, 1.61	12.71, 12.81, 12.91, 13.01, 13.11, 13.21, 13.31, 13.41, 13.51, 13.61, 13.71, 13.81, 13.91, 13.99	0.97, 0.98, 0.98, 0.99, 1.00, 1.01, 1.02, 1.03, 1.03, 1.04, 1.05, 1.06, 1.07, 1.15
Strawberry	1.43, 1.45, 147, 1.49, 1.51, 1.53, 1.55, 1.57, 1.59, 1.61, 1.63, 1.65, 1.67, 1.75	0.37, 0.38, 0.39, 0.40, 0.41, 0.42, 0.43, 0.44, 0.45, 0.46, 0.47, 0.48, 0.49, 0.57	4.88, 4.94, 5.00, 5.06, 5.12, 5.18, 5.24, 5.30, 5.36, 5.42, 5.48, 5.54, 5.60, 5.68	8.62, 8.63, 8.64, 8.65, 8.66, 8.67, 8.68, 8.69, 8.70, 8.71, 8.72, 8.73, 8.74, 8.82	0.68, 0.68, 0.69, 0.69, 0.70, 0.70, 0.70, 0.71, 0.71, 0.71, 0.72, 0.72, 0.73, 0.81
Sapota	0.51, 0.53, 0.55, 0.57, 0.59, 0.61, 0.63, 0.65, 0.67, 0.69, 0.71, 0.73, 0.75, 0.83	0.22, 0.22, 0.22, 0.22, 0.22, 0.22, 0.22, 0.22, 0.22, 0.22, 0.22, 0.22, 0.22, 0.30	3.42, 3.44, 3.46, 3.48, 3.50, 3.52, 3.54, 3.56, 3.58, 3.60, 3.62, 3.64, 3.66, 3.74	8.35, 8.54, 8.73, 8.92, 9.11, 9.30, 9.49, 9.68, 9.87, 10.06, 10.25, 10.44, 10.63, 10.71	0.93, 0.95, 0.97, 0.98, 1.00, 1.01, 1.03, 1.05, 1.06, 1.08, 1.09, 1.11, 1.13, 1.21
Pomegranate	0.59, 0.61, 0.63, 0.65, 0.67, 0.69, 0.71, 0.73, 0.75, 0.77, 0.79, 0.81, 0.83, 0.91	0.32, 0.35, 0.38, 0.41, 0.44, 0.47, 0.50, 0.53, 0.56, 0.59, 0.62, 0.65, 0.68, 0.76	1.79, 1.85, 1.91, 1.97, 2.03, 2.09, 2.15, 2.21, 2.27, 2.33, 2.39, 2.45, 2.51, 2.59	10.71, 10.96, 11.21, 11.46, 11.71, 11.96, 12.21, 12.46, 12.71, 12.96, 13.21, 13.46, 13.71, 13.79	1.26, 1.29, 1.32, 1.36, 1.39, 1.42, 1.45, 1.49, 1.52, 1.55, 1.58, 1.62, 1.65, 1.73

Fruits	Protein	Fat	Total Fibre	Carbohydrates	Supply
Demand	0.35, 0.36, 0.37, 0.37, 0.38, 0.39, 0.40, 0.41, 0.42, 0.43, 0.43, 0.44, 0.45, 0.53	0.17, 0.18, 0.18, 0.19, 0.19, 0.19, 0.20, 0.20, 0.21, 0.21, 0.21, 0.22, 0.22, 0.30	1.04, 1.05, 1.06, 1.07, 1.08, 1.09, 1.10, 1.11, 1.12, 1.13, 1.14, 1.15, 1.16, 1.24	3.49, 3.54, 3.59, 3.63, 3.68, 3.73, 3.78, 3.83, 3.88, 3.92, 3.97, 4.02, 4.07, 4.15	

Let $\tilde{C}_T$ Be an epitomized tetradecagonal number of uncertain sets. The foremost ranking of $\tilde{C}_T$ is implied by R ($\tilde{C}_T$)And determined as pursued [9]:

$$R(\tilde{C}_T) = \left[\frac{c_1+c_2+c_3+c_4+c_5+c_6+c_7+c_8+c_9+c_{10}+c_{11}+c_{12}+c_{13}+c_{14}}{14}\right]$$

$R(\tilde{C}_T) = \frac{1}{14}[22.58] = 1.61$	$R(\tilde{C}_T) = \frac{1}{14}[9.02] = 0.64$	**Supply**
$R(\tilde{C}_T) = \frac{1}{14}[7.84] = 0.56$	$R(\tilde{C}_T) = \frac{1}{14}[3.16] = 0.23$	$R(\tilde{C}_T) = \frac{1}{14}[19.18] = 1.37$
$R(\tilde{C}_T) = \frac{1}{14}[31] = 2.21$	$R(\tilde{C}_T) = \frac{1}{14}[49.76] = 3.55$	$R(\tilde{C}_T) = \frac{1}{14}[13.35] = 0.95$
$R(\tilde{C}_T) = \frac{1}{14}[167.54] = 11.97$	$R(\tilde{C}_T) = \frac{1}{14}[134.08] = 9.58$	$R(\tilde{C}_T) = \frac{1}{14}[9.95] = 0.71$
$R(\tilde{C}_T) = \frac{1}{14}[11.82] = 0.84$	$R(\tilde{C}_T) = \frac{1}{14}[10.14] = 0.72$	$R(\tilde{C}_T) = \frac{1}{14}[14.60] = 1.04$
$R(\tilde{C}_T) = \frac{1}{14}[5.4] = 0.39$	$R(\tilde{C}_T) = \frac{1}{14}[7.26] = 0.52$	$R(\tilde{C}_T) = \frac{1}{14}[20.63] = 1.47$
$R(\tilde{C}_T) = \frac{1}{14}[19.94] = 1.42$	$R(\tilde{C}_T) = \frac{1}{14}[30.54] = 2.18$	
$R(\tilde{C}_T) = \frac{1}{14}[187.02] = 13.36$	$R(\tilde{C}_T) = \frac{1}{14}[172.52] = 12.32$	**Demand**
$R(\tilde{C}_T) = \frac{1}{14}[21.9] = 1.56$		$R(\tilde{C}_T) = \frac{1}{14}[5.73] = 0.41$
$R(\tilde{C}_T) = \frac{1}{14}[6.16] = 0.44$		$R(\tilde{C}_T) = \frac{1}{14}[2.87] = 0.21$
$R(\tilde{C}_T) = \frac{1}{14}[73.8] = 5.27$		$R(\tilde{C}_T) = \frac{1}{14}[15.54] = 1.11$
$R(\tilde{C}_T) = \frac{1}{14}[121.66] = 8.69$		$R(\tilde{C}_T) = \frac{1}{14}[53.28] = 3.81$

After applying ranking technology for fuzzy tetradecagonal numbers, we get data and form a table to apply for further investigations [10].

Table (**2**) uses fuzzy logic to analyze the nutritional content of different fruits like Blackberry, Litchi, Strawberry, Sapota, and Pomegranate, along with their supply and demand figures [11].

Table 2. Fuzzy logic with healthcare data.

Fruits	Protein	Fat	Total Fibre	Carbohydrates	Supply
Blackberry	1.61	0.56	2.21	11.97	1.37
Litchi	0.84	0.39	1.42	13.36	0.95
Strawberry	1.56	0.44	5.27	8.69	0.71
Sapota	0.64	0.23	3.55	9.58	1.04
Pomegranate	0.72	0.52	2.18	12.32	1.47
Demand	0.41	0.21	1.11	3.81	5.54

In healthcare, allocation is often solved by fuzzy transportation problems. Since there are a lot of potential techniques, VAM is superior in solving this fuzzy transportation problem [12]. Because it acts on clarity in operation and computational efficiency compared to more complex methods, while still providing near-optimal solutions. VAM improves the accuracy of the optimization process in healthcare applications [13]. VAM handles uncertainties while accommodating constraints in a fuzzy setting, such as demand and supply. VAM is an excellent method to solve transportation problems in fuzzy environments [14].

The data presented in Table (**3**), based on Vogel's Approximation Method for healthcare, outlines the nutritional values of protein, fat, total fiber, and carbohydrates of different fruits, including blackberry, litchi, strawberry, sapota, and pomegranate, alongside their supply and demand figures [15]

Table 3. Vogel's approximation method for the healthcare.

Fruits	Protein	Fat	Total Fiber	Carbohydrates	Supply
Blackberry	1.61	0.56	**1.02** 2.21	**0.35** 11.97	1.37
Litchi	0.84	0.39	1.42	**0.95** 13.36	0.95
Strawberry	**0.41** 1.56	**0.21** 0.44	**0.09** 5.27	8.69	0.71
Sapota	0.64	0.23	3.55	**1.04** 9.58	1.04
Pomegranate	0.72	0.52	2.18	**1.47** 12.32	1.47
Demand	0.41	0.21	1.11	3.81	5.54

The gross minimal amount for fruits is given by:

Minimum Z = (2.21) (1.02) + (11.97) (0.35) + (13.36) (0.95) + (1.56) (0.41) + (0.44) (0.21) +

(5.27) (0.09) + (9.58) (1.04) + (12.32) (1.47)

Minimum Z = Rs. 48.40.

Fig. (**1**) outlines the nutritional values of protein, fat, total fiber, and carbohydrates of different fruits, including blackberry, litchi, strawberry, sapota, and pomegranate, alongside their supply and demand figures [16].

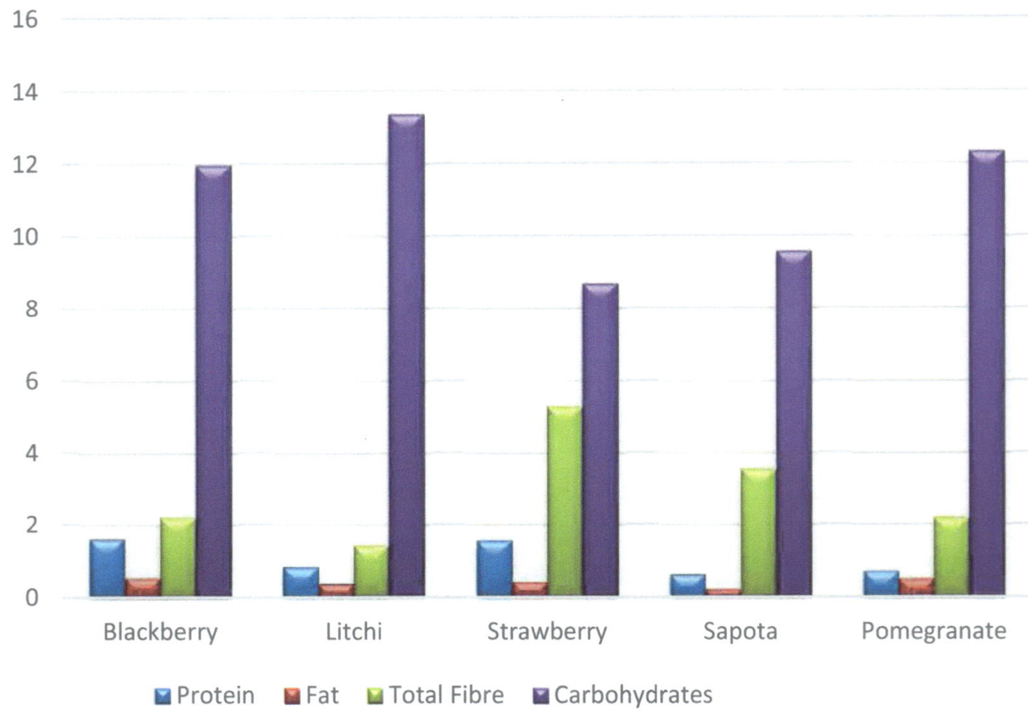

Fig. (1). Nutrient content of fruits for healthcare.

CONCLUSION

By ranking generalities tetradecagonal fuzzy numbers, an ostensible rate is obtained for the fruit diet. We are often engrossed in our activity. The food mix we posited in this paper is frequently used in India because fruit yields are the imperative cause of macronutrients and micronutrients. The vital intent of the research is to forge aliveness around the fruit in society [17] due to fruits being less starchy and high in fiber. Fruits are a dominant part of a well-balanced diet and surely benefit the population by controlling obesity. The analysis enlivened us by outlining the regime division of dietary products. With the complication of uncertain sets of problems in transportation, we draw a satisfactory and active, well-balanced dietary element.

REFERENCES

[1] B. Manoj A, S. T, B. R, B. M, and K. P N, "A mathematical model for green leaves diet using ranking of tridecagonal fuzzy numbers", *Malaysian Journal of Fundamental and Applied Sciences,* vol. 20, no. 4, pp. 946-955, 2024. [http://dx.doi.org/10.11113/mjfas.v20n4.3580]

[2] D. Dubois, and H. Prade, "Operations on fuzzy numbers", *Int. J. Syst. Sci.,* vol. 9, no. 6, pp. 613-626, 1978. [http://dx.doi.org/10.1080/00207727808941724]

[3] E.R. Mathew, and S.J. Kalayathankal, "A new ranking method using dodecagonal fuzzy number to solve fuzzy transportation problem", *International Journal of Applied Engineering Research, Vol,* vol. 14, no. 4, pp. 948-951, 2019.

[4] C Gopalan, B.V. Rama Sastri, and S.C. Balasubramanian, "Nutritive value of indian foods", *National Institute of Nutrition (NIN), Indian Council of Medical Research (ICMR), Hyderabad..*

[5] T. Longvah, R. Ananthan, and K. Bhaskarachary Venkaiah, "Indian food composition tables", *National Institute of Nutrition (NIN), Indian Council of Medical Research, Indian Council of Medical Research (ICMR), Hyderabad.*

[6] R. Saneifard, "A modified method for defuzzification by probability density function", *Journal of Applied Sciences Research, Vol,* vol. 7, no. 2, pp. 102-110, 2011.

[7] A. Venkatesh, and A. Britto Manoj, "A mathematical model for stabilized fruit diet using ranking of tridecagonal fuzzy number", *Journal of the Maharaja Sayajirao University of Baroda, Vol,* vol. 54, no. 2, pp. 138-143, 2020.

[8] A. Venkatesh, and A. Britto Manoj, "A fuzzy mathematical transportation problem model for well balanced oil seeds diet plan", *Sambodhi,* vol. 43, no. 4, pp. 85-90, 2020.

[9] A. Venkatesh, and A.B. Manoj, "A fuzzy mathematical model for vegetable diet plan using ranking of pentagonal fuzzy number", *Malaya Journal of Matematik,* vol. 8, no. 4, pp. 1995-1999, 2020. [http://dx.doi.org/10.26637/MJM0804/0113]

[10] A. Venkatesh, and A. Britto Manoj, "A fuzzy mathematical model for balanced green leaves diet plan", *Journal of Xidian University,* vol. 14, no. 7, pp. 390-398, 2020.

[11] A. Venkatesh, and A. Britto Manoj, "A mathematical model for diet control using ranking of decagonal fuzzy number", *Journal of Xi'an University of Architecture & Technology,* vol. XII, no. VII, pp. 945-951, 2020.

[12] A. Venkatesh, and A. Britto Manoj, "An application of fuzzy transportation problem for diet control", *International Journal of Applied Engineering Research, Vol,* vol. 14, no. 4, pp. 13-19, 2019.

[13] Z. Wang, and Y. Mo, "Ranking fuzzy numbers based on ideal solution", *Fuzzy Information and Engineering,* vol. 2, no. 1, pp. 27-36, 2010. [http://dx.doi.org/10.1007/s12543-010-0035-8]

[14] L.A. Zadeh, "Fuzzy sets", *Inf. Control,* vol. 8, no. 3, pp. 338-353, 1965. [http://dx.doi.org/10.1016/S0019-9958(65)90241-X]

[15] Z. Wang, and L. Zhang-Westmant, "New ranking method for fuzzy numbers by their expansion center", *J. Artif. Intell. Soft Comput. Res.,* vol. 4, no. 3, pp. 181-187, 2014.

[http://dx.doi.org/10.1515/jaiscr-2015-0007]

[16] S. Meti, S. Razauddin, R. Nallakumar, and P.M. Benson Mansingh, "An empirical IoT and cloud-based customizable healthcare surveillance system", *Int. j. inf. tecnol,* vol. 16, pp. 5317-5323, 2024. [http://dx.doi.org/10.1007/s41870-024-01939-2]

[17] Mohana, J., Yakkala, Bhaskarrao, Vimalnath, S., Benson Mansingh, P. M., Yuvaraj, N., Srihari, K., Sasikala, G., Mahalakshmi, V., Yasir Abdullah, R., Sundramurthy, Venkatesa Prabhu, "Application of internet of things on the healthcare field using convolutional neural network processing, journal of healthcare engineering", 2022, 1892123, 7 pages, 2022. [http://dx.doi.org/10.1155/2022/1892123]

CHAPTER 10

Innovative Approaches in Drug Discovery: Target Identification, Computational Strategies, and Emerging Trends in ML and AI Integration

Sneha Subramaniyan[1], **Karthika Alagesan**[1], **Raji Rajmichael**[1], **Veerapandiyan Malaisamy**[1] and **Jeyaraman Jeyakanthan**[1,*]

[1] *Department of Bioinformatics (4th Floor), Science Block, Alagappa University, Karaikudi – 630003, Tamil Nadu, India*

Abstract: In modern pharmaceutical research, drug discovery is the cornerstone that drives the development of new drugs for life-threatening diseases. A growing amount of evidence suggests the promising applications and benefits of Machine Learning (ML) and Artificial Intelligence (AI) in drug discovery. The ideal of personalized medicine in drug discovery is currently being realized through neural network approaches that tailor therapeutic strategies to patients based on their genomic profiles. Combining modern, sophisticated computational algorithms with high-throughput biomedical research is the current gold standard for drug discovery. Since AI and ML are still in their infancy, these scientific paradigms offer significant opportunities for massive technological innovations. Besides the apparent scientific benefits, the expenditure, manpower, and time required for traditional drug discovery are significantly reduced. In this chapter, we have implemented a comprehensive case study review strategy to explore and uncover the potential intricacies and probable limitations of learning algorithms in drug discovery research. The advent of bioinformatics and its subsidiary computational methodologies has revitalized crucial phases of drug discovery, such as the discovery of novel drug targets, screening, candidate molecule validation, and preclinical testing. Thus, this chapter explores the latest innovations and benefits of self-learning algorithms in pharmaceutical research and development, highlighting their potential future opportunities in drug design and drug discovery.

Keywords: Artificial Intelligence (AI), Machine Learning (ML), Computer-aided drug design, Structure-based drug design, Ligand-based drug design, Personalized medicine.

* **Corresponding Author Jeyaraman Jeyakanthan:** Department of Bioinformatics (4th Floor), Science Block, Alagappa University, Karaikudi – 630003, Tamil Nadu, India; E-mail: jjbioinformatics@gmail.com

A. Shankar, Saranya Jayapalan, & Basant. K. Tiwary (Eds.)

INTRODUCTION

The global healthcare landscape is being transformed by Artificial Intelligence (AI) and Machine Learning (ML), revolutionizing diagnostic and treatment processes. Conventional drug discovery techniques relied heavily on human expertise and manual procedures, which resulted in errors, delays, and inadequacies. This process requires extensive experiments, including *in vitro* and *in vivo*, with drug development taking 10-15 years and costing $1-2 billion per drug. Conversely,

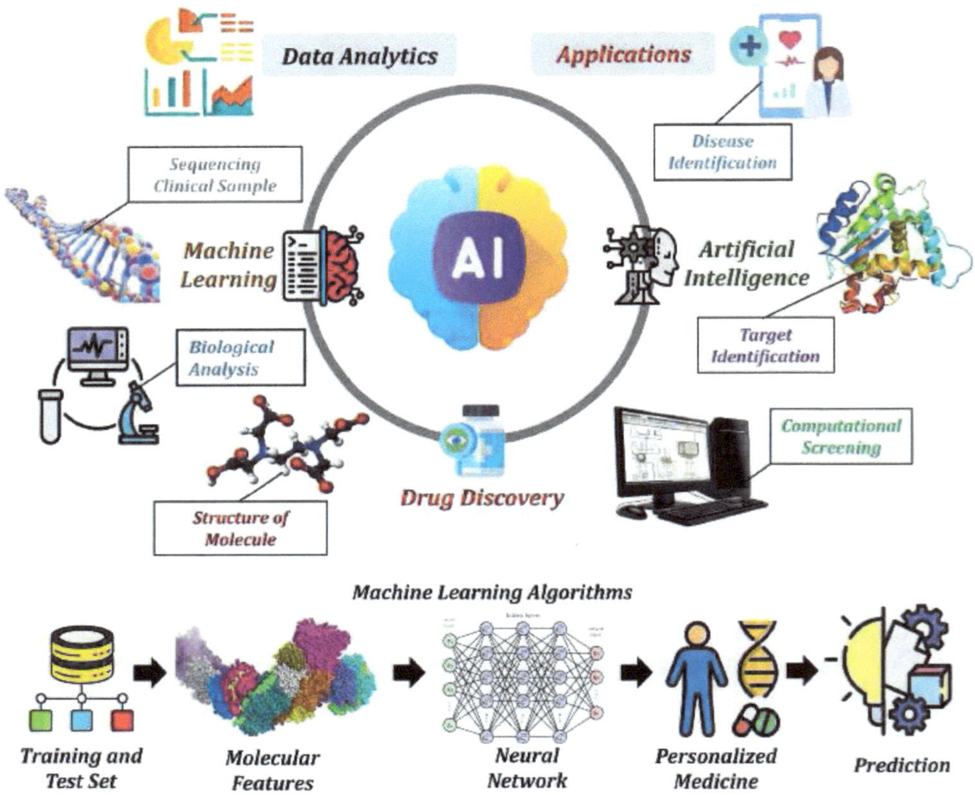

Fig. (1). Schematic representation of artificial intelligence and machine learning integrated in drug development and discovery.

Computer-Aided Drug Design (CADD) provides a more efficient alternative, substantially reducing the time and cost required to discover new therapeutic compounds [1]. In recent decades, AI has played a transformative role in drug design by streamlining precision and speed. This enhances the accuracy of drug discovery while lowering the expenses in clinical trials [2, 3]. AI is the ultimate goal, with ML acting as the brain and DL as the driving force. This system deals with unorganized data, such as text and images. AI, ML, and DL are interconnected through a complex system, using mathematical processes and algorithms to manage data in ways that mimic the human brain. This advanced approach requires substantial computing power and data (Fig. **1**).

In the realm of AI, Machine Learning (ML) is a discipline that leverages statistical techniques to learn, either with or without substantial human involvement. ML can be categorized into three types: supervised, unsupervised, and Reinforcement Learning (RL) [4]. Supervised learning utilizes input and output data to develop predictive models, applying methods such as regression and classification. The classification output determines if a molecule is biologically active, while the regression output predicts the binding affinity score. Categorizing and analyzing data without external guidance is the aim of unsupervised learning, which includes clustering and feature-finding techniques. Through unsupervised ML, disease subtypes can be clustered, and disease targets can be identified using feature-finding methods. RL is utilized to make decisions and take action in a given context.

In the present scientific landscape, the explosion of medical data has coincided with innovation in computational technologies such as cloud computing, GPUs, and TPUs, alongside the emergence of deep learning. The enormous datasets generated from molecular screening, personal health records, and public health databases can be efficiently analyzed using AI, facilitating drug discovery and diminishing failure rates [5]. AI is a revolutionary tool that bridges the knowledge gap between disease diagnosis and the identification of potential treatment agents. Its ability to analyze large datasets and perceive patterns is crucial for optimizing drug discovery processes, intensifying the accuracy of predictive models, and improving effectiveness across the drug discovery pipeline, including clinical trial management. In light of these factors, AI holds the potential to revolutionize drug discovery, providing extensive benefits to patients and the healthcare industry [6]. This chapter highlights modern strategies in drug discovery, focusing on target identification, computational methodologies, and the incorporation of ML and AI. These innovations enhance efficiency, accuracy, and prognostic capabilities, driving the development of novel therapeutics and transforming the pharmaceutical landscape.

DRUG DISCOVERY PIPELINE AND COMPUTATIONAL INTEGRATION

The pipeline of drug discovery comprises multiple stages that can be broadly categorized as follows: preclinical development, clinical trials, hit-to-lead optimization, target identification, and hit identification [7].

- **Target identification:** Understanding and analyzing the biological pathways and identifying molecular targets.
- **Hit identification:** Identifying compounds that show potential binding to targets by screening large compound libraries.
- **Lead optimization:** Improve the efficacy, selectivity, and pharmacokinetics of hit compounds by refining their chemical structures.
- **Preclinical studies:** Preclinical trials evaluate a drug's safety, efficacy, and toxicity through cell and animal testing before moving to human clinical trials, using predictive models to evaluate lead compounds' pharmacokinetics and toxicity profiles.
- **Clinical Trials:** To evaluate novel medications or therapies' efficacy, safety, and possible adverse effects. Phase I, Phase II, Phase III, Phase IV, and post-approval monitoring to guarantee the drug's suitability for public distribution and widespread application [8].

The computational strategies are virtually integrated into most phases of the drug discovery process (Fig. **2**).

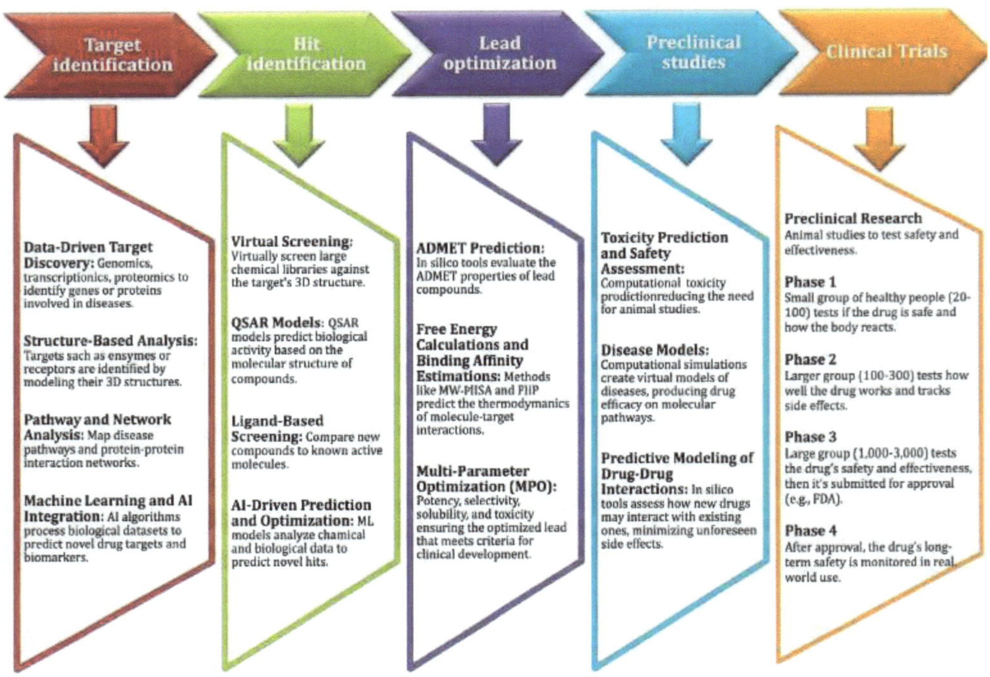

Fig. (2). Computational strategies integrated into the drug discovery pipeline.

Target Identification for Drug Development

Target identification is one of the most important steps in the intricate and multi-phase drug discovery process [9]. Typically, a target is an RNA molecule, gene, or protein that contributes to the pathophysiology of an illness. By identifying these biomolecules, researchers aim to develop therapeutics that produce potent pharmaceutical effects, leading to therapeutic benefits [9, 10]. Understanding the principles of target identification and the tools used to discover and validate these targets is essential for innovation in the healthcare industry. Target identification aims to elucidate the biological pathways involved in diseases, which is critical for developing effective treatments [11]. By knowing the specific molecular targets, more specific drugs can be developed, thereby reducing potential side effects and improving efficacy [12]. Early and effective target identification can mitigate failures in late-stage clinical trials by ensuring that the selected targets are relevant to the disease [11, 13].

Role of Genomics and Proteomics in Target Identification

Genomic Approaches

Genomics plays a crucial role in target identification for drug development, leveraging genetic information to uncover potential therapeutic targets linked to various diseases [14]. The rapid advances in genomics, proteomics, and bioinformatics have revolutionized target identification. Genomic data enables researchers to explore the relationship between genes and diseases, identify molecular pathways that might be disrupted, and discover potential therapeutic targets [15].

Genome-Wide Association Studies (GWAS)

GWAS is one of the most potent genomic tools for target identification. GWAS systematically compares the genomes of large populations to identify Single Nucleotide Polymorphisms (SNPs) that are more common in individuals with a specific disease [16]. GWAS provides insights into the biological pathways involved in disease progression by linking specific SNPs to disease. Once disease-associated variants are identified, this paves the way for investigating the genes and biological pathways in which these variants are located [17]. Furthermore, GWAS helps estimate the heritability of diseases and traits, allowing researchers to understand the trait's variation with specific disease attributes.

GWAS results often point to genes that encode proteins in disease processes, thus providing a basis for developing targeted therapies [18]. This method has revealed numerous genetic associations across various diseases, enhancing our understanding of their genetic architecture. The findings from GWAS extend beyond identifying disease risk factors [18 - 20]. These findings are also utilized to assess an individual's genetic predisposition to disease through epidemiological studies, gene-environment interaction analyses, and polygenic risk score calculations [21].

Functional Genomics

Understanding the functions of genes, RNA, and protein in biological mechanisms is a primary focus of functional genomics [22]. Using multiple genomic techniques, functional genomics assists in identifying genes critical to disease development and can guide targeted therapeutic interventions. This approach leverages high-throughput molecular, genetic, and cellular technologies to assess gene function and its implications [22, 23].

- **CRISPR/Cas9 screening:** This revolutionary genome-editing technology allows for systematically knocking out genes across the genome for large-scale, loss-of-function screens. Additionally, researchers can investigate their function by precisely modifying DNA sequences by creating knockouts or activating specific genes. Knockout genes that lead to a change in disease phenotype can be prioritized as a potential target [24, 25].
- **RNA Interference (RNAi):** RNAi is another functional genomics tool used to silence gene expression [26]. Like CRISPR, RNAi can be used for large-scale screens to identify genes essential for disease processes. The difference is that RNAi suppresses gene expression at the mRNA level, temporarily decreasing the production of a specific protein. It is beneficial for target identification in early drug discovery phases [27].

Proteomic Approach

Genomics provides critical information on the genetic blueprint of an organism, while proteomics elucidates the dynamic and functional characteristics of proteins. In drug development, target identification emphasizes locating proteins directly associated with disease processes or therapeutic responses. Proteomics enables researchers to study expression levels of proteins, post-translational modifications, protein-protein interactions, and changes in response to drug treatments or disease states [14, 28].

Protein Expression Profiling

A key application of proteomics is comparing protein expression levels between healthy and diseased states [29]. Identifying differentially expressed proteins in disease conditions helps researchers pinpoint potential drug targets.

- **Differential Expression Analysis:** In diseases like cancer, cardiovascular disorders, and neurodegenerative conditions, proteomic profiling can identify upregulated and downregulated proteins that may serve as therapeutic targets [30]. For instance, cancer cells often express specific proteins at much higher levels than normal cells, and these overexpressed proteins can be prioritized as drug targets.
- **Proteomic Biomarker:** Proteomics also helps in identifying protein biomarkers that not only serve as disease indicators but also as therapeutic targets [31]. For example, increased levels of specific proteins in patients' blood, tissues, or urine can indicate the presence of a disease. They may be involved in its progression, making them potential drug targets.

Protein-Protein Interaction (PPIs)

Most cellular functions are performed by proteins that act within complex networks, interacting with each other in a highly regulated manner. Understanding Protein-Protein Interactions (PPIs) is essential for identifying key nodes in disease pathways that drugs can target [32].

- **Interactomics:** The branch of proteomics that studies protein interactions, known as interactomics, helps map the physical interactions between proteins within cells [33]. Researchers can uncover new targets in critical pathways by identifying proteins interacting with disease-associated proteins.
- **Drugging the Undruggable:** Many proteins involved in diseases, particularly those involved in protein-protein interactions, are often considered "undruggable" because they lack well-defined binding pockets for small molecules [34]. However, proteomics-driven insights into these interactions have opened new avenues for developing drugs that target PPIs.

Assay in High Throughput Screening (HTS) for Target Identification

HTS relies on creating robust, reliable, and reproducible assays to evaluate the interaction between a target and a compound. Different assays are used in HTS depending on the nature of the target and the screening goal [35].

Biochemical Assays

Biochemical assays measure the activity of isolated enzymes, receptors, or other proteins in a cell-free environment. Additionally, they are employed to evaluate the direct interaction between a compound and a purified target protein or enzyme. They are often used in target-based HTS to assess the effect of compounds on enzyme activity, protein-protein interactions, or receptor binding.

Biochemical assays have low variability and can be easily miniaturized for HTS [36].

Cell-Based Assays

Cell-based assays are performed in living cells and measure cellular responses to compounds, such as changes in gene expression, signaling pathways, or cell viability. Cell-based assays are helpful for phenotypic screening and evaluating compounds' effects on more complex biological systems [37]. Cell-based assays provide a more physiologically relevant system, accounting for cell permeability, metabolism, and signaling cascades.

Phenotypic Assays

Phenotypic assays measure observable effects, such as changes in cell shape, proliferation, or differentiation, in response to compound treatment. These essays are especially valuable for unknown targets, as they enable the identification of compounds based on their impact on disease-relevant phenotypes [38]. Phenotypic assays are unbiased, frequently identifying new drug targets and their novel mechanisms.

TRADITIONAL DRUG DISCOVERY

Traditional drug discovery methodologies were dependent on structure and ligand-based approaches. They are enhanced by AI and machine learning, enabling more accurate and efficient predictions.

Structure-Based Drug Design (SBDD)

The 3D structure of the protein or nucleic acid is used to design drug candidates in structure-based drug design [39]. SBDD highly depends on X-ray crystallography, NMR, or cryo-Electron Microscopy (cryo-EM) structures with higher resolution [40]. Due to the structural revolution, from automated crystallography to micro-crystallography to cryo-electron microscopy, the most clinically relevant targets can now be visualized in 3D [41 - 43]. SBDD involves docking small molecules into macromolecular structures and predicting [44] their affinity for binding.

Structure-Based Virtual Screening (SBVS)

The SBVS technique screens a virtual library of compounds against a known target structure. This technique is essential for identifying lead compounds that maybind to a target and exhibit significant biological activity (Fig. **3**) [44].

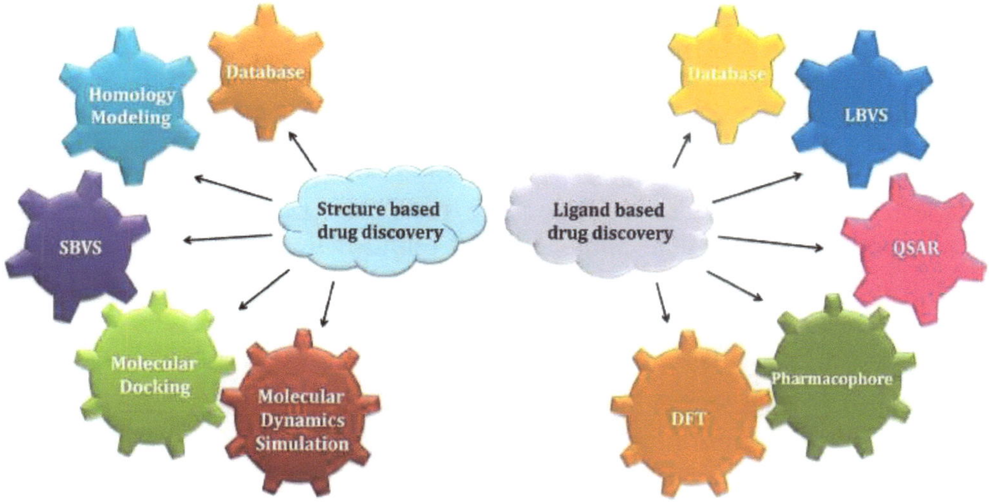

Fig. (3). The framework of Structure-Based Drug Design (SBDD) and Ligand-Based Drug Design (LBDD).

- **Library Screening:** Docking allows millions of compounds to be virtually screened, eliminating the need for wet laboratory testing. In the next step, the highest-ranked results from the virtual screen are synthesized and tested experimentally [45].
- **Integration with AI:** As a result of recent advances, machine learning models are being incorporated into scoring functions to improve scoring accuracy and optimize hit rates for virtual screening [46].

Molecular Docking

The molecular docking process simulates the interaction between a ligand and its receptor during drug discovery [47]. Based on scoring functions, the docking algorithm estimates how strong an interaction between a ligand and its target will be. Molecular docking is utilized for screening against a vast library of compounds and evaluating their binding affinity to a target, thereby decreasing the number of compounds for future synthesis and experimental procedures [48].

Molecular Dynamics (MD) Simulations

The simulation of macromolecules through molecular dynamics will provide insight into the dynamic behaviour of biological molecules [49]. While docking provides static snapshots of protein-ligand interactions, MD simulations examine both the protein and the ligand's flexibility and conformational changes taking place over time [50]. An MD simulation is helpful for studying protein flexibility, ligand-induced conformational changes, and binding thermodynamics. They can be used to refine docking results or predict the stability of protein-ligand complexes [51].

Ligand-Based Drug Design (LBDD)

LBDD relies on known ligands with potential binding properties, which are highly effective when there is inadequate structural information for the target. This approach uses chemical and structural features to guide the design of new compounds, with similarity metrics (Fig. **3**) [52, 53].

Ligand-Based Virtual Screening (LBVS)

Ligand-Based Virtual Screening (LBVS) is a technique utilized in computational drug discovery to predict potential bioactive compounds. This approach focuses on existing ligands instead of the 3D structure of a target protein to search for similar compounds that exhibit comparable biological activity. LBVS involves ligand preparation, feature extraction, similarity search, pharmacophore modeling, database screening, scoring and ranking, filtering, evaluation, and experimental validation. Applications include drug repurposing, lead identification, optimization of known compounds, and natural product screening. Common tools used in LBVS include AutoDock and PyRx for docking-based similarity scoring, ChemistryMine for 2D similarity searches, Open Babel for molecular fingerprinting, Ligand Scout for pharmacophore modeling, and ROCS for 3D shape-based screening. LBVS proves efficient; however, it relies on minimal structural information about the target [52].

Quantitative Structure-Activity Relationship (QSAR)

Quantitative Structure-Activity Relationships (QSARs) serve as essential components of LBDD, linking the compounds' chemical structures to their biological activities. These generated models elucidate the structural features that influence biological activity by facilitating the prediction of the efficacy of novel compounds [54].

- **2D QSAR:** Uses topological descriptors derived from the molecular structure [55].
- **3D QSAR:** Incorporates spatial and geometric features of the ligands, allowing a more detailed understanding of structure-activity relationships [56].

By combining machine learning techniques with QSAR models, large datasets can be handled, and nonlinear relationships between molecular features and biological activity can be identified.

Pharmacophore Modeling

A pharmacophore defines the molecular features essential for a compound to bind to a precise target. It involves identifying essential characteristics, including hydrophobic regions and hydrogen bond donors, that contribute to the compound's biological activity. Pharmacophore models are utilized for virtual screening, where compounds that match the pharmacophore are predicted to have similar biological activity [57].

Density Functional Theory (DFT)

Density Functional Theory (DFT) is an essential tool in computational drug discovery, offering detailed information on the chemical properties and electronic structure of small molecules and drug candidates. It offers high accuracy for studying binding interactions, reaction mechanisms, and molecular properties at the quantum level. Applications include optimizing ligands and drug candidates, determining stable 3D structures, analyzing drug-target binding mechanisms, and predicting metabolic reactions. DFT is a commonly applied computational method, used in case studies such as COVID-19 targets, anticancer drugs, and metal-drug complexes [58].

EMERGING TRENDS IN MACHINE LEARNING (ML) AND ARTIFICIAL INTELLIGENCE (AI) IN DRUG DISCOVERY

To address these challenges, ML and deep learning algorithms, key subsets of AI, offer promising solutions for more accurate and efficient drug discovery. Improvements in ML and the increasing availability of drug-related data have made AI an indispensable tool in various aspects of drug design. The healthcare sector may experience significant changes due to advancing technology. As healthcare data continues to grow exponentially, it offers an opportunity for revolutionizing the current healthcare setting, making it more efficient, cost-effective, and personalized. AI helps with tasks like modeling, virtual screening, scoring the effectiveness of drug candidates, analyzing the relationship between a compound's structure and its activity (QSAR), designing new drugs from scratch, and predicting ADME/T properties [59, 60]. ML algorithms widely used in drug discovery include Deep Learning (DL), Random Forests (RF), clustering, Bayesian Networks (BN), and Support Vector Machines (SVM). For instance, DL models are effective at processing and analyzing large datasets, with applications in clinical imaging, Virtual Screening (VS), and prediction of bioactivity [61, 62]. BNs are used to forecast bioactivity, toxicity, and patient response to therapy. RF models assist in identifying molecular targets and selecting important features from data [63]. SVM, a supervised learning algorithm, classifies data into categories and is applied in pharmacokinetic property prediction, virtual screening, and toxicity prediction [64].

Machine Learning in Drug Discovery

ML has transformed computational drug discovery, enhancing efficiency through its capability to analyze large and complex datasets. The activity of new compounds can be anticipated with ML models on numerous sets of biological and chemical data, including chemical structures, high-throughput screening results, and biological assays [65].

Applications of ML in Compound Screening

ML algorithms, particularly deep learning, are used for virtual screening by determining the binding affinity of compounds to target proteins. These models learn patterns from existing screening data and can generalize to new chemical spaces [65].

De Novo Drug Design

De novo drug design is one of the key methods in Structure-Based Drug Design (SBDD), in which new compounds are generated from scratch based on target protein structures in three dimensions [66]. Generative Adversarial Networks (GANs) and Variational Autoencoders (VAEs) are tools that learn from chemical data and help design new compounds with the desired biological activity [67].

Predicting ADMET Properties

In addition to identifying active compounds, ML is instrumental in predicting ADMET (Absorption, Distribution, Metabolism, Excretion, and Toxicity) properties. Accurate ADMET predictions are vital for analyzing whether a compound will be suitable for further development, helping avoid costly failures in later stages [68]. The use of Deep Learning (DL) and data-driven ML methods for predicting PK and ADMET properties underscores the essentiality of computational approaches [2].

Multi-Target Drug Design and Polypharmacology

Drug discovery is increasingly shifting from the conventional "one target, one drug" paradigm to embrace multiple-target drug development [69]. Many diseases, especially complex ones like cancer and neurodegenerative disorders, involve multiple biological pathways. To increase therapeutic effectiveness, polypharmacology aims to design drugs that act on multiple targets at once [70].

- **Network Pharmacology:** Computational tools can be used to design or repurpose drugs that modulate multiple nodes within the network underlying a disease by understanding the molecular interactions that underlie the disease [71]. In polypharmacology, computational strategies like network analysis and machine learning are used to identify secondary or off-target effects, turning potential side effects into therapeutic advantages [72].

These innovative strategies are crucial in tackling complex diseases and enhancing drug development timelines, thereby enhancing the speed and accuracy of these efforts.

Machine Learning for Protein-Ligand Binding Affinity Prediction

Virtual screening methods, including structure and ligand-based approaches, improve compound analysis and expedite the identification of drug molecules. Molecular fingerprints and Coulomb matrices are used in drug design algorithms to select lead compounds according to their physicochemical and toxicological profiles. Reinforcement Learning (RL) is widely applied in *de novo* drug design for molecular optimization [73].

Binding properties can be predicted using algorithms such as SMILES. A molecule's properties can be predicted more accurately by using these algorithms, allowing correlations between a molecular structure and properties to be identified. Estimation Program Interfaces (EPIs) are utilized to demonstrate how physicochemical properties, including boiling points, solubility, partition coefficients, vapor pressure, melting points, and bioconcentrations, can be evaluated using a Quantitative Structure–Property Relationship (QSPR) method. EPIs have shown promising results in various *in silico* strategies, including molecular docking (using software such as rDOCK, AutoDock, ZDOCK, HEX, and Flex-Aid), *de novo* molecular design (with tools like lvaBuilder, ChemTSv2, AIDDISON, and GenUI), drug repurposing (applications such as SAveRUNNER, DRviaSPCN, and ADMET Predictor), retrosynthesis (using tools like AiZynthFinder, SYNTHIA, and CAS SciFinder n), target identification, and the prediction of bioactivity.

Chemical compounds and bimolecular drugs form a combination within the human body, targeting proteins and other substances. By utilizing computational AI, we can improve traditional drug development methods and address their inherent inefficiencies and uncertainties. Conventional prediction techniques and technical limitations have been surpassed by AI, which has also contributed significantly to mitigating bias, minimizing human involvement, and managing economic aspects. Drug-Target Interactions (DTI) currently utilizes various computational approaches such as docking simulations, ligand-based methods, machine learning/deep learning, chemogenomic approaches, text mining, sequence-based deep learning, transformer methods, and network-based methods. The literature contains multiple documented methods for drug target identification, including omics and machine learning approaches. High-throughput technologies provide omics data, which allows for widespread analysis. Information about the proteins and metabolites in a biological sample is obtained from the proteome and metabolome. Furthermore, the interactome provides information about the interactions involving DNA, RNA, proteins, and other small molecules. ANPELA, ConSIG, POSREG, NOREVA, SingPro, and other AI/ML technologies are applied to evaluate the extensive data generated by the entities [74, 75].

***AI in Target Identification*:** Neural networks and Support Vector Machines (SVMs) can rank potential targets according to their importance in the disease under study. AI-based target identification leverages machine learning algorithms to analyze vast datasets and pinpoint potential drug interaction targets. By incorporating data from sources like protein-protein interaction networks, gene expression profiles, and biological pathways, this approach generates a list of promising targets for further investigation [76].

***AI in Structure Predictions*:** When the experimental data is unavailable, researchers would use computational methods to predict the tertiary structure of proteins. Modeller is an extensively used tool that uses a process called homology modeling [77]. It predicts protein structure by comparing it to one or more proteins whose structures are already known, using them as templates. AlphaFold is designed for the structure prediction of proteins using a deep learning algorithm developed by DeepMind [78]. AlphaFold relies exclusively on AI techniques and algorithms to predict the structure of a protein target, and recent case studies about AI structure prediction have demonstrated the high accuracy and precision of the predicted structures. However, the referred study has also emphasized the importance of optimizing AI technologies and improving the overall AI architecture and infrastructure to further improve the existing areas of membrane protein science [79].

***AI in Virtual Screening*:** Several machine learning techniques are utilized in virtual screening, including Naïve Bayes classifiers (NB), k-Nearest Neighbors (kNN), random forests (RF), Support Vector Machines (SVM), and Artificial Neural Networks (ANN). Among these methods, SVMs and ANNs are commonly considered the most precise. Each machine learning technique has its pros and cons. For example, Naïve Bayesian (NB) is good at finding functional building blocks in molecules, Random Forests (RFs) can run multiple tasks at once and be improved upon, and k-Nearest Neighbors (kNN) are easy to use and can handle

Multiple Types of Learning (MTL). Often, combining several ML models into an ensemble is preferred because it can improve the overall performance [80]. For Ligand-Based Virtual Screening (LBVS), Naïve Bayesian (NB) classifiers are commonly used and perform very well [81, 82]. Another straightforward machine learning method is k-Nearest Neighbors (kNN), which can be easily understood. In a study by Luo and colleagues on G-Protein-Coupled Receptor ligands, they found that uing kNN with variable selection (kNN-QSAR) performed better than traditional LBVS methods without machine learning [83].

AI in Drug Toxicity Prediction: Predicting drug toxicity is crucial for minimizing failures and enhancing efficiency. Many drug candidates are eliminated during clinical trials because of unforeseen side effects. Traditional methods often depend on small datasets and simplified models, which limit their effectiveness. AI-based approaches, using ML and large, diverse data, offer more accurate toxicity predictions. This helps lower risks in clinical trials, reduces development costs, and leads to better patient outcomes [84 - 87]. FP-ADMET and Interpretable-ADMET are tools used to predict the LD50, the median lethal dose, indicating toxicity. Toxicologists rely on the LD50 to assess toxicity levels, and it is commonly used as a key first step in the drug screening process. These models help streamline toxicity predictions, improving the efficiency of early drug discovery by providing quick, interpretable insights into a compound's potential risks [88, 89].

INTEGRATION OF AI/ML WITH COMPUTATIONAL DRUG DISCOVERY TOOLS

AI in Structure-Based Drug Design (SBDD)

The amalgamation of AI has revolutionized drug discovery, offering a promising way to accelerate the development of new therapeutic compounds. The success of AI models in this field heavily depends on using reliable datasets for training and testing. AI requires a dynamic fusion of chemical, biological, and clinical data to uncover insights into molecular structures, disease pathways, and interactions [90].

In drug discovery, computational models are crucial for pinpointing potential lead compounds. In AI, active learning, also called "selective sampling," involves choosing data points for testing and integration into the model using various strategies. Categorization of compound selection methodologies is based on the characteristics of these pinpointed data points [91]. Algorithms that extract compounds with targeted properties from existing data are described as "exploitation". Alternatively, some methods aim to refine the model by a process called exploration. Predictive models and design strategies address multiple factors when evaluating the drug-likeliness of the compound. Instead of sequential optimization, we aim to achieve simultaneous optimization of different properties through multidimensional optimization [92]. The pharmaceutical industry is being transformed by AI, revolutionizing drug development and delivery, from identifying drug candidates accurately to optimizing pharmaceutical formulations for better bioavailability.

Computer-Aided Drug Discovery (CADD) has been broadly adopted by the pharmaceutical industry in recent decades, utilizing both structure- and ligand-based design strategies [93]. However, CADD encounters several challenges and limitations. These factors include the complex nature of biological systems, the challenges in accurately depicting target flexibility, and the restricted analysis scope of traditional methods for closely related compounds. The emergence of AI in the present era has significantly transformed the conventional techniques used in identifying, developing, and delivering potential therapeutics. The ability of AI to analyze extensive data is a significant catalyst in carrying out this transformation [90, 91].

AI-ENHANCED PREDICTIVE ANALYTICS IN DRUG DEVELOPMENT

A drug designer works to develop new chemical compounds that can specifically identify target molecules without relying on existing templates from a compound library. This process involves formulating compounds using computational algorithms, which can significantly aid drug discovery and development. One key technology used in this domain is Generative Adversarial Networks (GANs), an AI-based strategy that can be employed in drug design and compound optimization. The applications of GANs in drug discovery are diverse, encompassing the development of new molecules, the search for novel peptides, and the design of innovative proteins. Once a lead compound with desirable characteristics is identified, the drug development process progresses to the lead optimization phase. During this phase, the structure of the compound is refined to enhance its potency, selectivity, and pharmacokinetic properties, aiming to discover the most promising candidate for clinical use. Incorporating AI into lead optimization offers significant advantages, such as reducing human bias, facilitating ongoing chemical exploration, and overcoming data limitations through transfer learning and semi-supervised learning. Numerous studies have leveraged Generative Deep Learning (GDL) models, including recurrent neural networks, variational autoencoders, GANs, graph convolutional networks, and transformer models, all of which utilize deep neural networks in their methodologies.

CASE STUDIES OF ML AND AI IN DRUG DISCOVERY

An increasing number of researchers are employing ML and AI algorithms in drug discovery research, which is discussed in detail in this section. Drug research ventures have been mainly aimed at designing novel drugs to treat both communicable and non-communicable diseases, with particular emphasis on lifestyle diseases such as cancer, diabetes, *etc.*

AI in Cancer Research: AI is transforming cancer research by using high-dimensional data, advanced computing, and deep learning in areas like detection, drug discovery, and prognosis. It holds great potential to revolutionize oncology, from diagnosis to personalized treatments [99]. One study explored the use of ML techniques in cancer diagnostics and therapy, focusing on predictive models using high-throughput data such as gene expression and biomarker data. This study was aimed at identifying new therapeutic targets and optimizing treatment strategies, highlighting the transformative role of ML in personalized medicine, despite challenges in model interpretability and data quality [95]. Another study employed a discriminative Structure-Based Virtual Screening (SBVS) method to identify IRAK1 inhibitors; however, only one active compound was found. The low hit rate of 2.63% was attributed to weak docking capabilities. Hence, an AI method was introduced to enhance the traditional IRAK1-VS protocol, which led to the exclusion of over 50% of inactive compounds from the screening of IRAK1 inhibitors, significantly improving prediction accuracy. Four active molecules were pinpointed from analogs that exhibited good selectivity against IRAk4. This AI-driven workflow holds great promise as an effective tool for advancing SBVS results [101]. In a similar study, FGF receptors, key members of the tyrosine kinase family, were reported as promising drug targets for cancer studies. Using AI, researchers were able to identify inhibitors for FGF receptors. The combination of AI and drug repositioning methodologies can aid in selecting suitable drug targets for future cancer treatment [99].

AI in Infectious Diseases Research: Within the paradigm of infectious disease research, the report by Shahab *et al.* (2024) explores the application of ML in designing novel inhibitors against thymidylate kinase as a potential treatment for drug resistance in Mycobacterium tuberculosis. In this study, widely implemented ML algorithms, including K-Nearest Neighbors, Support Vector Machines (SVMs), and Random Forest Algorithms, were employed to repurpose those drugs. Among 307 compounds, the model identified several promising candidates, which were further validated by molecular docking and simulations. These inhibitors demonstrate incredible promise in combating tuberculosis by inhibiting key enzymatic activity [93]. Another study explored ML and deep learning models to analyze the interactions between bitter molecules and TAS2R receptors.

This receptor plays a significant role beyond taste perception, holding significance in drug design. In this study, a combination of traditional ML models and deep learning techniques was used to ensure the accuracy, interpretability, and reliability of the receptor-ligand binding interactions [9]. A similar study explored machine learning in identifying biological targets and predicting molecular interactions in drug discovery against HIV infection. To reduce experimental workloads and potentially enhance lead optimization, advanced AI algorithms were utilized. The study also addresses data complexity and model validation challenges, emphasizing the model elucidation throughout the AI-driven approach [96]. A research study identified 26 potential phytochemicals targeting the SARS-CoV-2 3CLPRO enzyme using ML-based virtual screening. The random forest algorithm achieved an accuracy of nearly 98% among 4000 phytochemicals. The top candidates showed strong binding affinity and stable interaction within the active site, suggesting they could be effective COVID-19 inhibitors [97]. In addition, a study used ML to identify potential antimicrobial agents for Staphylococcus aureus strains, including MRSA and MSSA. Six compounds showed antibacterial activity, with MICs ranging from 12.5 to 200 μM. The research highlights the effectiveness of ML models in screening novel MRSA antibiotics [98].

Recently, Chung *et al.* (2024) developed an ensemble model to predict the minimum inhibitory concentration (MIC) of antimicrobial peptides (AMPs) for three bacterial strains: Escherichia coli, Staphylococcus aureus, and Pseudomonas aeruginosa. This model integrates AMP sequence-based and genomic features, employing eight AI architectures for thorough evaluation and training. The CNN, BiLSTM, and MBM models constantly demonstrated high performance over other approaches. This research highlights the prominence of integrating numerous biological data sources and the synergistic effect of combining sequence and genomic features in predicting MIC [100]. The studies discussed in this section demonstrate the effectiveness and cumulative benefits of employing ML and AI techniques for Drug Discovery research.

TRENDS SHAPING THE FUTURE OF DRUG DISCOVERY

Advancements in AI are changing the field and accelerating development, securing the creation of new therapies. Some notable developments taking place in AI include methods to use AI in expediting drug development, expanding accessibility to biosimilars, and using more representative real-world data, illustrating the continuously changing pharmaceutical landscape. AI tools and ongoing advancements strive to alleviate the obstacles encountered by the pharmaceutical sector, potentially impacting drug development and discovery [94].

The healthcare sector is currently grappling with several complex challenges, including rising costs of drugs and therapies. To address these issues, significant changes are needed. By integrating AI into pharmaceutical manufacturing, personalized medications can be produced that are tailored to individual patient needs, including specific dosages, release parameters, and other essential factors [95]. Employing the cutting-edge AI technologies will accelerate product quality and increase safety in the manufacturing process. Additionally, it will optimize resource utilization, making the process more streamlined and further highlighting the importance of automation in the pharmaceutical industry [96]. The main concerns regarding the adoption of these technologies are manpower reductions and stringent regulations for AI implementation. However, these systems are designed to complement human work by making tasks more efficient, rather than replacing humans entirely [97]. AI can facilitate the quick and efficient identification of hit compounds and assist in suggesting synthesis routes for these molecules. Additionally, it can predict the desired chemical structures and provide insights into drug–target interactions, as well as Structure-Activity Relationships (SAR).

AI plays a vital role in determining the optimal drug dosage form, enabling the safety and efficacy of products during clinical trials. Additionally, it can assist with pricing, pre, and post-marketing progress, and predictive modeling. While AI-based drug development has not yet led to market-ready products, there are still specific challenges to overcome in implementation. Soon, AI will invade as a precious tool in the healthcare sector [98].

THE ROLE OF AI IN PERSONALIZED MEDICINE AND DRUG DEVELOPMENT

The rapidly developing field of personalized medicine seeks to customize medical interventions and therapies for each patient by taking into consideration their distinct physiological, environmental, and genetic traits. However, incorporating personalized medicine into clinical practice presents several challenges. A key concern in this field is the ethical issues surrounding patient confidentiality and privacy. The use of personal genetic and health data raises significant privacy risks [99].

Personalized medicine is being revolutionized by AI, which makes it possible for computer systems to carry out normal human-intelligence-dependent tasks like decision-making and pattern recognition. ML in healthcare is a crucial domain that is useful for predicting health outcomes and analyzing patient data (*e.g.*, genetics, medical history) [100]. Personalized medicine benefits greatly from deep learning to process intricate data relationships. These algorithms are excellent at identifying images, which makes it possible to accurately diagnose MRI scans. Based on extensive datasets, AI-powered systems can also suggest successful treatments and forecast patient outcomes. However, data privacy, algorithmic bias, and ethical regulation remain a critical issue in the pharmaceutical industry. The responsible application of AI in medicine requires cooperation between data scientists, regulatory agencies, and healthcare professionals. AI can predominantly transform personalized medicine by enhancing the treatment outcomes with progressive advancements [101, 102]. By leveraging big data and artificial intelligence, healthcare providers can evaluate extensive amounts of diverse data, which includes genetic profiles, information from wearable devices, medical records, and patient-reported outcomes [103]. AI is revolutionizing disease detection by improving diagnostic accuracy and reducing errors for healthcare professionals. AI enhances surgical outcomes by providing real-time analysis during procedures, while its data-processing capabilities enable the creation of predictive models that facilitate early interventions for high-risk individuals. Overall, AI is transforming healthcare, with its potential in personalized medicine continuing to unfold. As data grows, AI will enable more precise treatments, expand precision medicine, and support real-time patient monitoring *via* wearables, ultimately enhancing treatment accuracy, reducing errors, and improving outcomes [104, 105].

CURRENT CHALLENGES AND LIMITATIONS

AI and ML, in modern pharmaceutical research, present a plethora of opportunities to optimize the drug discovery pipeline and minimize the overall financial workload imposed on these companies to deliver a novel drug to the market. However, looking at the present state of AI in drug discovery, massive strides in technological development need to take place. One of the main concerns pertaining to the widespread implementation of AI in drug discovery pipelines is the issue of data privacy and the reliability of the models employed to execute the screening approaches. Since most AI models are currently reliant on cloud computing, there is also a risk of data breach and data exploitation. Another issue that is not widely discussed with the utilization of AI approaches in drug development is the lack of diversity in the models used to train AI. Since a significant portion of the data is received from developed and first-world nations, scientists risk not accounting for a diverse variety of people, which severely limits the potential use-case scenarios of these self-learning algorithms. This phenomenon, widely known as algorithmic bias among the scientific community, is a well-known concern regarding the vast applicability of AI. Researchers also encounter ethical issues regarding the use of AI in drug discovery, since the data used to train the AI models needs to be obtained ethically, with the consent of the people who provided the data. All these concerns ultimately affect the interpretability of the AI model, raising questions about the model's quality and operability in a diverse range of scenarios. Therefore, without continuous optimization and innovations in AI architecture, AI models will be bottlenecked and remain stagnant. Hence, these concerns need to be addressed around the world in order to achieve the widespread applicability of AI in drug design and development [106 - 108].

CONCLUSION

The current generation of scientific research is exploring the realms of Artificial Intelligence, amid an exponential increase in information. Technological advancements in AI algorithms have driven unprecedented breakthroughs in early diagnosis, personalized precision therapy, and prevention. The pharmaceutical industry is well positioned to continue leading the adoption of new technology. However, the key question is whether these approaches should be incorporated into current pipelines and processes, or if the processes themselves should be restructured to fully leverage these advancements. In general, integrating AI and ML has the potential to significantly improve public health outcomes and associated costs, making preventive healthcare more sustainable and accessible for everyone. Nevertheless, it is crucial to be considerate of ethics, ensuring that these innovations do not widen healthcare gaps and inequalities in healthcare outcomes. The key to successfully integrating AI and ML is engaging all researchers and healthcare professionals' stakeholders. Massive monetary and intellectual investments are required to transform literacy and educational policies, paving the way for capacity growth in integrating AI into widespread healthcare practices. This chapter sustains ongoing AI research in developing effective tools for diagnosing and treating diseases and significantly contributes to pharmaceutical drug development and research.

CONSENT FOR PUBLICATION

None Declared

CONFLICT OF INTEREST

The authors declare no competing financial interest.

ACKNOWLEDGEMENT

This book chapter was supported by TANSCHE (RGP/2019-20/ALU/HECP-0049 dated: 27/04/2021), DBT-NNP No.BT /PR40156 /BTIS /137/54/2023, Department of Biotechnology-Bioinformatics Centre (DBT-BIC) No.BT/PR40154/BTIS/137/34/2021, DSTINDO-TAIWAN (GITA /DST/

TWN/P-86/2019), ST-Fund for Improvement of S &T Infrastructure in Universities Higher Educational Institutions (FIST) (SR/FST/LSI-667/2016) (C), and MHRD-RUSA 2.0, New Delhi (F.24e51/2014-U, MoE-STARS (No.MoE-STARS/STARS-2/2023-0966 dt:29-05-2024), RR acknowledges Indian Council of Medical Research, New Delhi (ICMR) for providing financial assistance through ICMR/SRF Fellowship (AMR/Fellowship/24/2022-ECD-II).

REFERENCES

[1] S.K. Niazi, and Z. Mariam, "Computer-aided drug design and drug discovery: a prospective analysis", *Pharmaceuticals (Basel),* vol. 17, no. 1, p. 22, 2023. [http://dx.doi.org/10.3390/ph17010022] [PMID: 38256856]

[2] A.V. Sadybekov, and V. Katritch, "Computational approaches streamlining drug discovery", *Nature,* vol. 616, no. 7958, pp. 673-685, 2023. [http://dx.doi.org/10.1038/s41586-023-05905-z] [PMID: 37100941]

[3] I.V. Hinkson, B. Madej, and E.A. Stahlberg, "Accelerating therapeutics for opportunities in medicine: a paradigm shift in drug discovery", *Front. Pharmacol.,* vol. 11, p. 770, 2020. [http://dx.doi.org/10.3389/fphar.2020.00770] [PMID: 32694991]

[4] A. Sethi, and B. Rathi, "Artificial intelligence in drug discovery: A mirage or an oasis?", *Drug Discov. Today,* vol. 29, no. 6, 2024.103994 [http://dx.doi.org/10.1016/j.drudis.2024.103994] [PMID: 38663577]

[5] T. Davenport, and R. Kalakota, "The potential for artificial intelligence in healthcare", *Future Healthc. J.,* vol. 6, no. 2, pp. 94-98, 2019. [http://dx.doi.org/10.7861/futurehosp.6-2-94] [PMID: 31363513]

[6] K.H. Yu, A.L. Beam, and I.S. Kohane, "Artificial intelligence in healthcare", *Nat. Biomed. Eng.,* vol. 2, no. 10, pp. 719-731, 2018. [http://dx.doi.org/10.1038/s41551-018-0305-z] [PMID: 31015651]

[7] F.E. Agamah, G.K. Mazandu, R. Hassan, C.D. Bope, N.E. Thomford, A. Ghansah, and E.R. Chimusa, "Computational/*in silico* methods in drug target and lead prediction", *Brief. Bioinform.,* vol. 21, no. 5, pp. 1663-1675, 2020. [http://dx.doi.org/10.1093/bib/bbz103] [PMID: 31711157]

[8] G. Sliwoski, S. Kothiwale, J. Meiler, and E.W. Lowe Jr, "Computational methods in drug discovery", *Pharmacol. Rev.,* vol. 66, no. 1, pp. 334-395, 2014. [http://dx.doi.org/10.1124/pr.112.007336] [PMID: 24381236]

[9] A. Rasul *et al.*, "Target Identification Approaches in Drug Discovery," in Drug Target Selection and Validation, M. T. Scotti and C. L. Bellera, Eds., Computer-Aided Drug Discovery and Design, vol. 1. Cham, Switzerland: Springer, 2022. [http://dx.doi.org/10.1007/978-3-030-95895-4_3]

[10] Y. Tabana, D. Babu, R. Fahlman, A.G. Siraki, and K. Barakat, "Target identification of small molecules: an overview of the current applications in drug discovery", *BMC Biotechnol.,* vol. 23, no. 1, p. 44, 2023. [http://dx.doi.org/10.1186/s12896-023-00815-4] [PMID: 37817108]

[11] R.L. Davis, "Mechanism of action and target identification: a matter of timing in drug discovery", *iScience,* vol. 23, no. 9, 2020.101487 [http://dx.doi.org/10.1016/j.isci.2020.101487] [PMID: 32891054]

[12] E.L. Korn, J.A. Moscow, and B. Freidlin, "Dose optimization during drug development: whether and when to optimize", *J. Natl. Cancer Inst.,* vol. 115, no. 5, pp. 492-497, 2023. [http://dx.doi.org/10.1093/jnci/djac232] [PMID: 36534891]

[13] D. Sun, W. Gao, H. Hu, and S. Zhou, "Why 90% of clinical drug development fails and how to improve it?", *Acta Pharm. Sin. B,* vol. 12, no. 7, pp. 3049-3062, 2022. [http://dx.doi.org/10.1016/j.apsb.2022.02.002] [PMID: 35865092]

[14] J. Sundarasekar and G. Sahgal, "Role of genomics and proteomics in drug discovery," in Concepts in Pharmaceutical Biotechnology and Drug Development, S. Bose, A. C. Shukla, M. R. Baig, and S. Banerjee, Eds., Interdisciplinary Biotechnological Advances. Singapore: Springer, 2024. [Online]. Available: [http://dx.doi.org/10.1007/978-981-97-1148-2_11]

[15] R. Spreafico, L.B. Soriaga, J. Grosse, H.W. Virgin, and A. Telenti, "Advances in genomics for drug development", *Genes (Basel),* vol. 11, no. 8, p. 942, 2020. [http://dx.doi.org/10.3390/genes11080942] [PMID: 32824125]

[16] C. Finan, A. Gaulton, F.A. Kruger, R.T. Lumbers, T. Shah, J. Engmann, L. Galver, R. Kelley, A. Karlsson, R. Santos, J.P. Overington, A.D. Hingorani, and J.P. Casas, "The druggable genome and support for target identification and validation in drug development", *Sci. Transl. Med.,* vol. 9, no. 383, 2017.eaag1166 [http://dx.doi.org/10.1126/scitranslmed.aag1166] [PMID: 28356508]

[17] S. Namba, T. Konuma, K.H. Wu, W. Zhou, and Y. Okada, "A practical guideline of genomics-driven drug discovery in the era of global biobank meta-analysis", *Cell Genomics,* vol. 2, no. 10, 2022.100190 [http://dx.doi.org/10.1016/j.xgen.2022.100190] [PMID: 36778001]

[18] C. Cao, and J. Moult, "GWAS and drug targets", *BMC Genomics,* vol. 15, no. S4, suppl. Suppl. 4, p. S5, 2014. [http://dx.doi.org/10.1186/1471-2164-15-S4-S5] [PMID: 25057111]

[19] L. Shu, M. Blencowe, and X. Yang, "Translating GWAS findings to novel therapeutic targets for coronary artery disease", *Front. Cardiovasc. Med.,* vol. 5, p. 56, 2018. [http://dx.doi.org/10.3389/fcvm.2018.00056] [PMID: 29900175]

[20] E. Uffelmann, Q.Q. Huang, N.S. Munung, J. de Vries, Y. Okada, A.R. Martin, H.C. Martin, T. Lappalainen, and D. Posthuma, "Genome-wide association studies", *Nat. Rev. Methods Primers,* vol. 1, no. 1, p. 59, 2021. [http://dx.doi.org/10.1038/s43586-021-00056-9]

[21] W.Y. Lin, C.C. Huang, Y.L. Liu, S.J. Tsai, and P.H. Kuo, "Polygenic approaches to detect gene–environment interactions when external information is unavailable", *Brief. Bioinform.,* vol. 20, no. 6, pp. 2236-2252, 2019. [http://dx.doi.org/10.1093/bib/bby086] [PMID: 30219835]

[22] S. Carpenter, and R. Conlan, "Clinical functional genomics", *Cancers (Basel),* vol. 13, no. 18, p. 4627, 2021. [http://dx.doi.org/10.3390/cancers13184627] [PMID: 34572854]

[23] E.M. Bunnik, and K.G. Le Roch, "An introduction to functional genomics and systems biology", *Adv. Wound Care (New Rochelle),* vol. 2, no. 9, pp. 490-498, 2013. [http://dx.doi.org/10.1089/wound.2012.0379] [PMID: 24527360]

[24] M. Jost, and J.S. Weissman, "CRISPR approaches to small molecule target identification", *ACS Chem. Biol.,* vol. 13, no. 2, pp. 366-375, 2018. [http://dx.doi.org/10.1021/acschembio.7b00965] [PMID: 29261286]

[25] J.E. Neggers, B. Kwanten, T. Dierckx, H. Noguchi, A. Voet, L. Bral, K. Minner, B. Massant, N. Kint, M. Delforge, T. Vercruysse, E. Baloglu, W. Senapedis, M. Jacquemyn, and D. Daelemans, "Target identification of small molecules using large-scale CRISPR-Cas mutagenesis scanning of essential genes", *Nat. Commun.,* vol. 9, no. 1, p. 502, 2018. [http://dx.doi.org/10.1038/s41467-017-02349-8] [PMID: 29402884]

[26] A.L. Jackson, and P.S. Linsley, "Recognizing and avoiding siRNA off-target effects for target

identification and therapeutic application", *Nat. Rev. Drug Discov.,* vol. 9, no. 1, pp. 57-67, 2010. [http://dx.doi.org/10.1038/nrd3010] [PMID: 20043028]

[27] W. Xu, X. Jiang, and L. Huang, "RNA interference technology," in Comprehensive Biotechnology, 3rd ed., M. Moo-Young, Ed. Oxford, UK: Pergamon, 2019, pp. 560–575. [Online]. Available: [http://dx.doi.org/10.1016/B978-0-444-64046-8.00282-2]

[28] K.K. Kopec, D. Bozyczko-Coyne, and M. Williams, "Target identification and validation in drug discovery: the role of proteomics", *Biochem. Pharmacol.,* vol. 69, no. 8, pp. 1133-1139, 2005. [http://dx.doi.org/10.1016/j.bcp.2005.01.004] [PMID: 15794933]

[29] V. Murty, [http://dx.doi.org/10.2174/138920207781386942]

[30] D. Rosati, M. Palmieri, G. Brunelli, A. Morrione, F. Iannelli, E. Frullanti, and A. Giordano, "Differential gene expression analysis pipelines and bioinformatic tools for the identification of specific biomarkers: A review", *Comput. Struct. Biotechnol. J.,* vol. 23, pp. 1154-1168, 2024. [http://dx.doi.org/10.1016/j.csbj.2024.02.018] [PMID: 38510977]

[31] T.J. Hedl, R. San Gil, F. Cheng, S.L. Rayner, J.M. Davidson, A. De Luca, M.D. Villalva, H. Ecroyd, A.K. Walker, and A. Lee, "Proteomics approaches for biomarker and drug target discovery in ALS and FTD", *Front. Neurosci.,* vol. 13, p. 548, 2019. [http://dx.doi.org/10.3389/fnins.2019.00548] [PMID: 31244593]

[32] H. Lu, Q. Zhou, J. He, Z. Jiang, C. Peng, R. Tong, and J. Shi, "Recent advances in the development of protein–protein interactions modulators: mechanisms and clinical trials", *Signal Transduct. Target. Ther.,* vol. 5, no. 1, p. 213, 2020. [http://dx.doi.org/10.1038/s41392-020-00315-3] [PMID: 32968059]

[33] J. Loscalzo, "Molecular interaction networks and drug development: Novel approach to drug target identification and drug repositioning", *FASEB J.,* vol. 37, no. 1, 2023.e22660 [http://dx.doi.org/10.1096/fj.202201683R] [PMID: 36468661]

[34] C.V. Dang, E.P. Reddy, K.M. Shokat, and L. Soucek, "Drugging the 'undruggable' cancer targets", *Nat. Rev. Cancer,* vol. 17, no. 8, pp. 502-508, 2017. [http://dx.doi.org/10.1038/nrc.2017.36] [PMID: 28643779]

[35] V. Blay, B. Tolani, S.P. Ho, and M.R. Arkin, "High-Throughput Screening: today's biochemical and cell-based approaches", *Drug Discov. Today,* vol. 25, no. 10, pp. 1807-1821, 2020. [http://dx.doi.org/10.1016/j.drudis.2020.07.024] [PMID: 32801051]

[36] M. Schenone, V. Dančík, B.K. Wagner, and P.A. Clemons, "Target identification and mechanism of action in chemical biology and drug discovery", *Nat. Chem. Biol.,* vol. 9, no. 4, pp. 232-240, 2013. [http://dx.doi.org/10.1038/nchembio.1199] [PMID: 23508189]

[37] W.F. An, and N. Tolliday, "Cell-based assays for high-throughput screening", *Mol. Biotechnol.,* vol. 45, no. 2, pp. 180-186, 2010. [http://dx.doi.org/10.1007/s12033-010-9251-z] [PMID: 20151227]

[38] F. Vincent, P.M. Loria, A.D. Weston, C.M. Steppan, R. Doyonnas, Y.M. Wang, K.L. Rockwell, and M.C. Peakman, "Hit triage and validation in phenotypic screening: considerations and strategies", *Cell Chem. Biol.,* vol. 27, no. 11, pp. 1332-1346, 2020. [http://dx.doi.org/10.1016/j.chembiol.2020.08.009] [PMID: 32888500]

[39] G. Klebe, "Recent developments in structure-based drug design", *J. Mol. Med. (Berl.),* vol. 78, no. 5, pp. 269-281, 2000. [http://dx.doi.org/10.1007/s001090000084] [PMID: 10954199]

[40] J.P. Renaud, A. Chari, C. Ciferri, W. Liu, H.W. Rémigy, H. Stark, and C. Wiesmann, "Cryo-EM in drug discovery: achievements, limitations and prospects", *Nat. Rev. Drug Discov.,* vol. 17, no. 7, pp. 471-492, 2018. [http://dx.doi.org/10.1038/nrd.2018.77] [PMID: 29880918]

[41] R. Fernandez-Leiro, and S.H.W. Scheres, "Unravelling biological macromolecules with cryo-electron microscopy", *Nature,* vol. 537, no. 7620, pp. 339-346, 2016. [http://dx.doi.org/10.1038/nature19948] [PMID: 27629640]

[42] N. Jones, "Crystallography: Atomic secrets", *Nature,* vol. 505, no. 7485, pp. 602-603, 2014. [http://dx.doi.org/10.1038/505602a] [PMID: 24476871]

[43] B.L. Nannenga, and T. Gonen, "The cryo-EM method microcrystal Electron Diffraction (MicroED)", *Nat. Methods,* vol. 16, no. 5, pp. 369-379, 2019. [http://dx.doi.org/10.1038/s41592-019-0395-x] [PMID: 31040436]

[44] E.H.B. Maia, L.C. Assis, T.A. de Oliveira, A.M. da Silva, and A.G. Taranto, "Structure-based virtual screening: from classical to artificial intelligence", *Front Chem.,* vol. 8, p. 343, 2020. [http://dx.doi.org/10.3389/fchem.2020.00343] [PMID: 32411671]

[45] N.M. Tripathi, and A. Bandyopadhyay, "High Throughput Virtual Screening (HTVS) of peptide library: Technological advancement in ligand discovery", *Eur. J. Med. Chem.,* vol. 243, 2022.114766 [http://dx.doi.org/10.1016/j.ejmech.2022.114766] [PMID: 36122548]

[46] M. Wójcikowski, P.J. Ballester, and P. Siedlecki, "Performance of machine-learning scoring functions in structure-based virtual screening", *Sci. Rep.,* vol. 7, no. 1, p. 46710, 2017. [http://dx.doi.org/10.1038/srep46710] [PMID: 28440302]

[47] X.Y. Meng, H.X. Zhang, M. Mezei, and M. Cui, "Molecular docking: a powerful approach for structure-based drug discovery", *Curr. Computeraided Drug Des.,* vol. 7, no. 2, pp. 146-157, 2011. [http://dx.doi.org/10.2174/157340911795677602] [PMID: 21534921]

[48] A. Lavecchia, and C. Giovanni, "Virtual screening strategies in drug discovery: a critical review", *Curr. Med. Chem.,* vol. 20, no. 23, pp. 2839-2860, 2013. [http://dx.doi.org/10.2174/09298673113209990001] [PMID: 23651302]

[49] D.J. Huggins, P.C. Biggin, M.A. Dämgen, J.W. Essex, S.A. Harris, R.H. Henchman, S. Khalid, A. Kuzmanic, C.A. Laughton, J. Michel, A.J. Mulholland, E. Rosta, M.S.P. Sansom, and M.W. van der Kamp, "Biomolecular simulations: From dynamics and mechanisms to computational assays of biological activity", *Wiley Interdiscip. Rev. Comput. Mol. Sci.,* vol. 9, no. 3, 2019.e1393 [http://dx.doi.org/10.1002/wcms.1393]

[50] R. Shukla and T. Tripathi, "Molecular dynamics simulation of protein and protein–ligand complexes," in Computer-Aided Drug Design, D. B. Singh, Ed. Singapore: Springer, 2020. [Online]. Available: [http://dx.doi.org/10.1007/978-981-15-6815-2_7]

[51] M. Amaral, D.B. Kokh, J. Bomke, A. Wegener, H.P. Buchstaller, H.M. Eggenweiler, P. Matias, C. Sirrenberg, R.C. Wade, and M. Frech, "Protein conformational flexibility modulates kinetics and thermodynamics of drug binding", *Nat. Commun.,* vol. 8, no. 1, p. 2276, 2017. [http://dx.doi.org/10.1038/s41467-017-02258-w] [PMID: 29273709]

[52] S. S. Bhunia, M. Saxena, and A. K. Saxena, "Ligand- and structure-based virtual screening in drug discovery," in Biophysical and Computational Tools in Drug Discovery, A. K. Saxena, Ed., Topics in Medicinal Chemistry, vol. 37. Cham, Switzerland: Springer, 2021. [Online]. Available: [http://dx.doi.org/10.1007/7355_2021_130]

[53] V. Yadav, and J. Reang, Vinita, and R. K. Tonk, "Ligand-Based Drug Design (LBDD).*Computer Aided Drug Design (CADD): From Ligand-Based Methods to Structure-Based Approaches.* Elsevier, 2022, pp. 57-99. [http://dx.doi.org/10.1016/B978-0-323-90608-1.00009-5]

[54] R. Perkins, H. Fang, W. Tong, and W.J. Welsh, "Quantitative structure-activity relationship methods: Perspectives on drug discovery and toxicology", *Environ. Toxicol. Chem.,* vol. 22, no. 8, pp. 1666-1679, 2003. [http://dx.doi.org/10.1897/01-171] [PMID: 12924569]

[55] T. Wang, M.B. Wu, J.P. Lin, and L.R. Yang, "Quantitative structure–activity relationship: promising

advances in drug discovery platforms", *Expert Opin. Drug Discov.,* vol. 10, no. 12, pp. 1283-1300, 2015.
[http://dx.doi.org/10.1517/17460441.2015.1083006] [PMID: 26358617]

[56] F. Hassanzadeh, S. Sadeghian-Rizi, and A. Sakhteman, "A Quantitative Structure-Activity Relationship (QSAR) study of some diaryl urea derivatives of B-RAF inhibitors", *Res. Pharm. Sci.,* vol. 11, no. 6, pp. 445-453, 2016.
[http://dx.doi.org/10.4103/1735-5362.194869] [PMID: 28003837]

[57] H. Sun, "Pharmacophore-based virtual screening", *Curr. Med. Chem.,* vol. 15, no. 10, pp. 1018-1024, 2008.
[http://dx.doi.org/10.2174/092986708784049630] [PMID: 18393859]

[58] F. Wu, Y. Zhou, L. Li, X. Shen, G. Chen, X. Wang, X. Liang, M. Tan, and Z. Huang, "Computational approaches in preclinical studies on drug discovery and development", *Front Chem.,* vol. 8, p. 726, 2020.
[http://dx.doi.org/10.3389/fchem.2020.00726] [PMID: 33062633]

[59] F. Zhong, J. Xing, X. Li, X. Liu, Z. Fu, Z. Xiong, D. Lu, X. Wu, J. Zhao, X. Tan, F. Li, X. Luo, Z. Li, K. Chen, M. Zheng, and H. Jiang, "Artificial intelligence in drug design", *Sci. China Life Sci.,* vol. 61, no. 10, pp. 1191-1204, 2018.
[http://dx.doi.org/10.1007/s11427-018-9342-2] [PMID: 30054833]

[60] N. Brown, P. Ertl, R. Lewis, T. Luksch, D. Reker, and N. Schneider, "Artificial intelligence in chemistry and drug design", *J. Comput. Aided Mol. Des.,* vol. 34, no. 7, pp. 709-715, 2020.
[http://dx.doi.org/10.1007/s10822-020-00317-x] [PMID: 32468207]

[61] Y. Ding, J.H. Sohn, M.G. Kawczynski, H. Trivedi, R. Harnish, N.W. Jenkins, D. Lituiev, T.P. Copeland, M.S. Aboian, C. Mari Aparici, S.C. Behr, R.R. Flavell, S.Y. Huang, K.A. Zalocusky, L. Nardo, Y. Seo, R.A. Hawkins, M. Hernandez Pampaloni, D. Hadley, and B.L. Franc, "A deep learning model to predict a diagnosis of alzheimer disease by using 18 F-FDG PET of the brain", *Radiology,* vol. 290, no. 2, pp. 456-464, 2019.
[http://dx.doi.org/10.1148/radiol.2018180958] [PMID: 30398430]

[62] A. Narin, C. Kaya, and Z. Pamuk, "Automatic detection of coronavirus disease (COVID-19) using X-ray images and deep convolutional neural networks", *Pattern Anal. Appl.,* vol. 24, no. 3, pp. 1207-1220, 2021.
[http://dx.doi.org/10.1007/s10044-021-00984-y] [PMID: 33994847]

[63] C. Berzuini, R. Bellazzi, S. Quaglini, and D.J. Spiegelhalter, "Bayesian networks for patient monitoring", *Artif. Intell. Med.,* vol. 4, no. 3, pp. 243-260, 1992.
[http://dx.doi.org/10.1016/0933-3657(92)90030-S]

[64] K. Heikamp, and J. Bajorath, "Support vector machines for drug discovery", *Expert Opin. Drug Discov.,* vol. 9, no. 1, pp. 93-104, 2014.
[http://dx.doi.org/10.1517/17460441.2014.866943] [PMID: 24304044]

[65] K.A. Carpenter, D.S. Cohen, J.T. Jarrell, and X. Huang, "Deep learning and virtual drug screening", *Future Med. Chem.,* vol. 10, no. 21, pp. 2557-2567, 2018.
[http://dx.doi.org/10.4155/fmc-2018-0314] [PMID: 30288997]

[66] S.R. Krishnan, N. Bung, S.R. Vangala, R. Srinivasan, G. Bulusu, and A. Roy, "*De Novo* Structure-Based Drug Design Using Deep Learning", *J. Chem. Inf. Model.,* vol. 62, no. 21, pp. 5100-5109, 2022.
[http://dx.doi.org/10.1021/acs.jcim.1c01319] [PMID: 34792338]

[67] D.D. Martinelli, "Generative machine learning for *de novo* drug discovery: A systematic review", *Comput. Biol. Med.,* vol. 145, 2022.105403
[http://dx.doi.org/10.1016/j.compbiomed.2022.105403] [PMID: 35339849]

[68] V.G. Maltarollo, J.C. Gertrudes, P.R. Oliveira, and K.M. Honorio, "Applying machine learning techniques for ADME-Tox prediction: a review", *Expert Opin. Drug Metab. Toxicol.,* vol. 11, no. 2, pp. 259-271, 2015.

[http://dx.doi.org/10.1517/17425255.2015.980814] [PMID: 25440524]

[69] J.L. Medina-Franco, M.A. Giulianotti, G.S. Welmaker, and R.A. Houghten, "Shifting from the single to the multitarget paradigm in drug discovery", *Drug Discov. Today,* vol. 18, no. 9-10, pp. 495-501, 2013.
[http://dx.doi.org/10.1016/j.drudis.2013.01.008] [PMID: 23340113]

[70] A. Kabir, and A. Muth, "Polypharmacology: The science of multi-targeting molecules", *Pharmacol. Res.,* vol. 176, 2022.106055
[http://dx.doi.org/10.1016/j.phrs.2021.106055] [PMID: 34990865]

[71] C. Nogales, Z.M. Mamdouh, M. List, C. Kiel, A.I. Casas, and H.H.H.W. Schmidt, "Network pharmacology: curing causal mechanisms instead of treating symptoms", *Trends Pharmacol. Sci.,* vol. 43, no. 2, pp. 136-150, 2022.
[http://dx.doi.org/10.1016/j.tips.2021.11.004] [PMID: 34895945]

[72] J. Tang, and T. Aittokallio, "Network pharmacology strategies toward multi-target anticancer therapies: from computational models to experimental design principles", *Curr. Pharm. Des.,* vol. 20, no. 1, pp. 23-36, 2014.
[http://dx.doi.org/10.2174/13816128113199990470] [PMID: 23530504]

[73] A. Gangwal, A. Ansari, I. Ahmad, A.K. Azad, and W.M.A. Wan Sulaiman, "Current strategies to address data scarcity in artificial intelligence-based drug discovery: A comprehensive review", *Comput. Biol. Med.,* vol. 179, 2024.108734
[http://dx.doi.org/10.1016/j.compbiomed.2024.108734] [PMID: 38964243]

[74] A.I. Odugbemi, C. Nyirenda, A. Christoffels, and S.A. Egieyeh, "Artificial intelligence in antidiabetic drug discovery: The advances in QSAR and the prediction of α-glucosidase inhibitors", *Comput. Struct. Biotechnol. J.,* vol. 23, pp. 2964-2977, 2024.
[http://dx.doi.org/10.1016/j.csbj.2024.07.003] [PMID: 39148608]

[75] L.K. Vora, A.D. Gholap, K. Jetha, R.R.S. Thakur, H.K. Solanki, and V.P. Chavda, "Artificial intelligence in pharmaceutical technology and drug delivery design", *Pharmaceutics,* vol. 15, no. 7, p. 1916, 2023.
[http://dx.doi.org/10.3390/pharmaceutics15071916] [PMID: 37514102]

[76] B.S. Yadav, and V. Tripathi, "Recent advances in the system biology-based target identification and drug discovery", *Curr. Top. Med. Chem.,* vol. 18, no. 20, pp. 1737-1744, 2018.
[http://dx.doi.org/10.2174/1568026618666181025112344] [PMID: 30360719]

[77] B. Webb, and A. Sali, "Comparative protein structure modeling using MODELLER", *Curr. Protoc. Bioinformatics,* vol. 54, no. 1, pp. 6.1-, 37, 2016.
[http://dx.doi.org/10.1002/cpbi.3] [PMID: 27322406]

[78] J. Jumper, R. Evans, A. Pritzel, T. Green, M. Figurnov, O. Ronneberger, K. Tunyasuvunakool, R. Bates, A. Žídek, A. Potapenko, A. Bridgland, C. Meyer, S.A.A. Kohl, A.J. Ballard, A. Cowie, B. Romera-Paredes, S. Nikolov, R. Jain, J. Adler, T. Back, S. Petersen, D. Reiman, E. Clancy, M. Zielinski, M. Steinegger, M. Pacholska, T. Berghammer, S. Bodenstein, D. Silver, O. Vinyals, A.W. Senior, K. Kavukcuoglu, P. Kohli, and D. Hassabis, "Highly accurate protein structure prediction with AlphaFold", *Nature,* vol. 596, no. 7873, pp. 583-589, 2021.
[http://dx.doi.org/10.1038/s41586-021-03819-2] [PMID: 34265844]

[79] S.B. Guo, Y. Meng, L. Lin, Z.Z. Zhou, H.L. Li, X.P. Tian, and W.J. Huang, "Artificial intelligence alphafold model for molecular biology and drug discovery: a machine-learning-driven informatics investigation", *Mol. Cancer,* vol. 23, no. 1, p. 223, 2024.
[http://dx.doi.org/10.1186/s12943-024-02140-6] [PMID: 39369244]

[80] K.A. Carpenter, and X. Huang, "Machine learning-based virtual screening and its applications to alzheimer's drug discovery: a review", *Curr. Pharm. Des.,* vol. 24, no. 28, pp. 3347-3358, 2018.
[http://dx.doi.org/10.2174/1381612824666180607124038] [PMID: 29879881]

[81] W. Lian, J. Fang, C. Li, X. Pang, A.L. Liu, and G.H. Du, "Discovery of Influenza A virus

neuraminidase inhibitors using support vector machine and Naïve Bayesian models", *Mol. Divers.*, vol. 20, no. 2, pp. 439-451, 2016.
[http://dx.doi.org/10.1007/s11030-015-9641-z] [PMID: 26689205]

[82] L. Wang, X. Le, L. Li, Y. Ju, Z. Lin, Q. Gu, and J. Xu, "Discovering new agents active against methicillin-resistant *Staphylococcus aureus* with ligand-based approaches", *J. Chem. Inf. Model.*, vol. 54, no. 11, pp. 3186-3197, 2014.
[http://dx.doi.org/10.1021/ci500253q] [PMID: 25375651]

[83] M. Mochizuki, S.D. Suzuki, K. Yanagisawa, M. Ohue, and Y. Akiyama, "QEX: target-specific druglikeness filter enhances ligand-based virtual screening", *Mol. Divers.*, vol. 23, no. 1, pp. 11-18, 2019.
[http://dx.doi.org/10.1007/s11030-018-9842-3] [PMID: 29971617]

[84] A.O. Basile, A. Yahi, and N.P. Tatonetti, "Artificial intelligence for drug toxicity and safety", *Trends Pharmacol. Sci.*, vol. 40, no. 9, pp. 624-635, 2019.
[http://dx.doi.org/10.1016/j.tips.2019.07.005] [PMID: 31383376]

[85] E. Pérez Santín, R. Rodríguez Solana, M. González García, M.D.M. García Suárez, G.D. Blanco Díaz, M.D. Cima Cabal, J.M. Moreno Rojas, and J.I. López Sánchez, "Toxicity prediction based on artificial intelligence: A multidisciplinary overview", *Wiley Interdiscip. Rev. Comput. Mol. Sci.*, vol. 11, no. 5, 2021.e1516
[http://dx.doi.org/10.1002/wcms.1516]

[86] A.H. Vo, T.R. Van Vleet, R.R. Gupta, M.J. Liguori, and M.S. Rao, "An overview of machine learning and big data for drug toxicity evaluation", *Chem. Res. Toxicol.*, vol. 33, no. 1, pp. 20-37, 2020.
[http://dx.doi.org/10.1021/acs.chemrestox.9b00227] [PMID: 31625725]

[87] X. Yang, Y. Wang, R. Byrne, G. Schneider, and S. Yang, "Concepts of artificial intelligence for computer-assisted drug discovery", *Chem. Rev.*, vol. 119, no. 18, pp. 10520-10594, 2019.
[http://dx.doi.org/10.1021/acs.chemrev.8b00728] [PMID: 31294972]

[88] V. Venkatraman, "FP-ADMET: a compendium of fingerprint-based ADMET prediction models", *J. Cheminform.*, vol. 13, no. 1, p. 75, 2021.
[http://dx.doi.org/10.1186/s13321-021-00557-5] [PMID: 34583740]

[89] Y. Wei, S. Li, Z. Li, Z. Wan, and J. Lin, "Interpretable-ADMET: a web service for ADMET prediction and optimization based on deep neural representation", *Bioinformatics,* vol. 38, no. 10, pp. 2863-2871, 2022.
[http://dx.doi.org/10.1093/bioinformatics/btac192] [PMID: 35561160]

[90] S. Singh, N. Kaur, and A. Gehlot, "Application of artificial intelligence in drug design: A review", *Comput. Biol. Med.,* vol. 179, 2024.108810
[http://dx.doi.org/10.1016/j.compbiomed.2024.108810] [PMID: 38991316]

[91] J.A. Weller, and R. Rohs, "Structure-based drug design with a deep hierarchical generative model", *J. Chem. Inf. Model.,* vol. 64, no. 16, pp. 6450-6463, 2024.
[http://dx.doi.org/10.1021/acs.jcim.4c01193] [PMID: 39058534]

[92] R. Özçelik, D. van Tilborg, J. Jiménez-Luna, and F. Grisoni, "Structure-based drug discovery with deep learning", *ChemBioChem,* vol. 24, no. 13, 2023.e202200776
[http://dx.doi.org/10.1002/cbic.202200776] [PMID: 37014633]

[93] A. Fluetsch, E. Di Lascio, G. Gerebtzoff, and R. Rodríguez-Pérez, "Adapting deep learning QSPR models to specific drug discovery projects", *Mol. Pharm.,* vol. 21, no. 4, pp. 1817-1826, 2024.
[http://dx.doi.org/10.1021/acs.molpharmaceut.3c01124] [PMID: 38373038]

[94] H.C.S. Chan, H. Shan, T. Dahoun, H. Vogel, and S. Yuan, "Advancing drug discovery *via* artificial intelligence", *Trends Pharmacol. Sci.,* vol. 40, no. 8, pp. 592-604, 2019.
[http://dx.doi.org/10.1016/j.tips.2019.06.004] [PMID: 31320117]

[95] J. Rantanen, and J. Khinast, "The future of pharmaceutical manufacturing sciences", *J. Pharm. Sci.,*

vol. 104, no. 11, pp. 3612-3638, 2015.
[http://dx.doi.org/10.1002/jps.24594] [PMID: 26280993]

[96] S.L. Jämsä-Jounela, "Future trends in process automation", *Annu. Rev. Contr.,* vol. 31, no. 2, pp. 211-220, 2007.
[http://dx.doi.org/10.1016/j.arcontrol.2007.08.003]

[97] S. Ghosh, and A. Singh, "The scope of Artificial Intelligence in mankind: A detailed review", *J. Phys. Conf. Ser.,* vol. 1531, 2020.012045
[http://dx.doi.org/10.1088/1742-6596/1531/1/012045]

[98] D. Paul, G. Sanap, S. Shenoy, D. Kalyane, K. Kalia, and R.K. Tekade, "Artificial intelligence in drug discovery and development", *Drug Discov. Today,* vol. 26, no. 1, pp. 80-93, 2021.
[http://dx.doi.org/10.1016/j.drudis.2020.10.010] [PMID: 33099022]

[99] H. Taherdoost and A. Ghofrani, "AI's role in revolutionizing personalized medicine by reshaping pharmacogenomics and drug therapy," Intelligent Pharmacy, vol. 2, no. 5, pp. 643–650, 2024. [Online]. Available: [http://dx.doi.org/10.1016/j.ipha.2024.08.005]

[100] W. Abbaoui, S. Retal, B. El Bhiri, N. Kharmoum, and S. Ziti, "Towards revolutionizing precision healthcare: A systematic literature review of artificial intelligence methods in precision medicine", *Inform. Med. Unlocked,* vol. 46, 2024.101475
[http://dx.doi.org/10.1016/j.imu.2024.101475]

[101] S.A. Alowais, S.S. Alghamdi, N. Alsuhebany, T. Alqahtani, A.I. Alshaya, S.N. Almohareb, A. Aldairem, M. Alrashed, K. Bin Saleh, H.A. Badreldin, M.S. Al Yami, S. Al Harbi, and A.M. Albekairy, "Revolutionizing healthcare: the role of artificial intelligence in clinical practice", *BMC Med. Educ.,* vol. 23, no. 1, p. 689, 2023.
[http://dx.doi.org/10.1186/s12909-023-04698-z] [PMID: 37740191]

[102] L.A. Biesheuvel, D.A. Dongelmans, and P.W.G. Elbers, "Artificial intelligence to advance acute and intensive care medicine", *Curr. Opin. Crit. Care,* vol. 30, no. 3, pp. 246-250, 2024.
[http://dx.doi.org/10.1097/MCC.0000000000001150] [PMID: 38525882]

[103] T. Al-Quraishi, N. Al-Quraishi, H. AlNabulsi, H. AL-Qarishey, and A.H. Ali, "Big data predictive analytics for personalized medicine: perspectives and challenges", *Applied Data Science and Analysis,* vol. 2024, pp. 32-38, 2024.
[http://dx.doi.org/10.58496/ADSA/2024/004]

[104] C. Carini, and A.A. Seyhan, "Tribulations and future opportunities for artificial intelligence in precision medicine", *J. Transl. Med.,* vol. 22, no. 1, p. 411, 2024.
[http://dx.doi.org/10.1186/s12967-024-05067-0] [PMID: 38702711]

[105] K.B. Johnson, W.Q. Wei, D. Weeraratne, M.E. Frisse, K. Misulis, K. Rhee, J. Zhao, and J.L. Snowdon, "Precision medicine, AI, and the future of personalized health care", *Clin. Transl. Sci.,* vol. 14, no. 1, pp. 86-93, 2021.
[http://dx.doi.org/10.1111/cts.12884] [PMID: 32961010]

[106] A.E. Rhatrif, B. Bouihi, and M. Mestari, "Challenges and limitations of artificial intelligence implementation in modern power grid", *Procedia Comput. Sci.,* vol. 236, pp. 83-92, 2024.
[http://dx.doi.org/10.1016/j.procs.2024.05.008]

[107] M. Ennab, and H. Mcheick, "Enhancing interpretability and accuracy of AI models in healthcare: a comprehensive review on challenges and future directions", *Front. Robot. AI,* vol. 11, 2024.1444763
[http://dx.doi.org/10.3389/frobt.2024.1444763] [PMID: 39677978]

[108] H. Askr, E. Elgeldawi, H. Aboul Ella, Y.A.M.M. Elshaier, M.M. Gomaa, and A.E. Hassanien, "Deep learning in drug discovery: an integrative review and future challenges", *Artif. Intell. Rev.,* vol. 56, no. 7, pp. 5975-6037, 2023.
[http://dx.doi.org/10.1007/s10462-022-10306-1] [PMID: 36415536]

CHAPTER 11

AI and NLP in Drug Discovery and Target Identification: Focus on COVID-19

Guneswar Sethi[1] and **Jeong Ho Hwang**[1,*]

[1] *Center for Companion Animal New Drug Development, Korea Institute of Toxicology, 30 Baehak 1-gil, Jeongeup, Jeollabuk-do - 56212, Republic of Korea*

Abstract: The integration of Artificial Intelligence (AI) and Natural Language Processing (NLP) is evidently accelerating the processes of drug discovery and target identification. The conventional techniques employed in these domains have been characterized by high labor intensity and cost, frequently resulting in extended timelines and substantial financial outlays. AI and NLP provide innovative solutions to streamline and enhance these processes by automating and improving accuracy. AI technologies, including Machine Learning (ML) and Deep Learning (DL), facilitate predictive modeling of drug activity, design novel drug molecules, and optimize lead compounds for improved efficacy and safety. Concurrently, NLP processing techniques facilitate the extraction of actionable insights from extensive biomedical literature and databases. This enables uncovering gene-disease associations, potential drug repurposing opportunities, and relevant biomolecular interactions. The combination of AI-driven predictive analytics with NLP-extracted knowledge enables researchers to achieve more accurate identification of therapeutic targets and promising drug candidates. This integrative approach accelerates the drug development timeline and enhances the precision of target identification. Despite these advancements, challenges such as data quality, model interpretability, and the necessity for experimental validation persist. Future developments in AI and NLP promise to refine drug discovery processes, leading to more effective and targeted therapeutic interventions and ultimately improving patient outcomes.

Keywords: Artificial Intelligence (AI), Natural Language Processing (NLP), Drug discovery, Target identification, Machine Learning (ML), Deep Learning (DL).

INTRODUCTION

Drug discovery and target identification are very pivotal for the pharmaceutical industry. However, the traditional approaches are often slow, expensive, and

* **Corresponding author Jeong Ho Hwang:** Center for Companion Animal New Drug Development, Korea Institute of Toxicology, 30 Baehak 1-gil, Jeonguep, Jeollabuk-do, 56212, Republic of Korea;
E-mail: jeongho.hwang@kitox.re.kr

A. Shankar, Saranya Jayapalan, & Basant. K. Tiwary (Eds.)

incompetent. Drug discovery is a laborious process that involves identifying disease-related genes, followed by experimental validation, high-throughput screening, lead optimization, preclinical testing, and clinical trials, which can take up to 15 years and cost \$1 to \$2 billion to bring a single drug to market [1, 2]. Due to prolonged clinical trial durations, nearly 90% of drug candidates failed to advance past phase I [3]. The difficulties of bringing drug candidates from the lab to the clinic are highlighted by the substantial financial support required, which is important for pharmaceutical corporations and academic organizations. Due to its poor success rate, there is an increasing demand for cutting-edge technologies to expedite and simplify this process. Thus, to increase the success rates of lead identifications in clinical trials, researchers increasingly use large-scale computational screening and molecular docking techniques [4]. However, traditional methodologies often suffer from inefficiencies and inaccuracies in predictive outcomes. The integration of DL and ML, both subsets of AI, has emerged as a promising solution to these challenges [5]. AI tools can accurately predict complex properties and relationships within biological systems while maintaining low computational costs, leading to their adoption in the pharmaceutical landscape [6]. ML has become an integral part of modern drug discovery, leveraging various algorithms such as DL, Bayesian Networks (BN), Random Forests (RF), clustering methods, and Support Vector Machines (SVM). Each of these algorithms has specialized functions: DL models are particularly effective at handling large datasets, supporting tasks like clinical imaging [7, 8], Virtual Screening (VS) [9, 10], and predicting bioactivity [11]. Bayesian networks contribute by predicting toxicity levels and patient responses to treatments, while RF is employed to identify molecular targets and select critical features [12, 13]. Clustering methods, including k-means and hierarchical clustering, help group drugs or patients with similar molecular or clinical characteristics. Other techniques like Principal Component Analysis (PCA) further simplify complex, high-dimensional data, revealing patterns that enhance understanding of toxicity risks and pharmacokinetic properties [14]. SVMs are particularly valuable for classifying data into distinct categories, essential for accurately predicting pharmacokinetic behaviors and assessing potential toxicity [15].

The convergence of AI and ML within drug discovery has already begun to streamline the R&D pipeline, easing access, reducing costs, and improving the efficiency of drug development. By adopting these technologies, the pharmaceutical industry is poised to overcome the limitations of traditional methodologies and bring effective treatments to market more rapidly.

AI in Drug Discovery

The AI-based computational modeling approach has transformed drug discovery by improving drug identification, target discovery, and prediction of toxicity and efficacy. ML algorithms have played an important role in expediting the discovery of lead compounds from large chemical libraries, including over 106 million molecules, further effectively addressing off-target toxicity [16]. Innovative tools such as AlphaFold, developed by Google's DeepMind, have transformed protein structure prediction, a crucial aspect of drug development.

Moreover, recent advancements have enabled AI to predict novel drug candidates and discover therapeutic peptides. Platforms, such as Deep-AmPEP30 [17] and ACP-DL [18], leverage DL methodologies to identify antimicrobial and anticancer peptides. Additionally, AI technologies are increasingly utilized to optimize drug dosages; for instance, the AI-PRS platform employs neural networks to correlate drug combinations and dosages with therapeutic efficacy. Various ML and statistical techniques also forecast potential disruptions in protein-protein interactions, enhancing our understanding of drug dynamics. AI's influence extends across multiple stages of drug discovery, from lead compound identification to structure-based drug design, drug repurposing, and dosage optimization. Table **1** summarizes the key AI techniques and their roles in drug discovery.

Table 1. Roles of AI techniques in drug discovery.

AI Technique	Role in Drug Discovery	Key Application
Machine Learning (ML)	Prediction of drug-target interaction	Lead compound identification
Deep Learning (DL)	Protein-ligand docking, virtual screening	Structure-based drug design
Natural Language Processing (NLP)	Text mining from biomedical literature for target identification	Biomedical literature mining
Reinforcement Learning (RL)	Optimization of drug design and synthesis process	Drug synthesis pathways

AI in drug screening enables researchers to dramatically reduce the number of compounds that require experimental testing, saving time and resources while increasing the probability of success. Furthermore, AI-driven drug discovery encompasses four major categories: drug design, polypharmacology, chemical synthesis, and drug screening. Fig. (**1**) illustrates these categories, highlighting AI's distinct roles.

AI in Drug Design

AI is revolutionizing medication design by significantly speeding the identification of possible therapeutic candidates. The initial step is collecting massive amounts of genomic, proteomic, and chemical data from many sources, including experimental research and literature. This data is then utilized to train AI models, allowing ML algorithms to detect complex relationships between chemical structures and biological processes. By analyzing Structure-Activity Relationships (SAR), AI can predict how specific molecular alterations affect biological processes. Based on these findings, AI algorithms can predict new medication candidates, focusing on molecules most likely to bind successfully to certain biological targets. But AI does not stop there; it goes one step further, suggesting changes to these lead compounds. This enables increased drug efficacy, reduced toxicity, and improved pharmacokinetic features, ultimately optimizing drug discovery [6]. The result is a more rapid, precise, and efficient strategy for generating novel treatments.

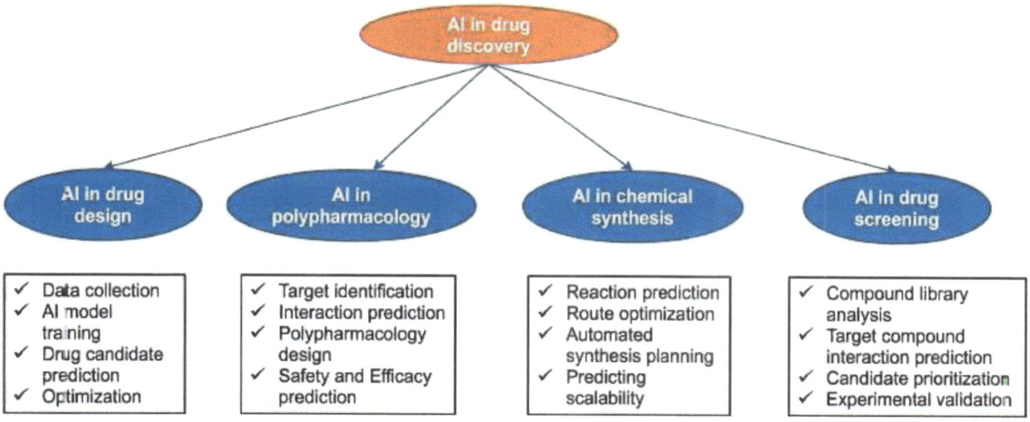

Fig. (1). Overview of AI applications in drug discovery.

AI in Polypharmacology

Polypharmacology focuses on developing therapeutics that engage multiple biological targets, providing a holistic approach to treatment. AI is instrumental in predicting these interactions, enabling the development of drugs with broader effects, particularly for challenging diseases like cancer and neurodegenerative diseases. AI improves the process of generating multi-target pharmaceuticals by streamlining each workflow phase. It starts by analyzing molecular structures and biological networks to uncover various pharmacological targets inside illness pathways, broadening the therapeutic interventions [19]. Using ML algorithms and molecular docking simulations, AI predicts how a single therapeutic molecule may interact with several targets simultaneously, providing a better knowledge of multi-target interactions. Furthermore, AI helps develop medications with synergistic effects, allowing for the regulation of many disease-related pathways to optimize therapeutic outcomes. Finally, AI evaluates the safety and efficacy of these multi-target medications by anticipating off-target effects and assessing interactions with other biological systems, resulting in a more thorough approach to drug safety assessment.

AI in Chemical Synthesis

AI has revolutionized the chemical synthesis process in drug development by making it more efficient and cost-effective. Traditionally, optimizing the synthesis of complex molecules requires multiple iterations, but AI models now streamline this process by predicting the most suitable synthetic pathways. By analyzing existing data on chemical reactions and their outcomes, AI algorithms can suggest the most likely routes for synthesizing a target compound. These predictions are then used to identify the most efficient reaction sequence, helping maximize yield, minimize costs, and reduce the occurrence of unwanted side reactions. Additionally, AI-powered retrosynthesis tools break down complex molecules into simpler components, offering detailed plans for laboratory synthesis. This automation speeds up the entire synthesis planning process, saving time and resources. Beyond planning, AI also evaluates the scalability of these synthetic routes, ensuring that they are not only feasible on a small scale but also practical for large-scale industrial production, thus optimizing the drug development process from lab to market [20].

AI in Drug Screening

AI plays a transformative role in drug screening by significantly speeding up the identification of compounds with therapeutic potential. Traditional methods involve testing thousands of compounds to find candidates, but AI enhances this by virtually simulating the interaction between drug candidates and their target proteins. AI can estimate the binding affinities of known and unknown compounds by processing large chemical libraries, allowing it to narrow down the most promising ones for further study. AI models replicate drug-target interactions using molecular docking and ML techniques to determine binding strength, stability, and biological activity. This enables AI to choose the most effective therapeutic candidates based on anticipated efficacy, eliminating those unlikely to succeed and allowing researchers to concentrate on the most promising compounds [21]. Once the best candidates have been identified, they are subjected to experimental testing to evaluate their efficacy through *in vitro* and *in vivo* investigations, speeding the discovery and development process from virtual screening to experimental validation.

NLP in Drug Discovery

NLP has emerged as a vital technology in drug discovery, enabling researchers to analyze unstructured textual data and uncover novel insights. NLP automates the extraction of critical insights from various sources, including scientific literature, patents, clinical trials, and health records. NLP applications can be categorized into four key areas: NLP for knowledge extraction, target identification, drug repurposing, and clinical trial analysis. The workflow of NLP in drug discovery, from data collection to knowledge extraction, is outlined in Fig. (**2**).

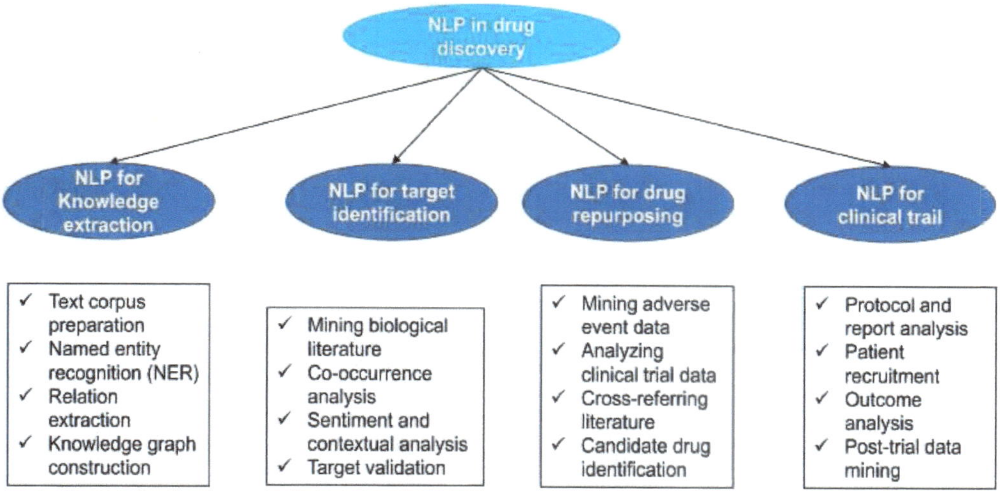

Fig. (2). Overview of NLP applications in drug discovery.

Knowledge Extraction

Knowledge extraction is crucial for navigating vast scientific literature and keeping up with the latest research developments in drug discovery. NLP streamlines this process by automating the extraction and synthesis of data from diverse textual resources. The process begins by curating a comprehensive collection of biomedical texts, such as research articles, patents, and clinical reports, from databases like PubMed and ClinicalTrials.gov. NLP algorithms then employ Named Entity Recognition (NER) techniques to identify key biological entities, such as genes, proteins, diseases, and drug compounds. Once these entities are identified, NLP further maps their relationships, revealing connections like drug-target interactions and gene-disease associations [22]. These relationships are then visualized as knowledge graphs, which provide a structured view of the complex interplay among biological components. This enables researchers to uncover new drug targets or gain insights into mechanisms of action, significantly advancing the efficiency and accuracy of drug discovery.

Target Identification

A significant challenge in drug discovery is identifying the correct biological targets for therapeutic intervention. NLP plays a crucial role by mining vast amounts of biomedical literature to discover potential targets associated with diseases and their molecular pathways. The approach starts with text mining, where NLP systems analyze large repositories of scientific literature to extract information on disease mechanisms and relevant therapeutic targets, such as genes and proteins. NLP identifies correlations between these biological entities through pattern recognition, detecting associations that may indicate potential drug targets. NLP does not just stop at extraction; it performs contextual analysis to evaluate how these targets are discussed and whether they are implicated in disease progression or play a role in therapeutic responses. This allows researchers to focus on the most promising candidates. Once these potential targets are identified, further validation is carried out by cross-referencing them with experimental data or using complementary computational models. This ensures that these candidates are viable options in the drug discovery pipeline [23].

Drug Repurposing

Drug repurposing presents a highly efficient strategy for discovering new therapeutic applications for existing drugs, significantly reducing both time and cost in drug development. NLP plays a vital role in this process by analyzing vast amounts of clinical and scientific data to uncover hidden opportunities. NLP systems mine clinical data, such as adverse event reports, electronic health records, and clinical trial outcomes, to detect patterns suggesting new drug uses. By scanning clinical trial reports, NLP identifies off-target effects or unexpected therapeutic benefits, which can be a rich source of insights for repurposing [22]. Additionally, NLP cross-references scientific literature and patents to discover novel drug-disease associations, which might not have been evident from initial studies. After gathering and analyzing this information, NLP can prioritize the most promising drug candidates for repurposing, flagging them for further experimental validation [22]. This approach enhances efficiency and broadens the scope of potential therapeutic interventions.

Clinical Trial Analysis

Clinical trials are vital for ensuring the safety and efficacy of new drugs; until now, the vast amount of unstructured text data generated from trial protocols, reports, and patient records has made it challenging to derive meaningful insights. NLP offers a practical solution by automating the analysis of clinical trial data, making the process more efficient. NLP systems can parse clinical trial protocols and reports, extracting essential details such as study objectives, treatment plans, patient eligibility, and outcomes [24]. This allows for quick access to critical information. Additionally, NLP can help optimize patient recruitment by analyzing electronic health records and identifying patients who match the eligibility criteria, thus speeding up the recruitment process. Once trials are completed, NLP can extract key findings from results, including signals of efficacy and patterns of adverse events, helping researchers evaluate the overall impact of the drug. Moreover, post-trial data, such as post-marketing studies and pharmacovigilance reports, can be analyzed using NLP to provide insights into a drug's long-term safety and efficacy, offering a comprehensive understanding of its performance even after clinical trials.

AI-Driven Target Identification

Identifying a biological target, typically a protein or gene implicated in a disease, is a crucial first step in drug development. AI and ML algorithms, particularly neural networks, have demonstrated impressive capabilities for predicting Drug-Target Interactions (DTIs), revealing potential targets that might not have been considered using traditional methods.

AI-based target identification typically involves:

Genomic Data Analysis

AI-based target identification frequently starts with analyzing genomic data, particularly gene expression profiles. ML techniques, such as clustering, regression models, and neural networks, are utilized to analyze large-scale transcriptomic data and detect genes exhibiting differential expression. These DEGs are often associated with disease conditions, allowing insights into which genes are upregulated or downregulated in disease states. The significance of AI in this context lies in its ability to handle high-dimensional data, identify hidden patterns, and predict gene functions or their involvement in disease pathways [25]. For example, Support Vector Machines (SVMs) or random forests can classify disease vs. healthy samples based on gene expression data. At the same time, DL models further help predict novel gene-disease associations. AI also excels in analyzing scRNA-seq data, which provides gene expression profiles at a single-cell level [26]. This allows researchers to understand disease heterogeneity at a cellular resolution and identify target genes specific to particular cell types.

Network Biology

AI and ML algorithms analyze complex biomolecular interactions in network biology, focusing on protein interaction networks. These networks map the physical and functional interactions between proteins in a cell, often offering insights into disease mechanisms. AI-based approaches, such as graph-based models or network embeddings, allow for prioritizing disease-associated proteins based on their connectivity, centrality, or roles in specific subnetworks (modules) [27]. The rationale is that proteins at the core of disease-related networks or those interacting with multiple disease-associated proteins may represent ideal drug targets. AI can refine these analyses by integrating other biological information, such as genetic mutations or pathway data, to create more nuanced models. DL models have been successfully employed to predict which proteins in PPI networks are likely critical in disease progression and good drug targets. Network-based AI approaches also help uncover functional module clusters of interacting proteins involved in disease pathways, thereby aiding the discovery of potential treatment targets.

Multi-omics Integration

AI also plays a crucial role in combining diverse omics datasets, such as genomics, proteomics, and metabolomics, to gain a comprehensive understanding of complex biological systems and diseases. Each omics layer provides different insights: genomics reveals DNA sequences and mutations, proteomics gives information about proteins and their interactions, and metabolomics focuses on cellular metabolic changes. Integrating these layers provides a systems-level understanding of disease mechanisms [28].

AI techniques, such as Bayesian networks, multi-view learning, and autoencoders, are commonly used to combine these diverse datasets. The ability of AI to merge multi-omics data offers a more holistic view of biological processes. It helps identify biomarkers and potential drug targets that might be missed when analyzing a single data layer. This integrative approach often uncovers novel disease-associated targets by correlating genetic mutations with changes in protein expression and metabolic shifts, leading to more effective and personalized therapies [29].

NLP-Driven Target Identification

NLP plays a significant role in identifying therapeutic targets within drug development and biomedicine. It utilizes AI to process and derive insights from extensive unstructured text sources. Here is how NLP-driven approaches contribute to target identification:

Mining Scientific Literature and Databases

NLP is highly effective at processing vast amounts of biomedical literature, such as research papers, clinical trials, and drug patents. Traditionally, the identification of potential drug targets relied heavily on manual curation, which is time-consuming and labor-intensive. NLP algorithms can automate this process from text data by identifying biomedical entities (genes, proteins, diseases) and their relationships, such as disease-gene associations or protein interactions. For instance, NLP-based tools like text mining for drug discovery or BioBERT are trained on biomedical literature to recognize key biological entities and relationships [26]. By extracting gene or protein mentions from millions of articles, these algorithms accelerate the identification of novel drug targets. NLP can also identify co-occurrences between disease symptoms and specific genetic mutations or proteins, suggesting new targets for drug development.

Gene-Disease Association and Drug Repositioning

NLP models can be applied to identify gene-disease associations, a key step in target identification. By extracting disease-related genes from existing literature, NLP can help prioritize which genes or proteins are most relevant to a particular condition. The PubMed database, for example, contains millions of research articles rich in such associations, and NLP models can efficiently sift through this information to identify novel connections.

NLP techniques have also been leveraged to aid drug repositioning, which involves discovering new therapeutic applications for already-approved medications. NLP models can detect potential off-label drug use by processing various data sources such as clinical reports, DrugBank databases, and real-world evidence [30]. These advanced models examine the intricate networks connecting diseases, targets, and drugs, revealing underlying relationships that may not be immediately apparent through conventional research approaches.

Knowledge Graphs and Ontology-Based Target Discovery

NLP also plays a key role in generating biomedical knowledge graphs and networks of interconnected biological entities such as genes, proteins, diseases, and drugs. Knowledge graphs, powered by NLP techniques, offer a visual and data-driven approach to exploring complex biological relationships [14]. In drug discovery, these graphs are used to find connections between diseases and molecular targets by integrating data from multiple sources.

Moreover, ontology-based NLP links textual data with structured biological databases, improving the accuracy of identifying biological terms and relationships. For example, tools like NCBO BioPortal [31] or UMLS Metathesaurus enable NLP-driven integration of disease ontologies with unstructured data, helping identify potential drug targets by associating genes or proteins with specific diseases [32].

NER in Biomedical Texts

NLP models often use NER to identify and classify biological terms like proteins, drugs, and diseases in text. By automating the extraction of these entities, NLP systems can analyze large volumes of biomedical literature and create datasets of potential drug targets. NLP-based NER systems trained on biomedical datasets (like Medline or PubMed Central) can pinpoint emerging therapeutic targets, accelerating the drug discovery pipeline [33]. Additionally, Machine Reading Comprehension (MRC) models such as BioASQ have been specifically trained to handle complex biomedical questions, assisting researchers in querying large text corpora for the most relevant gene-target or protein-disease relationships [34].

Case Study: ML and NLP Applications in Drug Discovery

COVID-19 Treatment and Vaccine Discovery Using AI

AI played a transformative role in the development of treatments and vaccines for COVID-19. ML algorithms analyzed diverse data sources to model virus-host interactions and predict effective treatment pathways. For instance, AI models assessed clinical trial data to forecast patient responses and optimize vaccine efficacy, especially for mRNA vaccines. Companies like Moderna and Pfizer used AI to streamline the design and validation phases of mRNA vaccines, fast-tracking clinical trials and aiding in the rapid vaccine rollout. Integrating AI-driven prediction models with clinical data enabled the swift identification of effective treatments and vaccine formulations, a crucial factor in containing the pandemic [35].

Protein-Based Drug Discovery for COVID-19

AI has been instrumental in accelerating the VS of repurposed drugs and new chemical compounds for COVID-19 treatments. By identifying existing drugs that interact with SARS-CoV-2 pathways, researchers aim to identify drugs that can quickly move into clinical trials due to established safety profiles. One notable early study by Gordon *et al.* reported 66 human proteins that interact with 26 viral proteins of SARS-CoV-2, laying the groundwork for drug repurposing efforts using these biological connections [36].

AI-driven network models have largely facilitated this analysis, focusing on the virus-host interactome. Companies like BenevolentAI and Atomwise have implemented knowledge graphs to explore these interactions and identified targets, such as the host protein AAK1, leading to the discovery of Baricitinib as a potential treatment [37, 38]. Initially approved for rheumatoid arthritis, Baricitinib was found to have promising effects against SARS-CoV-2 due to its modulation of pathways involved in viral infection [39].

Furthermore, multi-task DL models have identified several drugs by targeting critical viral proteins, including the main protease (3CLpro) and the spike protein [40, 41]. In addition, machine learning-aided molecular docking has been widely used to virtually screen databases of approved or druglike molecules. This approach requires high-quality structural information on the viral targets, such as crystal structures or homology models, and robust computational resources to evaluate drug binding. These AI-powered methodologies enable rapid assessment of large drug libraries, significantly shortening the timeline from virtual screening to potential COVID-19 therapies. The main protease, 3CLpro, is frequently targeted in COVID-19 virtual screening due to its essential role in viral replication and transcription. Since protease inhibitors have successfully treated other viral infections, they are an active area of research for SARS-CoV-2 [42]. Advanced DL approaches have been widely used to screen for 3CLpro inhibitors, relying on various datasets like the ZINC database, the FDA-approved LOPAC library [43], SWEETLEAD [44], and other comprehensive collections of purchasable drug compounds. By leveraging these resources, researchers can efficiently identify potential inhibitors that may be fast-tracked for COVID-19 therapy studies.

RNA-Based Therapeutics and Drug Discovery for COVID-19

Conserved structural elements are vital to coronaviruses' life cycles and add complexity layers to the regulatory information encoded in their RNA. Targeting these conserved elements makes it possible to reduce viral loads with minimal disruption to normal cellular functions. Recent progress in AI-driven computational modeling and large-scale RNA shape analysis techniques has been instrumental in addressing key challenges. Researchers have identified highly conserved RNA structural regions across various viral families, many of which have undergone functional validation. For instance, Rangan *et al.* pinpointed 106 structurally conserved regions as promising targets for potential antiviral agents [45]. Similarly, Park *et al.* discovered an RNA pseudoknot-binding molecule specifically against SARS-CoV-1 through target-based virtual screening [46]. Examining changes in RNA information enables the discovery of new and evolved therapeutic targets, such as Remdesivir, which recently received FDA approval, alongside other drug candidates [47].

Generative Approaches

AI has significantly transformed molecular generation in drug discovery, with Variational Autoencoders (VAEs) being notable models that enhance the diversity of data. For example, Chenthamarakshan *et al.*, in collaboration with IBM Research, developed a Variational Autoencoder (VAE) designed to encode molecular structures into a latent space, enabling the generation of molecular variants with tailored properties [48]. Similarly, Tang *et al.* introduced an enhanced deep Q-learning framework tailored for fragment-based drug design. This approach facilitates the stepwise construction of SARS-CoV-2-targeted molecules by sequentially adding individual fragments [49]. This method effectively designed novel compounds with strong binding affinities tailored to the structure of SARS-CoV-2's 3CLPro. Designing a drug-generative network involves several critical steps: first, collecting a dataset of drug-like molecules; next, representing these molecules in a computational format; then, modifying the molecules to enhance diversity; and finally, screening and adjusting the modified compounds for optimal characteristics. In *in silico* medicine, Generative Adversarial Networks (GANs) were explored to target the main protease, utilizing approaches like crystal structure-derived pocket generation, homology modeling, and ligand-based generation. These advancements highlight the growing intersection of AI and drug discovery, showcasing innovative methods to create effective therapeutic candidates against diseases like COVID-19.

COVID-19 Treatment and Vaccine Discovery Using NLP

The global pandemic led to the development of the CORD-19 dataset, a comprehensive resource designed to meet the urgent need for effective treatments. This comprehensive dataset compiled over 200,000 scientific articles on coronaviruses, their biological mechanisms, and potential therapeutic strategies. Researchers leveraged NLP techniques to efficiently navigate this vast repository of information.

NLP models played a crucial role in extracting pertinent data on the mechanisms of viral action, the immune responses elicited by the virus, and the identification of antiviral compounds with the potential to inhibit SARS-CoV-2. By analyzing existing literature on related viruses such as SARS and MERS, these models can predict candidate drugs for COVID-19 treatment based on similarities in viral behavior and potential therapeutic outcomes.

This NLP-driven literature mining process enhanced the efficiency of drug discovery and prioritized specific molecules for further investigation in laboratory settings (*in vitro* studies) and, eventually, clinical trials. This approach significantly accelerated the drug repurposing process, which is critical during a public health crisis when time is of the essence. Integrating NLP for information extraction, alongside Machine Learning (ML) algorithms, allowed researchers to refine their search and highlight promising treatments. For instance, well-known antiviral drugs like remdesivir and hydroxychloroquine were identified as potential candidates for inhibiting SARS-CoV-2, underscoring the effectiveness of AI-driven methodologies in rapidly addressing urgent health challenges [50]. In essence, the collaborative use of large-scale datasets and advanced computational techniques during the pandemic exemplified how innovative technologies could transform the landscape of drug discovery, enabling quicker responses to emerging infectious diseases.

Identifying Treatments for Rare Diseases Using AI and NLP

AI and NLP have made substantial contributions to rare disease research by enabling the identification of drug targets and therapeutic strategies through advanced data analysis. For instance, in Spinal Muscular Atrophy (SMA), AI models, complemented by NLP for literature review and data extraction, were used to analyze patient genetic and proteomic information, pinpointing neural pathways most impacted by SMA mutations [51]. A study employed AI to identify these specific pathways, allowing researchers to focus on potential therapeutic compounds that target these cellular mechanisms, providing key insights for treatment. AI and NLP's capacity to process and model interactions between compounds and disease pathways is essential for developing effective therapies for rare diseases, especially in scenarios with limited datasets. Additionally, by identifying relationships in vast scientific literature and patient data, AI can aid personalized medicine, potentially improving outcomes for rare diseases that lack targeted treatments [52, 53].

Predicting Drug-Target Interactions (DTIs) Using AI and NLP-Enhanced Models

AI, supported by NLP, has greatly advanced Drug-Target Interaction (DTI) prediction methodologies. In a recent study, NLP algorithms extracted chemical and pharmacological information from large-scale databases like PubChem [54] and ChEMBL [55], synthesizing insights for AI models trained to predict novel DTIs [56]. Chemical properties and known drug-target data were extracted using transformer-based NLP models to build comprehensive datasets. These were then analyzed by AI-driven models, including convolutional neural networks, to predict interactions for new drug classes, thereby reducing early-stage timelines. Previously, identifying effective DTIs required years. However, this NLP-AI hybrid approach enables the virtual screening of millions of compounds in mere weeks, highlighting the role of high-throughput, AI-powered analysis in optimizing drug discovery timelines. These examples showcase how integrating AI and NLP accelerates drug discovery and optimizes the identification of therapeutic targets, particularly for rare diseases and complex DTIs, laying a foundation for more targeted and efficient pharmaceutical research and development. These cases illustrate the transformative role of AI and NLP in expediting drug discovery and optimizing therapeutic strategies, particularly in crisis contexts and for diseases where traditional research is constrained by time and resources.

Challenges and Limitations of AI and NLP in Drug Discovery

AI and NLP are revolutionizing drug discovery by enhancing efficiency and data quality, yet they face significant challenges that hinder their full potential.

Data Quality and Availability

One of the most significant challenges in AI-driven drug discovery is the quality and availability of biomedical data. AI models, particularly ML and DL models, thrive on large datasets with high-quality labels. However, obtaining sufficient labeled biomedical data can be complex in drug discovery. Many datasets lack comprehensive annotations, and biomedical data, such as gene expression profiles or molecular interactions, are often fragmented across different studies and platforms. Furthermore, biological data may be biased toward well-studied diseases and targets, leaving rare diseases and novel targets underrepresented. Another problem is data noise. Experimental datasets can contain inconsistencies due to varying experimental conditions or differences in how data are recorded. This can lead to inaccurate models, reducing their ability to generalize effectively to unseen data. AI models trained on noisy or incomplete data might incorrectly identify drug targets, leading to erroneous conclusions. To mitigate these challenges, efforts are underway to create more structured and integrated databases. For instance, platforms like OMIM (Online Mendelian Inheritance in Man) [57] and DrugBank [58] provide valuable, curated information, but the diversity of sources still poses integration issues.

Domain-Specific Challenges

AI models' “black box” nature, particularly DL algorithms, presents another challenge. These models often lack transparency, making it difficult for researchers and regulatory bodies to understand how predictions are made. AI and NLP models face unique domain-specific challenges in biomedical sciences [59]. One of the most prominent issues is the lack of standardized vocabularies and terminologies across biomedical texts. Biomedical literature uses complex, often inconsistent genetic, protein, and disease terminologies. The same entity can be referred to by multiple names (*e.g.*, cancer *vs.* carcinoma), complicating text mining efforts. NLP models trained on general language data struggle with this complexity and require specialized corpora and ontologies such as UMLS (Unified Medical Language System) to improve accuracy [59]. Furthermore, biomedical data is inherently heterogeneous and multi-modal. For example, clinical data, genomic sequences, proteomics, and metabolomics datasets vary in format, scale, and measurement units. AI/NLP models trained on one data type may not readily generalize to another. Effective models must be capable of integrating these multi-modal datasets to provide meaningful insights, but this remains a major technical hurdle.

Regulatory and Ethical Issues

The generalizability of AI models is another concern; those developed using particular datasets may struggle to perform effectively on data from unfamiliar contexts, restricting their utility across varied clinical settings. In addition, ethical and privacy concerns are increasingly relevant as AI applications rely on sensitive personal data, including genetic and clinical records. Adherence to data protection laws, including GDPR and HIPAA, is crucial but can pose challenges to data accessibility for training AI systems. AI and NLP systems in drug discovery face several ethical and regulatory hurdles [60]. One key issue is bias within AI models. The effectiveness of ML models depends heavily on the quality of their training data; if the data is biased or unbalanced, the resulting model may perpetuate these biases. In drug discovery, this might mean that AI models could prioritize drug targets or therapies for more commonly studied populations, leaving underrepresented groups, such as patients with rare diseases, overlooked. Another challenge is ensuring patient privacy. As AI models increasingly rely on patient data, especially genomic and clinical data, maintaining the privacy and security of this information is critical. Regulations like GDPR in Europe and HIPAA in the U.S. govern the use of personal data. However, ensuring compliance can complicate the development of AI models [61]. Moreover, regulatory agencies like the FDA and EMA require robust evidence to support the clinical validity of AI-driven decisions. The lack of clear guidelines for validating AI systems in healthcare adds another layer of complexity, delaying the translation of AI research into clinical applications.

Finally, integrating multimodal data from various sources, such as genomics and clinical trials, poses technical challenges. Effective AI models must seamlessly process and analyze these diverse data types, often requiring complex and customized processing pipelines. Regulatory barriers can hinder the adoption of AI in drug discovery, as existing frameworks may not keep pace with rapid advances in AI technology. NLP faces its own set of challenges in extracting meaningful insights from biomedical literature. The lack of standardized vocabulary and terminology in medical texts can compromise the effectiveness of NLP models, making it difficult to accurately mine information from extensive, unstructured datasets.

Developing more transparent AI models and establishing standardized data protocols are crucial to overcoming these challenges. Fostering interdisciplinary collaboration among data scientists, biologists, and ethicists will be vital to ensuring that AI and NLP-driven approaches in drug discovery not only advance scientific knowledge but also remain ethical and equitable in their application. By addressing these limitations, the full potential of AI and NLP in revolutionizing drug discovery can be realized, leading to more effective and accessible healthcare solutions.

CONCLUSION AND FUTURE PROSPECTS

AI and NLP have made substantial strides in drug discovery and target identification, fundamentally transforming how novel therapeutic targets are identified. AI algorithms can process and interpret complex biological systems using extensive datasets derived from genomics, proteomics, and clinical records. This ability improves insights into intricate disease pathways and helps identify promising therapeutic targets. Notably, AI aids in drug repurposing, target validation, and identifying synergistic therapeutic combinations, leading to more effective treatment strategies.

NLP is critical for mining biomedical literature, enabling researchers to uncover disease-related genes and pathways that may have been overlooked. However, the field still faces significant challenges, particularly regarding data quality and availability. AI models require high-quality, labeled datasets to function optimally, and the scarcity of such data can impede progress. Moreover, DL models' "black box" complicates the interpretation of AI-generated decisions, which is particularly important in the highly regulated drug development environment. Ethical concerns also loom large, particularly regarding biases in AI algorithms, data privacy, and compliance with regulatory standards. Addressing these issues is crucial to ensuring that AI applications in drug discovery are both effective and equitable. Additionally, while AI can significantly enhance the target discovery process, it does not substantially reduce the lengthy timelines associated with clinical trials, which remain a significant barrier to bringing new therapies to market.

Looking ahead, advancements in Explainable AI (XAI) will be vital for enhancing model interpretability, which can foster greater trust and acceptance among researchers and regulatory bodies. By improving transparency, scientists can better understand the decision-making processes of AI models, thereby facilitating their integration into traditional drug development pathways. Furthermore, incorporating AI with automated robotic laboratories can streamline target validation and screening processes, accelerating the pace of discovery. For NLP, future innovations will need to address domain-specific challenges, including the standardization of biomedical vocabularies and the development of more sophisticated methods for processing heterogeneous data types. These advancements are essential for refining NLP's effectiveness in extracting actionable insights from unstructured biomedical literature.

In conclusion, the evolution of AI and NLP technologies holds immense potential for transforming drug discovery and target identification, particularly in addressing complex diseases and global health challenges. Ensuring safer and more effective therapies will require collaborative efforts across disciplines, along with robust ethical safeguards to protect patient interests. By harnessing the power of AI and NLP responsibly, the scientific community can enhance patient outcomes and drive significant advancements in healthcare.

REFERENCES

[1] U. Naithani, and V. Guleria, "Integrative computational approaches for discovery and evaluation of lead compound for drug design", *Front. Drug Discov. (Lausanne),* vol. 4, 2024.1362456 [http://dx.doi.org/10.3389/fddsv.2024.1362456]

[2] I.V. Hinkson, B. Madej, and E.A. Stahlberg, "Accelerating therapeutics for opportunities in medicine: a paradigm shift in drug discovery", *Front. Pharmacol.,* vol. 11, p. 770, 2020. [http://dx.doi.org/10.3389/fphar.2020.00770] [PMID: 32694991]

[3] D. Sun, W. Gao, H. Hu, and S. Zhou, "Why 90% of clinical drug development fails and how to improve it?", *Acta Pharm. Sin. B,* vol. 12, no. 7, pp. 3049-3062, 2022. [http://dx.doi.org/10.1016/j.apsb.2022.02.002] [PMID: 35865092]

[4] A.U. Rehman, M. Li, B. Wu, Y. Ali, S. Rasheed, S. Shaheen, X. Liu, R. Luo, and J. Zhang, "Role of artificial intelligence in revolutionizing drug discovery", *Fundamental Research,* vol. 5, no. 3, pp. 1273-1287, 2025. [http://dx.doi.org/10.1016/j.fmre.2024.04.021] [PMID: 40528990]

[5] F. Bianconi, and M. Filippucci, *Digital Wood Design: Innovative Techniques of Representation in Architectural Design.* Springer, 2019. [http://dx.doi.org/10.1007/978-3-030-03676-8]

[6] L.K. Vora, A.D. Gholap, K. Jetha, R.R.S. Thakur, H.K. Solanki, and V.P. Chavda, "Artificial intelligence in pharmaceutical technology and drug delivery design", *Pharmaceutics,* vol. 15, no. 7, p. 1916, 2023. [http://dx.doi.org/10.3390/pharmaceutics15071916] [PMID: 37514102]

[7] Y. Ding, J.H. Sohn, M.G. Kawczynski, H. Trivedi, R. Harnish, N.W. Jenkins, D. Lituiev, T.P. Copeland, M.S. Aboian, C. Mari Aparici, S.C. Behr, R.R. Flavell, S.Y. Huang, K.A. Zalocusky, L. Nardo, Y. Seo, R.A. Hawkins, M. Hernandez Pampaloni, D. Hadley, and B.L. Franc, "A deep learning model to predict a diagnosis of alzheimer disease by using 18 F-FDG PET of the brain", *Radiology,* vol. 290, no. 2, pp. 456-464, 2019. [http://dx.doi.org/10.1148/radiol.2018180958] [PMID: 30398430]

[8] A. Narin, C. Kaya, and Z. Pamuk, "Automatic detection of coronavirus disease (COVID-19) using X-ray images and deep convolutional neural networks", *Pattern Anal. Appl.,* vol. 24, no. 3, pp. 1207-1220, 2021. [http://dx.doi.org/10.1007/s10044-021-00984-y] [PMID: 33994847]

[9] G. Zhou, D.V. Rusnac, H. Park, D. Canzani, H.M. Nguyen, L. Stewart, M.F. Bush, P.T. Nguyen, H. Wulff, V. Yarov-Yarovoy, N. Zheng, and F. DiMaio, "An artificial intelligence accelerated virtual screening platform for drug discovery", *Nat. Commun.,* vol. 15, no. 1, p. 7761, 2024. [http://dx.doi.org/10.1038/s41467-024-52061-7] [PMID: 39237523]

[10] H. Wu, J. Liu, R. Zhang, Y. Lu, G. Cui, Z. Cui, and Y. Ding, "A review of deep learning methods for

ligand based drug virtual screening", *Fundamental Research,* vol. 4, no. 4, pp. 715-737, 2024. [http://dx.doi.org/10.1016/j.fmre.2024.02.011] [PMID: 39156568]

[11] Y. Yuan, C. Shi, and H. Zhao, "Machine learning-enabled genome mining and bioactivity prediction of natural products", *ACS Synth. Biol.,* vol. 12, no. 9, pp. 2650-2662, 2023. [http://dx.doi.org/10.1021/acssynbio.3c00234] [PMID: 37607352]

[12] C. Berzuini, R. Bellazzi, S. Quaglini, and D.J. Spiegelhalter, "Bayesian networks for patient monitoring", *Artif. Intell. Med.,* vol. 4, no. 3, pp. 243-260, 1992. [http://dx.doi.org/10.1016/0933-3657(92)90030-S]

[13] S. Kapsiani, and B.J. Howlin, "Random forest classification for predicting lifespan-extending chemical compounds", *Sci. Rep.,* vol. 11, no. 1, p. 13812, 2021. [http://dx.doi.org/10.1038/s41598-021-93070-6] [PMID: 34226569]

[14] S. Singh, R. Kumar, S. Payra, and S.K. Singh, "Artificial intelligence and machine learning in pharmacological research: bridging the gap between data and drug discovery", *Cureus,* vol. 15, no. 8, 2023.e44359 [http://dx.doi.org/10.7759/cureus.44359] [PMID: 37779744]

[15] R. Rodríguez-Pérez, and J. Bajorath, "Evolution of support vector machine and regression modeling in chemoinformatics and drug discovery", *J. Comput. Aided Mol. Des.,* vol. 36, no. 5, pp. 355-362, 2022. [http://dx.doi.org/10.1007/s10822-022-00442-9] [PMID: 35304657]

[16] N. Brown, P. Ertl, R. Lewis, T. Luksch, D. Reker, and N. Schneider, "Artificial intelligence in chemistry and drug design", *J. Comput. Aided Mol. Des.,* vol. 34, no. 7, pp. 709-715, 2020. [http://dx.doi.org/10.1007/s10822-020-00317-x] [PMID: 32468207]

[17] J. Yan, P. Bhadra, A. Li, P. Sethiya, L. Qin, H.K. Tai, K.H. Wong, and S.W.I. Siu, "Deep-AmPEP30: improve short antimicrobial peptides prediction with deep learning", *Mol. Ther. Nucleic Acids,* vol. 20, pp. 882-894, 2020. [http://dx.doi.org/10.1016/j.omtn.2020.05.006] [PMID: 32464552]

[18] H.C. Yi, Z.H. You, X. Zhou, L. Cheng, X. Li, T.H. Jiang, and Z.H. Chen, "ACP-DL: a deep learning long short-term memory model to predict anticancer peptides using high-efficiency feature representation", *Mol. Ther. Nucleic Acids,* vol. 17, pp. 1-9, 2019. [http://dx.doi.org/10.1016/j.omtn.2019.04.025] [PMID: 31173946]

[19] A. Cichońska, B. Ravikumar, and R. Rahman, "AI for targeted polypharmacology: The next frontier in drug discovery", *Curr. Opin. Struct. Biol.,* vol. 84, 2024.102771 [http://dx.doi.org/10.1016/j.sbi.2023.102771] [PMID: 38215530]

[20] J. Liu, and J.E. Hein, "Automation, analytics and artificial intelligence for chemical synthesis", *Nat. Synth.,* vol. 2, no. 6, pp. 464-466, 2023. [http://dx.doi.org/10.1038/s44160-023-00335-1]

[21] M.K.G. Abbas, A. Rassam, F. Karamshahi, R. Abunora, and M. Abouseada, "The role of AI in drug discovery", *ChemBioChem,* vol. 25, no. 14, 2024.e202300816 [http://dx.doi.org/10.1002/cbic.202300816] [PMID: 38735845]

[22] R. Bhatnagar, S. Sardar, M. Beheshti, and J.T. Podichetty, "How can natural language processing help model informed drug development?: a review", *JAMIA Open,* vol. 5, no. 2, 2022.ooac043 [http://dx.doi.org/10.1093/jamiaopen/ooac043] [PMID: 35702625]

[23] A.I. Visan, and I. Negut, "Integrating artificial intelligence for drug discovery in the context of revolutionizing drug delivery", *Life (Basel),* vol. 14, no. 2, p. 233, 2024. [http://dx.doi.org/10.3390/life14020233] [PMID: 38398742]

[24] K. Lee, Z. Liu, Y. Mai, T. Jun, M. Ma, T. Wang, L. Ai, E. Calay, W. Oh, G. Stolovitzky, E. Schadt, and X. Wang, "Optimizing clinical trial eligibility design using natural language processing models and real-world data: algorithm development and validation", *JMIR AI,* vol. 3, 2024.e50800 [http://dx.doi.org/10.2196/50800] [PMID: 39073872]

[25] S. Vadapalli, H. Abdelhalim, S. Zeeshan, and Z. Ahmed, "Artificial intelligence and machine learning approaches using gene expression and variant data for personalized medicine", *Brief. Bioinform.*, vol. 23, no. 5, 2022.bbac191
[http://dx.doi.org/10.1093/bib/bbac191] [PMID: 35595537]

[26] M. Brendel, C. Su, Z. Bai, H. Zhang, O. Elemento, and F. Wang, "Application of deep learning on single-cell RNA sequencing data analysis: a review", *Genomics Proteomics Bioinformatics,* vol. 20, no. 5, pp. 814-835, 2022.
[http://dx.doi.org/10.1016/j.gpb.2022.11.011] [PMID: 36528240]

[27] F. Soleymani, E. Paquet, H. Viktor, W. Michalowski, and D. Spinello, "Protein–protein interaction prediction with deep learning: A comprehensive review", *Comput. Struct. Biotechnol. J.*, vol. 20, pp. 5316-5341, 2022.
[http://dx.doi.org/10.1016/j.csbj.2022.08.070] [PMID: 36212542]

[28] J.H. Yoon, H. Lee, D. Kwon, D. Lee, S. Lee, E. Cho, J. Kim, and D. Kim, "Integrative approach of omics and imaging data to discover new insights for understanding brain diseases", *Brain Commun.*, vol. 6, no. 4, 2024.fcae265
[http://dx.doi.org/10.1093/braincomms/fcae265] [PMID: 39165479]

[29] L. Wei, D. Niraula, E.D.H. Gates, J. Fu, Y. Luo, M.J. Nyflot, S.R. Bowen, I.M. El Naqa, and S. Cui, "Artificial Intelligence (AI) and Machine Learning (ML) in precision oncology: a review on enhancing discoverability through multiomics integration", *Br. J. Radiol.*, vol. 96, no. 1150, 2023.20230211
[http://dx.doi.org/10.1259/bjr.20230211] [PMID: 37660402]

[30] R. Qureshi, M. Irfan, T.M. Gondal, S. Khan, J. Wu, M.U. Hadi, J. Heymach, X. Le, H. Yan, and T. Alam, "AI in drug discovery and its clinical relevance", *Heliyon,* vol. 9, no. 7, 2023.e17575
[http://dx.doi.org/10.1016/j.heliyon.2023.e17575] [PMID: 37396052]

[31] P. L. Whetzel, N. F. Noy, N. H. Shah, P. R. Alexander, C. Nyulas, T. Tudorache, and M. A. Musen, "BioPortal: enhanced functionality *via* new web services from the National Center for Biomedical Ontology to access and use ontologies in software applications," Nucleic Acids Research, vol. 39, suppl. 2, pp. W541–W545, Jul. 2011. [Online]. Available: https://doi.org/10.1093/nar/gkr469

[32] B.L. Humphreys, G. Del Fiol, and H. Xu, "The UMLS knowledge sources at 30: indispensable to current research and applications in biomedical informatics", *J. Am. Med. Inform. Assoc.*, vol. 27, no. 10, pp. 1499-1501, 2020.
[http://dx.doi.org/10.1093/jamia/ocaa208] [PMID: 33059366]

[33] N. Perera, M. Dehmer, and F. Emmert-Streib, "Named entity recognition and relation detection for biomedical information extraction", *Front. Cell Dev. Biol.*, vol. 8, p. 673, 2020.
[http://dx.doi.org/10.3389/fcell.2020.00673] [PMID: 32984300]

[34] G. Tsatsaronis, G. Balikas, P. Malakasiotis, I. Partalas, M. Zschunke, M.R. Alvers, D. Weissenborn, A. Krithara, S. Petridis, D. Polychronopoulos, Y. Almirantis, J. Pavlopoulos, N. Baskiotis, P. Gallinari, T. Artiéres, A.C.N. Ngomo, N. Heino, E. Gaussier, L. Barrio-Alvers, M. Schroeder, I. Androutsopoulos, and G. Paliouras, "An overview of the BIOASQ large-scale biomedical semantic indexing and question answering competition", *BMC Bioinformatics,* vol. 16, no. 1, p. 138, 2015.
[http://dx.doi.org/10.1186/s12859-015-0564-6] [PMID: 25925131]

[35] A. Sharma, T. Virmani, V. Pathak, A. Sharma, K. Pathak, G. Kumar, and D. Pathak, "Artificial intelligence-based data-driven strategy to accelerate research, development, and clinical trials of COVID vaccine", *BioMed Res. Int.*, vol. 2022, no. 1, 2022.7205241
[http://dx.doi.org/10.1155/2022/7205241] [PMID: 35845955]

[36] D.E. Gordon, "A SARS-CoV-2-human protein-protein interaction map reveals drug targets and potential drug-repurposing", *bioRxiv,* .2020.03.22.002386
[http://dx.doi.org/10.1101/2020.03.22.002386]

[37] D.P. Smith, O. Oechsle, M.J. Rawling, E. Savory, A.M.B. Lacoste, and P.J. Richardson, "Expert-augmented computational drug repurposing identified baricitinib as a treatment for COVID-19",

Front. Pharmacol., vol. 12, 2021.709856
[http://dx.doi.org/10.3389/fphar.2021.709856] [PMID: 34393789]

[38] J. Stebbing, A. Phelan, I. Griffin, C. Tucker, O. Oechsle, D. Smith, and P. Richardson, "COVID-19: combining antiviral and anti-inflammatory treatments", *Lancet Infect. Dis.,* vol. 20, no. 4, pp. 400-402, 2020.
[http://dx.doi.org/10.1016/S1473-3099(20)30132-8] [PMID: 32113509]

[39] S. Assadiasl, Y. Fatahi, B. Mosharmovahed, B. Mohebbi, and M.H. Nicknam, "Baricitinib: From Rheumatoid Arthritis to COVID-19", *J. Clin. Pharmacol.,* vol. 61, no. 10, pp. 1274-1285, 2021.
[http://dx.doi.org/10.1002/jcph.1874] [PMID: 33870531]

[40] O. Kadioglu, M. Saeed, H.J. Greten, and T. Efferth, "Identification of novel compounds against three targets of SARS CoV-2 coronavirus by combined virtual screening and supervised machine learning", *Comput. Biol. Med.,* vol. 133, 2021.104359
[http://dx.doi.org/10.1016/j.compbiomed.2021.104359] [PMID: 33845270]

[41] F. Hu, J. Jiang, and P. Yin, "Prediction of potential commercially available inhibitors against SARS-CoV-2 by multi-task deep learning model", *Biomolecules,* vol. 12, no. 8, p. 1156, 2022.
[http://dx.doi.org/10.3390/biom12081156] [PMID: 36009050]

[42] A.A.A. Abdusalam, and V. Murugaiyah, "Identification of potential inhibitors of 3CL protease of SARS-CoV-2 from ZINC database by molecular docking-based virtual screening", *Front. Mol. Biosci.,* vol. 7, 2020.603037
[http://dx.doi.org/10.3389/fmolb.2020.603037] [PMID: 33392261]

[43] S. Choudhary, Y.S. Malik, and S. Tomar, "Identification of SARS-CoV-2 Cell Entry Inhibitors by Drug Repurposing Using *in silico* Structure-Based Virtual Screening Approach", *Front. Immunol.,* vol. 11, p. 1664, 2020.
[http://dx.doi.org/10.3389/fimmu.2020.01664] [PMID: 32754161]

[44] P.A. Novick, O.F. Ortiz, J. Poelman, A.Y. Abdulhay, and V.S. Pande, "SWEETLEAD: an *in silico* database of approved drugs, regulated chemicals, and herbal isolates for computer-aided drug discovery", *PLoS One,* vol. 8, no. 11, 2013.e79568
[http://dx.doi.org/10.1371/journal.pone.0079568] [PMID: 24223973]

[45] R. Rangan, I.N. Zheludev, R.J. Hagey, E.A. Pham, H.K. Wayment-Steele, J.S. Glenn, and R. Das, "RNA genome conservation and secondary structure in SARS-CoV-2 and SARS-related viruses: a first look", *RNA,* vol. 26, no. 8, pp. 937-959, 2020.
[http://dx.doi.org/10.1261/rna.076141.120] [PMID: 32398273]

[46] S.J. Park, Y.G. Kim, and H.J. Park, "Identification of RNA pseudoknot-binding ligand that inhibits the -1 ribosomal frameshifting of SARS-coronavirus by structure-based virtual screening", *J. Am. Chem. Soc.,* vol. 133, no. 26, pp. 10094-10100, 2011.
[http://dx.doi.org/10.1021/ja1098325] [PMID: 21591761]

[47] C. Wu, Y. Liu, Y. Yang, P. Zhang, W. Zhong, Y. Wang, Q. Wang, Y. Xu, M. Li, X. Li, M. Zheng, L. Chen, and H. Li, "Analysis of therapeutic targets for SARS-CoV-2 and discovery of potential drugs by computational methods", *Acta Pharm. Sin. B,* vol. 10, no. 5, pp. 766-788, 2020.
[http://dx.doi.org/10.1016/j.apsb.2020.02.008] [PMID: 32292689]

[48] V. Chenthamarakshan, P. Das, S. C. Hoffman, H. Strobelt, I. Padhi, K. W. Lim, B. Hoover, M. Manica, J. Born, T. Laino, and A. Mojsilovic, “CogMol: Target-specific and selective drug design for COVID-19 using deep generative models,” arXiv preprint arXiv:2004.01215, 2020. [Online]. Available: https://arxiv.org/abs/2004.01215

[49] B. Tang, F. He, D. Liu, M. Fang, Z. Wu, and D. Xu, "AI-aided design of novel targeted covalent inhibitors against SARS-CoV-2", *bioRxiv,* .2020.03.03.972133
[http://dx.doi.org/10.1101/2020.03.03.972133]

[50] M. Wang, R. Cao, L. Zhang, X. Yang, J. Liu, M. Xu, Z. Shi, Z. Hu, W. Zhong, and G. Xiao, "Remdesivir and chloroquine effectively inhibit the recently emerged novel coronavirus (2019-nCoV)

in vitro", *Cell Res.,* vol. 30, no. 3, pp. 269-271, 2020.
[http://dx.doi.org/10.1038/s41422-020-0282-0] [PMID: 32020029]

[51] I. Tapken, D. Kuhn, N. Hoffmann, N.T. Detering, T. Schüning, J.N. Billaud, S. Tugendreich, N. Schlüter, J. Green, A. Krämer, and P. Claus, "From data to discovery: AI-guided analysis of disease-relevant molecules in Spinal Muscular Atrophy (SMA)", *Hum. Mol. Genet.,* vol. 33, no. 15, pp. 1367-1377, 2024.
[http://dx.doi.org/10.1093/hmg/ddae076] [PMID: 38704739]

[52] M. Wojtara, E. Rana, T. Rahman, P. Khanna, and H. Singh, "Artificial intelligence in rare disease diagnosis and treatment", *Clin. Transl. Sci.,* vol. 16, no. 11, pp. 2106-2111, 2023.
[http://dx.doi.org/10.1111/cts.13619] [PMID: 37646577]

[53] D. He, R. Wang, Z. Xu, J. Wang, P. Song, H. Wang, and J. Su, "The use of artificial intelligence in the treatment of rare diseases: A scoping review", *Intractable Rare Dis. Res.,* vol. 13, no. 1, pp. 12-22, 2024.
[http://dx.doi.org/10.5582/irdr.2023.01111] [PMID: 38404730]

[54] S. Kim, J. Chen, T. Cheng, A. Gindulyte, J. He, S. He, Q. Li, B.A. Shoemaker, P.A. Thiessen, B. Yu, L. Zaslavsky, J. Zhang, and E.E. Bolton, "PubChem 2023 update", *Nucleic Acids Res.,* vol. 51, no. D1, pp. D1373-D1380, 2023.
[http://dx.doi.org/10.1093/nar/gkac956] [PMID: 36305812]

[55] B. Zdrazil, E. Felix, F. Hunter, E.J. Manners, J. Blackshaw, S. Corbett, M. de Veij, H. Ioannidis, D.M. Lopez, J.F. Mosquera, M.P. Magarinos, N. Bosc, R. Arcila, T. Kizilören, A. Gaulton, A.P. Bento, M.F. Adasme, P. Monecke, G.A. Landrum, and A.R. Leach, "The ChEMBL Database in 2023: a drug discovery platform spanning multiple bioactivity data types and time periods", *Nucleic Acids Res.,* vol. 52, no. D1, pp. D1180-D1192, 2024.
[http://dx.doi.org/10.1093/nar/gkad1004] [PMID: 37933841]

[56] M. Bagherian, E. Sabeti, K. Wang, M.A. Sartor, Z. Nikolovska-Coleska, and K. Najarian, "Machine learning approaches and databases for prediction of drug–target interaction: a survey paper", *Brief. Bioinform.,* vol. 22, no. 1, pp. 247-269, 2021.
[http://dx.doi.org/10.1093/bib/bbz157] [PMID: 31950972]

[57] A. Hamosh, A.F. Scott, J. Amberger, C. Bocchini, D. Valle, and V.A. McKusick, "Online Mendelian Inheritance in Man (OMIM), a knowledge base of human genes and genetic disorders", *Nucleic Acids Res.,* vol. 30, no. 1, pp. 52-55, 2002.
[http://dx.doi.org/10.1093/nar/30.1.52] [PMID: 11752252]

[58] D. S. Wishart, C. Knox, A. C. Guo, S. Shrivastava, M. Hassanali, P. Stothard, Z. Chang, and J. Woolsey, "DrugBank: a comprehensive resource for in silico drug discovery and exploration," Nucleic Acids Research, vol. 34, suppl. 1, pp. D668–D672, Jan. 2006. [Online]. Available: https://doi.org/10.1093/nar/gkj067

[59] J. Wu, H. Dong, Z. Li, H. Wang, R. Li, A. Patra, C. Dai, W. Ali, P. Scordis, and H. Wu, "A hybrid framework with large language models for rare disease phenotyping", *BMC Med. Inform. Decis. Mak.,* vol. 24, no. 1, p. 289, 2024.
[http://dx.doi.org/10.1186/s12911-024-02698-7] [PMID: 39375687]

[60] M. Jeyaraman, S. Balaji, N. Jeyaraman, and S. Yadav, "Unraveling the ethical enigma: artificial intelligence in healthcare", *Cureus,* vol. 15, no. 8, 2023.e43262
[http://dx.doi.org/10.7759/cureus.43262] [PMID: 37692617]

[61] L. Bradford, M. Aboy, and K. Liddell, "International transfers of health data between the EU and USA: a sector-specific approach for the USA to ensure an 'adequate' level of protection", *J. Law Biosci.,* vol. 7, no. 1, 2020.lsaa055
[http://dx.doi.org/10.1093/jlb/lsaa055] [PMID: 34221424]

CHAPTER 12

AI-Assisted Public Health Surveillance of Gut Microbiome Health

Arockiyajainmary Michealsamy[1,*]

[1] *Independent Researcher, Chennai, Tamilnadu, India*

Abstract: Natural Language Processing plays a significant role in public health surveillance as it analyzes multimedia data to understand epidemics, forecast outbreaks, and address data-integration challenges. Syndromic surveillance systems that focus on symptoms rather than diagnoses provide immediate but less specific information for public health surveillance. By leveraging AI tools for surveillance, healthcare professionals can optimize interventions, identify gut microbiome modulation, and prevent chronic diseases. AI-driven approaches enable multi-omics data analysis, encompassing genomics, proteomics, and metabolomics, and provide extensive insights into the gut microbiome's influence on host metabolism and pathological conditions. Furthermore, AI can predict host phenotypes derived from gut microbiome characteristics, facilitating early identification of different disease states and improving human health outcomes. Generative AI can facilitate advanced analytics and provide new interventions for complex disease surveillance. For instance, unstructured clinical notes in medical examiners' case reports, social media activities, and news reports are potentially proper text signals currently inaccessible at the population level. This chapter highlights the diverse applications of AI in public health surveillance, emphasizing its role in optimizing decision-making, safety monitoring, and cognitive assessments across different contexts. We emphasize that the collaboration between AI and gut microbiome research has the potential to transform public health monitoring, personalized nutrition, and global metabolic health.

Keywords: AI-driven public health surveillance, Gut microbiome health, Local detection, Global epidemic monitoring, Early warning.

INTRODUCTION

Research on the human gut microbiome has evolved due to the rapid development of Artificial Intelligence (AI) techniques, particularly Machine Learning (ML) and Deep Learning (DL) [1]. AI possesses significant applications in advanced public health surveillance by enhancing data collection, analysis, and epidemic prediction capabilities [2]. Incorporating artificial intelligence into various

* **Corresponding author Arockiyajainmary Michealsamy:** Independent Researcher, Chennai, Tamilnadu, India; E-mail: -arockiyajainmary13@gmail.com

A. Shankar, Saranya Jayapalan, & Basant. K. Tiwary (Eds.)

information sources, including social networks, mobile health data, and digital health records, has revolutionized traditional surveillance systems by providing proactive interventions and real-time monitoring [3, 4]. However, in health surveillance, the widespread use of AI commenced recently with the onset of COVID-19. Gut microbiota is linked to several chronic diseases [5, 6], including Inflammatory Bowel Disease (IBD), diabetes, liver disease, chronic heart disease [7 - 9], cancers, HIV, and autism [10, 11]. By leveraging Natural Language Processing (NLP) techniques and diverse datasets, public health surveillance of gut ailments can be enhanced to better understand and respond to health challenges globally [12 - 14].

AI-assisted public health surveillance is feasible across various aspects of public health initiatives [15]. Furthermore, it enhances public health by enabling culture-fair and education-independent automated cognitive assessments in low- and middle-income nations. Integrating AI into public health surveillance holds immense promise for improving disease estimates, enabling early warning of outbreaks, and safeguarding public health through proactive measures, by utilizing data from the Emergency Medical Communication Centre (EMCC) to enhance active and passive surveillance efforts.

GUT MICROBIOME-RELATED DISEASE SURVEILLANCE USING AI

The gastrointestinal microbiome is a multifaceted and evolving ecological system that is integral to human well-being and the cause of various diseases [16 - 18]. Concerning surveillance of gut microbiome health, AI advances technologies to analyze microbial genomes, predict host phenotypes, and suggest personalized nutrition strategies [19]. The gut microbiome's dynamic nature, influenced by diet and disease, can lead to dysbiosis, impacting the immune system and overall health [17, 20, 21]. AI generates individualized gut microbiota profiles and possesses the capability to analyze extensive and diverse datasets that are associated with the health impacts of a community. Machine learning classifiers offer valuable insights regarding the link between microbial communities and diseases. Table (**1**) summarizes the application of machine learning approaches in microbiome research.

Metagenomics empowered by an AI framework provides a powerful approach to investigating microbial diversity [31], their genes, and gene products. The function- and sequence-based [32] analysis has provided a significant advantage in diagnosing infections by directly analyzing samples obtained from humans or their surroundings [33, 34]. Several AI-centred computational tools have adapted problem-solving techniques, including mathematical optimization, artificial neural networks, statistical methods, and logistic regression. Bzhalava *et al.* trained an ANN to taxonomically categorize the metagenomic sequences into virus and non-virus classes with a receiver operating characteristic curve of 0.79; the reported

Table 1. ML application in microbiome analysis guided by available scientific information.

ML method	Microbiome Research	Reference	Citation
Supervised Learning – Logistic Regression (LR) analysis.	Selecting 300 biomarkers from 13,990 microbial features, which include clinical data and gene abundance matrices from 806 Chinese microbiomes, enables a large-scale disease screening population.	H. Wu *et al.* (2018)	[22]
Linear Discriminant Analysis (LDA).	Described statistics, pattern recognition, and deep learning in microbiome data analysis.	Y. H. Zhou and P. Gallins (2019)	[23]
K-Nearest Neighbors (k-NN).	Generated a model that effectively predicts the postmortem interval.	H. R. Johnson *et al.* (2016)	[24]
Naïve Bayes probabilistic classifiers.	Enhances the accuracy of taxonomic classification for the 16S rRNA gene sequences.	J. J. Werner *et al.* (2012)	[25]
Artificial Neural Network (ANN).	ANN platform for classifying host phenotypes from metagenomic data.	C. Lo and R. Marculescu, (2019)	[26]
Random Forest (RF) - ensemble learning.	Random Forest classifiers and the Least Absolute Shrinkage and Selection Operator (LASSO) are commonly utilized for feature selection and patient analysis stratification.	S. Yachida *et al.* (2019)	[27]
ML classifiers: SVM, LR, and Naive Bayes.	Utility in Phy-PMRFI to demonstrate if phylogenetic relatedness accurately predicts functional similarity.	J. T. Wassan *et al.* (2019)	[28]
Bayesian Networks (BN).	Revealed an association between a specific taxon and enhanced therapeutic outcomes.	B. S. Jang *et al.* (2020)	[29]
Dynamic Bayesian Network (DBN).	DBN has been employed to examine longitudinal microbiome data sets to determine temporal correlations among various taxonomic levels and related clinical factors influencing the microbiome.	J. Lugo-Martinez *et al.* (2019)	[30]

accuracy was much higher than the chance level. The random forest has recently been preferred for its robustness and efficient classification, achieving more than 90% accuracy with 95% confidence [35, 36]. AI-driven integration of multi-omics data analysis provides comprehensive insights into the functional dynamics of the human gut microbiome and its impact on the host metabolism [37]. Recently, researchers at the Mayo Clinic have developed a computational tool called Gut Microbiome Wellness Index 2, which employs bioinformatics and machine learning methodologies to evaluate gastrointestinal health and track variations within the gut microbiome [38].

This book chapter explains how public health surveillance was used to treat gut microbiome-related diseases like obesity [39]. Public health officials are crucial in tackling this issue. The gut microbiome significantly influences obesity [40]. The gut microbiota composition varies between obese and lean individuals, determining energy metabolism. Dysbiosis, or bacterial imbalance, may lead to weight gain. The domains of artificial intelligence and robotics in healthcare encompass sequencing methodologies, telehealth services [41], mobile applications, biosensors for remote diagnostic evaluation and surveillance [42], speech recognition, and automated image analysis [43, 44]. Table (**2**) outlines the key resources for leveraging various ML methods concerning human gut microbiome health surveillance.

Table 2. Main studies on AI application in the various fields of gut microbiome-related illness surveillance.

Reference	Citation	Study Features	AI Techniques	Findings
J. Qin *et al.* (2010)	[46]	WGS data is utilized to discern genetic markers linked to IBD and Type II Diabetes (T2D) from faecal sample sequencing.	mRMR (minimum Redundancy Maximum Relevance)	Selected 50 marker genes for T2D and taxonomic abundance data to differentiate IBD from healthy individuals by PCoA analysis.
H. Cui and X. Zhang (2013)	[47]	To classify the IBD and non-IBD samples' metagenome dataset.	Recursive SVM.	Supervised classification method that does not require an alignment for categorizing metagenome samples based on sequence signatures.
P. E. Larsen and Y. Dail (2015)	[48]	Predicted metagenomic enzyme profiles from 16S rRNA microbiome structures were utilized to create metabolic pathway models.	SVM.	The human gut microbiome's metabolome may indicate host dysbiosis.
D. Fioravanti *et al.* (2018)	[49]	Phylogenetic CNN would facilitate the classification of the gut microbiome metagenomic data.	Convolutional neural network CNN.	The classification of gut microbiome metagenomic data associated with Crohn's Disease (CD) and Ulcerative Colitis (UC) into healthy or inflammatory bowel disease phenotypes culminates in a comprehensive total of six distinct classification endeavours.
G. M. Douglas *et al.* (2018)	[50]	Categorizing paediatric Crohn's patients according to their disease state and treatment responses. This categorization leverages the alpha diversity of samples alongside each patient's Genetic Risk Score (GRS).	RF.	16S rRNA datasets demonstrated higher classification accuracy than shotgun metagenomics.

(Table 2) cont.....

Reference	Citation	Study Features	AI Techniques	Findings
D. Travisany *et al.* (2015)	[51]	A dataset comprising 98 gastrointestinal tract genera from the Human Microbiome Project was utilized alongside another dataset featuring 17 previously studied gastrointestinal tract genera.	Multiple decision trees.	Ensemble method for microbial taxa prediction.
D. Zeevi *et al.* (2015)	[52]	A group of 800 overweight or obese non-diabetic individuals was studied to profile their gut microbiome using 16S rRNA amplicon analysis phyla.	Gradient boosting (GB).	Implemented a blinded randomized controlled dietary intervention utilizing ML-based predictions in a separate cohort.
Q. Zhu *et al.* (2020)	[53]	Performed microbiome-wide association studies (MWAS).	The DL ensemble feature selection model, Deep Forest, is based on the RF method.	Improved classification performance over SVMs, k-NNs, and CNNs.
E. B. Hollister *et al.*, (2019)	[54]	Assessed the connections between pediatric IBS, abdominal pain, intestinal microbes, and fecal matter metabolites.	LASSO feature selection, RF models, and SVM.	Microbiome-gut-brain axis to human health.
A. Mohammed and C. Guda (2015)	[55]	Predict enzymes encoded by the human gut microbiome in a hierarchical manner.	A consensus-driven ensemble includes k-NN, SVM, RF, decision stump, and Naive Bayes classifiers.	Utilized their approach to examine the enzyme profiles of lean versus obese and IBD versus non-IBD individuals.
L. Chen *et al.* (2016)	[56]	Investigated racial variations in gut microbiome gene expression among Asian, European, and American populations.	mRMR, RF, k-NN, sequential minimal optimization.	The accuracy surpassed 96% and underwent further analysis. The identified genes indicated variations among the examined populations, including dietary practices, environmental contexts, and metabolic rates, all recognized as factors affecting the gut microbiome.

(Table 2) cont.....

Reference	Citation	Study Features	AI Techniques	Findings
D. A. Hughes *et al.* (2020)	[57]	More than 3,800 participants and two German cohorts were involved in the Flemish Gut Flora Project.	Bidirectional Mendelian Randomization (MR).	MR employs human genetic variants, including SNPs, as proxies for significant clinical traits to assess causal relationships between traits and health outcomes, thereby mitigating confounding and reverse causation.

Early Detection and Prediction

Healthcare systems utilizing social media data, such as Twitter, relevant forums, and blogs, have shown strong correlations with actual outbreaks, providing timely alerts. Mobile health data, including geolocation and health indicators, allows for continuous monitoring and rapid response to emerging threats [58, 59]. The data analytics encompass outbreak detection, early warnings, spatiotemporal analytics, risk assessment, and trend forecasting. Additionally, integrating AI and ML systems allows for the monitoring and prediction of individual patient symptoms using digital biosensors. This fosters an adaptive clinical feedback process, facilitating real-time analysis and enhancing personalized healthcare delivery [60, 61]. Certain syndromic surveillance systems, including Websök and telehealth surveillance, demonstrate notable timeliness and predictive efficacy in identifying gastrointestinal infections [62]. The Office of Public Health Data, Surveillance, and Technology (OPHDST) improves access to public health data. It aims to enhance the efficiency of data and technology systems at every level of public health [63].

Real-Time Monitoring

The term mHealth (mobile health) involves using mobile applications, chatbots, social platforms, and wearable devices to monitor healthcare [64]. AI algorithms track disease transmission patterns, offering insights into how diseases spread, as demonstrated during the COVID-19 pandemic. The Indian government, in partnership with both public and private stakeholders, created "Arogya Setu" alongside the National Informatics Centre (NIC) within the Ministry of Electronics and Information Technology. This initiative offers individuals real-time contact tracing and self-assessment information, helping them stay informed during crucial times like the COVID-19 pandemic.

Using AI to track outbreaks necessitates epidemiological data to pinpoint the infection source. Epidemic modeling and simulation encompass agent-based modelling, multi-agent simulation, and response evaluation [65]. Zhang *et al.*

successfully identified *Salmonella typhimurium* as the genomic source for the major zoonotic outbreaks in the US between 1998 and 2013 by using an ML random forest classifier [66, 67]. Additionally, they discovered 50 essential genetic traits adequate for reliable livestock source prediction.

GIS enables the creation of dynamic maps and dashboards that visualize epidemiological data, such as case numbers and hotspots, facilitating an immediate understanding of outbreak dynamics. For instance, a GIS-enabled surveillance system for Lassa Fever demonstrated the ability to track and predict disease spread in real time, aiding in early containment efforts [4].

RESOURCE ALLOCATION

AI optimizes resource distribution by analyzing demographic and disease prevalence data, ensuring efficient use of healthcare resources during outbreaks. AI-based epidemiological surveillance is a potential strategy for monitoring and detecting disease transmission that uses machine learning to examine data collected from various sources, such as digital medical records and online communities [68]. While AI presents transformative potential for public health, data quality, privacy concerns, and algorithmic bias must be addressed to ensure effective implementation and equitable health outcomes. Integrating Geographic Information Systems (GIS) with wastewater data [69 - 71] enables the mapping of viral spread, facilitating targeted public health interventions [72]. Additionally, NLP methods combined with machine learning technologies facilitate the extraction of critical information from various sources like healthcare facilities, secondary data, and the web, aiding in detecting and monitoring disease outbreaks for more effective public health responses. Syndromic surveillance frameworks in England have exhibited effectiveness in promptly detecting seasonal Gastrointestinal Ailments (GI) [73], facilitating the analysis of their spatiotemporal distribution and permitting timely public health interventions [74].

Predictive Analytics

Machine learning models predict disease spread and severity, facilitating proactive resource allocation and intervention strategies. Innovative applications like predictive modelling and GIS have revolutionized outbreak prediction and resource management. AI algorithms process vast datasets, improving the accuracy of disease estimates and early warning systems for outbreaks. Support Vector Machines (SVMs) use kernel methods to infer the decision boundary within a high-dimensional space and for regression tasks. Amaan *et al.* unraveled a complex, bidirectional communication network of microbiome-gut-brain *via* predictive models that can forecast outcomes based on gut microbiome data [36]. This approach allows researchers to anticipate how changes in gut microbiota may influence mental health conditions. Bushra *et al.* developed an outbreak detection web application named OBDETECTOR [75]. It is designed to analyze data from disease surveillance systemson a weekly or daily basis. The application enhances the ability to identify disease outbreaks early.

COMBATING BIAS IN INTEGRATING THE DATA *VIA* IMPROVED NLP ALGORITHMS

Biases in deep learning algorithms can lead to misrepresentations, skewed results, and even exacerbated health disparities [76]. Researchers are working on strategies to combat these biases. How will AI improve current public health surveillance and facilitate new capabilities? Technically, there will be two challenges. One is the data sourcing, and the other is their analytics. First, the data sourcing should be accurate and easily operationalizable. The second analytics issue is the development of efficient computational frameworks to extract relevant information. Response approaches can be enhanced by advancing AI applications, such as deep learning, reinforcement learning, knowledge graphs, Bayesian networks, and multi-agent systems. This would streamline diagnostic accuracy and personalized health interventions. The progressive transformation of Automated Machine Learning (AutoML) in the healthcare sector, particularly concerning interpretative frameworks, enhances the accessibility and comprehensibility of machine learning models for clinicians [77, 78].

Begum *et al.* introduced a reusable open-source pipeline designed for training, validating, and interpreting machine learning models to identify disease-related microbial biomarkers. They emphasize that selecting an appropriate machine learning method should align with the study's objectives, as this decision will guide performance expectations and the interpretability of outcomes [39]. However, existing research often focuses on well-represented groups in developed nations, neglecting populations in developing countries with limited health surveillance capabilities.

In the last few decades, the emergence of inflammatory bowel disease has raised alarms as a global health threat, significantly challenging public health systems and healthcare costs. Conventional deep learning systems utilize CNNs reliant on clinician-derived subjective image assessments, while innovative methodologies have emerged that focus exclusively on algorithmic analysis of parameters like pixel colour and vascular patterns. These objective, computer-based, and operator-independent tools yield a dedicated score that correlates significantly with endoscopic and histological scoring systems.

CONCLUSION

This review underscores the necessity for additional rigorous research to substantiate the efficacy of AI surveillance in gastrointestinal infections. By combining AI with synthetic biology, researchers can engineer probiotics for therapeutic and nutritive value, enhancing gut health and overall well-being. This technological advancement is crucial for addressing the challenges posed by the diverse range of pathogens entering human communities due to various factors like climate change and global travel. We can propel microbiota research into a future of personalized, data-driven healthcare, employing AI as an essential asset for enhanced health and public health monitoring. AI facilitates the creation of personalized microbiota profiles to enhance individual health. Therefore, AI strengthens global health security by improving disease surveillance.

LIST OF ABBREVIATIONS

AI	Artificial Intelligence
ANN	Artificial Neural Network
BN	Bayesian Network
CD	Crohn's Disease
CNN	Convolutional Neural Network
DBN	Dynamic Bayesian network
DL	Deep Learning
GB	Gradient Boosting
GIS	Geographic Information Systems
GRS	Genetic Risk Score
IBD	Inflammatory Bowel Disease
LASSO	Least Absolute Shrinkage and Selection Operator
LDA	Linear Discriminant Analysis
LR	Logistic Regression
ML	Machine Learning
mRMR	minimum Redundancy Maximum Relevance
MWAS	Microbiome-wide Association Studies
NIC	National Informatics Centre
NLP	Natural Learning Programming
OTU	Operational Taxonomic Unit
PCoA	Principal Component Analysis
RF	Random Forest
SVM	Support Vector Machines

UC	Ulcerative Colitis
WGS	Whole Genome Sequencing

CONFLICT OF INTEREST

The author declares there is no conflict of interest.

ACKNOWLEDGEMENT

None Declared

REFERENCES

[1] B. Baddal, F. Taner, and D. Uzun Ozsahin, "Harnessing of artificial intelligence for the diagnosis and prevention of hospital-acquired infections: a systematic review", *Diagnostics (Basel),* vol. 14, no. 5, p. 484, 2024. [http://dx.doi.org/10.3390/diagnostics14050484] [PMID: 38472956]

[2] D.B. Olawade, O.J. Wada, A.C. David-Olawade, E. Kunonga, O. Abaire, and J. Ling, "Using artificial intelligence to improve public health: a narrative review", *Front. Public Health,* vol. 11, 2023.1196397 [http://dx.doi.org/10.3389/fpubh.2023.1196397] [PMID: 37954052]

[3] D. Quezada, S. Akwafuo, and A. Wattamwar, "Real-time hybrid dashboard and App for Mpox outbreak surveillance", *2023 IEEE Global Humanitarian Technology Conference, GHTC 2023,* 2023pp. 433-439 [http://dx.doi.org/10.1109/GHTC56179.2023.10355026]

[4] A. Wattamwar, S. Akwafuo, and V. Mistry, "Data-driven real-time surveillance system for tracking disease outbreaks: A case study of Lassa Fever outbreak," in 2024 IEEE 12th International Conference on Healthcare Informatics (ICHI), Orlando, FL, USA, 2024, pp. 344–349. [http://dx.doi.org/10.1109/ICHI61247.2024.00051]

[5] Y. Chen, J. Zhou, and L. Wang, "Role and mechanism of gut microbiota in human disease", *Front. Cell. Infect. Microbiol.,* vol. 11, 2021.625913 [http://dx.doi.org/10.3389/fcimb.2021.625913] [PMID: 33816335]

[6] Z.Y. Kho, and S.K. Lal, "The human gut microbiome - A potential controller of wellness and disease", *Front. Microbiol.,* vol. 9, no. AUG, p. 1835, 2018. [http://dx.doi.org/10.3389/fmicb.2018.01835] [PMID: 30154767]

[7] S. Aryal, A. Alimadadi, I. Manandhar, B. Joe, and X. Cheng, "Machine learning strategy for gut microbiome-based diagnostic screening of cardiovascular disease", *Hypertension,* vol. 76, no. 5, pp. 1555-1562, 2020. [http://dx.doi.org/10.1161/HYPERTENSIONAHA.120.15885] [PMID: 32909848]

[8] B. Vilne, J. Ķibilds, I. Siksna, I. Lazda, O. Valciņa, and A. Krūmiņa, "Could artificial intelligence/machine learning and inclusion of diet-gut microbiome interactions improve disease risk prediction? case study: coronary artery disease", *Front. Microbiol.,* vol. 13, 2022.627892 [http://dx.doi.org/10.3389/fmicb.2022.627892] [PMID: 35479632]

[9] M. Subramanian, A. Wojtusciszyn, L. Favre, S. Boughorbel, J. Shan, K.B. Letaief, N. Pitteloud, and L. Chouchane, "Precision medicine in the era of artificial intelligence: implications in chronic disease management", *J. Transl. Med.,* vol. 18, no. 1, p. 472, 2020. [http://dx.doi.org/10.1186/s12967-020-02658-5] [PMID: 33298113]

[10] T. Reynolds, S. Noorbakhsh, and R. Smith, "Microbiome contributions to health", *Surg. Infect. (Larchmt.),* vol. 24, no. 3, pp. 213-219, 2023. [http://dx.doi.org/10.1089/sur.2023.002] [PMID: 37010974]

[11] S. Robertson-Albertyn, E. Hardee, and N.R. Stanley-Wall, "Microbe motels: an interactive method to introduce the human microbiome", *J. Microbiol. Biol. Educ.,* vol. 17, no. 2, pp. 282-283, 2016. [http://dx.doi.org/10.1128/jmbe.v17i2.966] [PMID: 27158310]

[12] D. Todkill, A.J. Elliot, R. Morbey, J. Harris, J. Hawker, O. Edeghere, and G.E. Smith, "What is the utility of using syndromic surveillance systems during large subnational infectious gastrointestinal disease outbreaks? An observational study using case studies from the past 5 years in England", *Epidemiol. Infect.,* vol. 144, no. 11, pp. 2241-2250, 2016. [http://dx.doi.org/10.1017/S0950268816000480] [PMID: 27033409]

[13] H.E. Bays, A. Fitch, S. Cuda, S. Gonsahn-Bollie, E. Rickey, J. Hablutzel, R. Coy, and M. Censani, "Artificial intelligence and obesity management: An Obesity Medicine Association (OMA) Clinical Practice Statement (CPS) 2023", *Obesity Pillars,* vol. 6, 2023.100065 [http://dx.doi.org/10.1016/j.obpill.2023.100065] [PMID: 37990659]

[14] Y. Fu, Q. Dou, K. Smalla, Y. Wang, T.A. Johnson, K.K. Brandt, Z. Mei, M. Liao, S.A. Hashsham, A. Schäffer, H. Smidt, T. Zhang, H. Li, R. Stedtfeld, H. Sheng, B. Chai, M. Virta, X. Jiang, F. Wang, Y.G. Zhu, and J.M. Tiedje, "Gut microbiota research nexus: One Health relationship between human, animal, and environmental resistomes", *mLife,* vol. 2, no. 4, pp. 350-364, 2023. [http://dx.doi.org/10.1002/mlf2.12101] [PMID: 38818274]

[15] Topol E. "Preparing the healthcare workforce to deliver the digital future," 2019. [Online]. Available: https://digitalhealth.london/topol-1 [Accessed: Oct. 25, 2024].

[16] B. Madhogaria, P. Bhowmik, and A. Kundu, "Correlation between human gut microbiome and diseases", *Infect. Med.,* vol. 1, no. 3, pp. 180-191, 2022. [http://dx.doi.org/10.1016/j.imj.2022.08.004] [PMID: 38077626]

[17] J. Kuczynski, E.K. Costello, D.R. Nemergut, J. Zaneveld, C.L. Lauber, D. Knights, O. Koren, N. Fierer, S.T. Kelley, R.E. Ley, J.I. Gordon, and R. Knight, "Direct sequencing of the human microbiome readily reveals community differences", *Genome Biol.,* vol. 11, no. 5, p. 210, 2010. [http://dx.doi.org/10.1186/gb-2010-11-5-210] [PMID: 20441597]

[18] Z. Huang, K. Liu, W. Ma, D. Li, T. Mo, and Q. Liu, "The gut microbiome in human health and disease—Where are we and where are we going? A bibliometric analysis", *Front. Microbiol.,* vol. 13, 2022.1018594 [http://dx.doi.org/10.3389/fmicb.2022.1018594] [PMID: 36590421]

[19] M. Abavisani, A. Khoshrou, S.K. Foroushan, N. Ebadpour, and A. Sahebkar, "Deciphering the gut microbiome: The revolution of artificial intelligence in microbiota analysis and intervention", *Curr. Res. Biotechnol.,* vol. 7, 2024.100211 [http://dx.doi.org/10.1016/j.crbiot.2024.100211]

[20] P.J. Turnbaugh, V.K. Ridaura, J.J. Faith, F.E. Rey, R. Knight, and J.I. Gordon, "The effect of diet on the human gut microbiome: a metagenomic analysis in humanized gnotobiotic mice", *Sci. Transl. Med.,* vol. 1, no. 6, p. 6ra14, 2009. [http://dx.doi.org/10.1126/scitranslmed.3000322] [PMID: 20368178]

[21] J. Rajendhran, and P. Gunasekaran, "Human microbiomics", *Indian J. Microbiol.,* vol. 50, no. 1, pp. 109-112, 2010. [http://dx.doi.org/10.1007/s12088-010-0034-9] [PMID: 23100817]

[22] H. Wu, L. Cai, D. Li, X. Wang, S. Zhao, F. Zou, and K. Zhou, "Metagenomics biomarkers selected for prediction of three different diseases in chinese population", *BioMed Res. Int.,* vol. 2018, pp. 1-7, 2018. [http://dx.doi.org/10.1155/2018/2936257] [PMID: 29568746]

[23] Y.H. Zhou, and P. Gallins, "A review and tutorial of machine learning methods for microbiome host trait prediction", *Front. Genet.,* vol. 10, no. JUN, p. 579, 2019. [http://dx.doi.org/10.3389/fgene.2019.00579] [PMID: 31293616]

[24] H.R. Johnson, D.D. Trinidad, S. Guzman, Z. Khan, J.V. Parziale, J.M. DeBruyn, and N.H. Lents, "A machine learning approach for using the postmortem skin microbiome to estimate the postmortem interval", *PLoS One,* vol. 11, no. 12, 2016.e0167370 [http://dx.doi.org/10.1371/journal.pone.0167370] [PMID: 28005908]

[25] J.J. Werner, O. Koren, P. Hugenholtz, T.Z. DeSantis, W.A. Walters, J.G. Caporaso, L.T. Angenent, R. Knight, and R.E. Ley, "Impact of training sets on classification of high-throughput bacterial 16s rRNA gene surveys", *ISME J.,* vol. 6, no. 1, pp. 94-103, 2012. [http://dx.doi.org/10.1038/ismej.2011.82] [PMID: 21716311]

[26] C. Lo, and R. Marculescu, "MetaNN: accurate classification of host phenotypes from metagenomic data using neural networks", *BMC Bioinformatics,* vol. 20, no. S12, suppl. Suppl. 12, p. 314, 2019. [http://dx.doi.org/10.1186/s12859-019-2833-2] [PMID: 31216991]

[27] S. Yachida, S. Mizutani, H. Shiroma, S. Shiba, T. Nakajima, T. Sakamoto, H. Watanabe, K. Masuda, Y. Nishimoto, M. Kubo, F. Hosoda, H. Rokutan, M. Matsumoto, H. Takamaru, M. Yamada, T. Matsuda, M. Iwasaki, T. Yamaji, T. Yachida, T. Soga, K. Kurokawa, A. Toyoda, Y. Ogura, T. Hayashi, M. Hatakeyama, H. Nakagama, Y. Saito, S. Fukuda, T. Shibata, and T. Yamada, "Metagenomic and metabolomic analyses reveal distinct stage-specific phenotypes of the gut microbiota in colorectal cancer", *Nat. Med.,* vol. 25, no. 6, pp. 968-976, 2019. [http://dx.doi.org/10.1038/s41591-019-0458-7] [PMID: 31171880]

[28] J.T. Wassan, H. Wang, F. Browne, and H. Zheng, "Phy-PMRFI: phylogeny-aware prediction of metagenomic functions using random forest feature importance", *IEEE Trans. Nanobiosci.,* vol. 18, no. 3, pp. 273-282, 2019. [http://dx.doi.org/10.1109/TNB.2019.2912824] [PMID: 31021803]

[29] B.S. Jang, J.H. Chang, E.K. Chie, K. Kim, J.W. Park, M.J. Kim, E.J. Song, Y.D. Nam, S.W. Kang, S.Y. Jeong, and H.J. Kim, "Gut Microbiome Composition Is Associated with a Pathologic Response After Preoperative Chemoradiation in Patients with Rectal Cancer", *Int. J. Radiat. Oncol. Biol. Phys.,* vol. 107, no. 4, pp. 736-746, 2020. [http://dx.doi.org/10.1016/j.ijrobp.2020.04.015] [PMID: 32315676]

[30] J. Lugo-Martinez, D. Ruiz-Perez, G. Narasimhan, and Z. Bar-Joseph, "Dynamic interaction network inference from longitudinal microbiome data", *Microbiome,* vol. 7, no. 1, p. 54, 2019. [http://dx.doi.org/10.1186/s40168-019-0660-3] [PMID: 30940197]

[31] V.M. Markowitz, I.M.A. Chen, K. Chu, E. Szeto, K. Palaniappan, B. Jacob, A. Ratner, K. Liolios, I. Pagani, M. Huntemann, K. Mavromatis, N.N. Ivanova, and N.C. Kyrpides, "IMG/M-HMP: a metagenome comparative analysis system for the Human Microbiome Project", *PLoS One,* vol. 7, no. 7, 2012.e40151 [http://dx.doi.org/10.1371/journal.pone.0040151] [PMID: 22792232]

[32] A.K. Wani, P. Roy, V. Kumar, and T.G. Mir, "Metagenomics and artificial intelligence in the context of human health", *Infect. Genet. Evol.,* vol. 100, 2022.105267 [http://dx.doi.org/10.1016/j.meegid.2022.105267] [PMID: 35278679]

[33] X. Zhang, D. Zhang, X. Zhang, and X. Zhang, "Artificial intelligence applications in the diagnosis and treatment of bacterial infections", *Front. Microbiol.,* vol. 15, 2024.1449844 [http://dx.doi.org/10.3389/fmicb.2024.1449844] [PMID: 39165576]

[34] L. Zhang, F. Chen, Z. Zeng, M. Xu, F. Sun, L. Yang, X. Bi, Y. Lin, Y. Gao, H. Hao, W. Yi, M. Li, and Y. Xie, "Advances in metagenomics and its application in environmental microorganisms", *Frontiers in Microbiology,* vol. 12, p. 766364, 2021. [http://dx.doi.org/10.3389/fmicb.2021.766364]

[35] B.D. Topçuoğlu, N.A. Lesniak, M.T. Ruffin IV, J. Wiens, and P.D. Schloss, "A framework for effective application of machine learning to microbiome-based classification problems", *MBio,* vol. 11, no. 3, 2020.e00434-20 [http://dx.doi.org/10.1128/mBio.00434-20] [PMID: 32518182]

[36] A. Amaan, G. Prekshi, and S. Prachi, "Microbiome-gut-brain axis: AI insights," Insights in Biology and Medicine, vol. 8, no. 1, pp. 001–010, 2024. [Online]. Available: http://dx.doi.org/10.29328/journal.ibm.1001027

[37] So-Yeon Yang, "Advancing gut microbiome research: the shift from metagenomics to multi-omics and future perspectives", *J. Microbiol. Biotechnol.,* vol. 35, p. e2412001, 2025. [http://dx.doi.org/10.4014/jmb.2412.12001]

[38] https://newsnetwork.mayoclinic.org/discussion/mayo-researchers-develop-tool-that-measures--ealth-of-a-persons-gut-microbiome/

[39] E.T. Beyene, S. Cha, and Y. Jin, "Overweight and obesity trends and associated factors among reproductive women in Ethiopia", *Glob. Health Action,* vol. 17, no. 1, 2024.2362728 [http://dx.doi.org/10.1080/16549716.2024.2362728] [PMID: 38863400]

[40] J. Geng, Q. Ni, W. Sun, L. Li, and X. Feng, "The links between gut microbiota and obesity and obesity related diseases", *Biomed. Pharmacother.,* vol. 147, 2022.112678 [http://dx.doi.org/10.1016/j.biopha.2022.112678] [PMID: 35134709]

[41] J.R. Vasselli, S. Juray, and S.E. Trasino, "Success and failures of telehealth during COVID□19 should inform digital applications to combat obesity", *Obes. Sci. Pract.,* vol. 8, no. 2, pp. 254-258, 2022. [http://dx.doi.org/10.1002/osp4.551] [PMID: 34540264]

[42] K.A. Shastry, and A. Shastry, "An integrated deep learning and natural language processing approach for continuous remote monitoring in digital health", *Decision Analytics Journal,* vol. 8, 2023.100301 [http://dx.doi.org/10.1016/j.dajour.2023.100301]

[43] N. Hinchliffe, M.S. Capehorn, M. Bewick, and J. Feenie, "The potential role of digital health in obesity care", *Adv. Ther.,* vol. 39, no. 10, pp. 4397-4412, 2022. [http://dx.doi.org/10.1007/s12325-022-02265-4] [PMID: 35925469]

[44] U. Chaturvedi, S. B. Chauhan, and Indu Singh, "The impact of artificial intelligence on remote healthcare: Enhancing patient engagement, connectivity, and overcoming challenges", *Intell. Pharm.,* vol. 3, no. 5, pp. 323-329, 2025. [http://dx.doi.org/10.1016/j.ipha.2024.12.003]

[45] T. Zhou, and F. Zhao, "AI-empowered human microbiome research", *Gut,* 2025. [http://dx.doi.org/10.1136/gutjnl-2025-335946]

[46] J. Qin, R. Li, J. Raes, M. Arumugam, K.S. Burgdorf, C. Manichanh, T. Nielsen, N. Pons, F. Levenez, T. Yamada, D.R. Mende, J. Li, J. Xu, S. Li, D. Li, J. Cao, B. Wang, H. Liang, H. Zheng, Y. Xie, J. Tap, P. Lepage, M. Bertalan, J.M. Batto, T. Hansen, D. Le Paslier, A. Linneberg, H.B. Nielsen, E. Pelletier, P. Renault, T. Sicheritz-Ponten, K. Turner, H. Zhu, C. Yu, S. Li, M. Jian, Y. Zhou, Y. Li, X. Zhang, S. Li, N. Qin, H. Yang, J. Wang, S. Brunak, J. Doré, F. Guarner, K. Kristiansen, O. Pedersen, J. Parkhill, J. Weissenbach, P. Bork, S.D. Ehrlich, and J. Wang, "A human gut microbial gene catalogue established by metagenomic sequencing", *Nature,* vol. 464, no. 7285, pp. 59-65, 2010. [http://dx.doi.org/10.1038/nature08821] [PMID: 20203603]

[47] H. Cui, and X. Zhang, "Alignment-free supervised classification of metagenomes by recursive SVM", *BMC Genomics,* vol. 14, no. 1, p. 641, 2013. [http://dx.doi.org/10.1186/1471-2164-14-641] [PMID: 24053649]

[48] P.E. Larsen, and Y. Dai, "Metabolome of human gut microbiome is predictive of host dysbiosis", *Gigascience,* vol. 4, no. 1, 2015.s13742-015-0084-3 [http://dx.doi.org/10.1186/s13742-015-0084-3] [PMID: 25838885]

[49] D. Fioravanti, Y. Giarratano, V. Maggio, C. Agostinelli, M. Chierici, G. Jurman, and C. Furlanello, "Phylogenetic convolutional neural networks in metagenomics", *BMC Bioinformatics,* vol. 19, no. S2, suppl. Suppl. 2, p. 49, 2018. [http://dx.doi.org/10.1186/s12859-018-2033-5] [PMID: 29536822]

[50] G.M. Douglas, R. Hansen, C.M.A. Jones, K.A. Dunn, A.M. Comeau, J.P. Bielawski, R. Tayler, E.M.

El-Omar, R.K. Russell, G.L. Hold, M.G.I. Langille, and J. Van Limbergen, "Multi-omics differentially classify disease state and treatment outcome in pediatric Crohn's disease", *Microbiome,* vol. 6, no. 1, p. 13, 2018.
[http://dx.doi.org/10.1186/s40168-018-0398-3] [PMID: 29335008]

[51] D. Travisany, D. Galarce, A. Maass, and R. Assar, *Predicting the Metagenomics Content with Multiple CART Trees.* Mathematical Models in Biology, 2015, pp. 145-160.
[http://dx.doi.org/10.1007/978-3-319-23497-7_11]

[52] D. Zeevi, T. Korem, N. Zmora, D. Israeli, D. Rothschild, A. Weinberger, O. Ben-Yacov, D. Lador, T. Avnit-Sagi, M. Lotan-Pompan, J. Suez, J.A. Mahdi, E. Matot, G. Malka, N. Kosower, M. Rein, G. Zilberman-Schapira, L. Dohnalová, M. Pevsner-Fischer, R. Bikovsky, Z. Halpern, E. Elinav, and E. Segal, "Personalized nutrition by prediction of glycemic responses", *Cell,* vol. 163, no. 5, pp. 1079-1094, 2015.
[http://dx.doi.org/10.1016/j.cell.2015.11.001] [PMID: 26590418]

[53] Q. Zhu, B. Li, T. He, G. Li, and X. Jiang, "Robust biomarker discovery for microbiome-wide association studies", *Methods,* vol. 173, pp. 44-51, 2020.
[http://dx.doi.org/10.1016/j.ymeth.2019.06.012] [PMID: 31238097]

[54] E.B. Hollister, N. Oezguen, B.P. Chumpitazi, R.A. Luna, E.M. Weidler, M. Rubio-Gonzales, M. Dahdouli, J.L. Cope, T.A. Mistretta, S. Raza, G.A. Metcalf, D.M. Muzny, R.A. Gibbs, J.F. Petrosino, M. Heitkemper, T.C. Savidge, R.J. Shulman, and J. Versalovic, "Leveraging human microbiome features to diagnose and stratify children with irritable bowel syndrome", *J. Mol. Diagn.,* vol. 21, no. 3, pp. 449-461, 2019.
[http://dx.doi.org/10.1016/j.jmoldx.2019.01.006] [PMID: 31005411]

[55] A. Mohammed, and C. Guda, "Application of a hierarchical enzyme classification method reveals the role of gut microbiome in human metabolism", *BMC Genomics,* vol. 16, no. S7, suppl. Suppl. 7, p. S16, 2015.
[http://dx.doi.org/10.1186/1471-2164-16-S7-S16] [PMID: 26099921]

[56] L. Chen, Y.H. Zhang, T. Huang, and Y.D. Cai, "Gene expression profiling gut microbiota in different races of humans", *Sci. Rep.,* vol. 6, no. 1, p. 23075, 2016.
[http://dx.doi.org/10.1038/srep23075] [PMID: 26975620]

[57] D.A. Hughes, R. Bacigalupe, J. Wang, M.C. Rühlemann, R.Y. Tito, G. Falony, M. Joossens, S. Vieira-Silva, L. Henckaerts, L. Rymenans, C. Verspecht, S. Ring, A. Franke, K.H. Wade, N.J. Timpson, and J. Raes, "Genome-wide associations of human gut microbiome variation and implications for causal inference analyses", *Nat. Microbiol.,* vol. 5, no. 9, pp. 1079-1087, 2020.
[http://dx.doi.org/10.1038/s41564-020-0743-8] [PMID: 32572223]

[58] Samira Abdul, C.C. Maha, T.O. Kolawole, and S. Abdul, "Innovations in real-time infectious disease surveillance using AI and mobile data", *International Medical Science Research Journal,* vol. 4, no. 6, pp. 647-667, 2024.
[http://dx.doi.org/10.51594/imsrj.v4i6.1190]

[59] J.S. Brownstein, B. Rader, C.M. Astley, and H. Tian, "Advances in artificial intelligence for infectious-disease surveillance", *N. Engl. J. Med.,* vol. 388, no. 17, pp. 1597-1607, 2023.
[http://dx.doi.org/10.1056/NEJMra2119215] [PMID: 37099342]

[60] H. Kim, S. Park, I.G. Jeong, S.H. Song, Y. Jeong, C.S. Kim, and K.H. Lee, "Noninvasive precision screening of prostate cancer by urinary multimarker sensor and artificial intelligence analysis", *ACS Nano,* vol. 15, no. 3, pp. 4054-4065, 2021.
[http://dx.doi.org/10.1021/acsnano.0c06946] [PMID: 33296173]

[61] T. Wasilewski, W. Kamysz, and J. Gębicki, "AI-assisted detection of biomarkers by sensors and biosensors for early diagnosis and monitoring", *Biosensors (Basel),* vol. 14, no. 7, p. 356, 2024.
[http://dx.doi.org/10.3390/bios14070356] [PMID: 39056632]

[62] R.A. Morbey, A.J. Elliot, G.E. Smith, and A. Charlett, "Adapting syndromic surveillance baselines

after public health interventions", *Public Health Rep.,* vol. 135, no. 6, pp. 737-745, 2020. [http://dx.doi.org/10.1177/0033354920959080] [PMID: 33026959]

[63] "Office of Public Health Data, Surveillance, and Technology | OPHDST | CDC." Accessed: Jan. 05, 2026. [Online]. Available: https://www.cdc.gov/ophdst/index.html

[64] J. Zhu, H. Xie, Z. Yang, J. Chen, J. Yin, P. Tian, H. Wang, J. Zhao, H. Zhang, W. Lu, and W. Chen, "Statistical modeling of gut microbiota for personalized health status monitoring", *Microbiome,* vol. 11, no. 1, p. 184, 2023. [http://dx.doi.org/10.1186/s40168-023-01614-x] [PMID: 37596617]

[65] T. Shashkova, A. Popenko, A. Tyakht, K. Peskov, Y. Kosinsky, L. Bogolubsky, A. Raigorodskii, D. Ischenko, D. Alexeev, and V. Govorun, "Agent based modeling of human gut microbiome interactions and perturbations", *PLoS One,* vol. 11, no. 2, 2016.e0148386 [http://dx.doi.org/10.1371/journal.pone.0148386] [PMID: 26894828]

[66] S. Zhang, S. Li, W. Gu, H. den Bakker, D. Boxrud, A. Taylor, C. Roe, E. Driebe, D.M. Engelthaler, M. Allard, E. Brown, P. McDermott, S. Zhao, B.B. Bruce, E. Trees, P.I. Fields, and X. Deng, "Zoonotic source attribution of *Salmonella enterica* serotype *Typhimurium* using genomic surveillance data, United States", *Emerg. Infect. Dis.,* vol. 25, no. 1, pp. 82-91, 2019. [http://dx.doi.org/10.3201/eid2501.180835] [PMID: 30561314]

[67] M. Payne, S. Octavia, L.D.W. Luu, C. Sotomayor-Castillo, Q. Wang, A.C.Y. Tay, V. Sintchenko, M.M. Tanaka, and R. Lan, "Enhancing genomics-based outbreak detection of endemic *Salmonella enterica* serovar *Typhimurium* using dynamic thresholds", *Microb. Genom.,* vol. 7, no. 6, 2021.000310 [http://dx.doi.org/10.1099/mgen.0.000310] [PMID: 31682222]

[68] P. Anjaria, V. Asediya, P. Bhavsar, A. Pathak, D. Desai, and V. Patil, "Artificial intelligence in public health: Revolutionizing epidemiological surveillance for pandemic preparedness and equitable vaccine access," Vaccines, vol. 11, no. 7, p. 1154, 2023. [Online]. Available: http://dx.doi.org/10.3390/vaccines11071154

[69] H.A. Carleton, J. Besser, A.J. Williams-Newkirk, A. Huang, E. Trees, and P. Gerner-Smidt, "Metagenomic approaches for public health surveillance of foodborne infections: opportunities and challenges", *Foodborne Pathog. Dis.,* vol. 16, no. 7, pp. 474-479, 2019. [http://dx.doi.org/10.1089/fpd.2019.2636] [PMID: 31170005]

[70] J. I. Levy, K. G. Andersen, R. Knight, and S. Karthikeyan, "Wastewater surveillance for public health: Wastewater contains information on pathogen spread, evolution, and outbreak risk," Science, vol. 379, no. 6627, pp. 26–27, Jan. 2023. [http://dx.doi.org/10.1126/science.ade2503]

[71] J. Wu, Y. Chen, J. Zhao, T.A. Prosun, J.W. O'Brien, L. Coin, F.I. Hai, M. Sanderson-Smith, P. Bi, and G. Jiang, "Associations between wastewater gut microbiome and community obesity rates: Potential microbial biomarkers for surveillance", *Soil & Environmental Health,* vol. 2, no. 2, 2024.100081 [http://dx.doi.org/10.1016/j.seh.2024.100081]

[72] B.T. Tierney, J. Foox, K.A. Ryon, D. Butler, N. Damle, B.G. Young, C. Mozsary, K.M. Babler, X. Yin, Y. Carattini, D. Andrews, A.G. Lucaci, N.S. Solle, N. Kumar, B. Shukla, D. Vidović, B. Currall, S.L. Williams, S.C. Schürer, M. Stevenson, A. Amirali, C.C. Beaver, E. Kobetz, M.M. Boone, B. Reding, J. Laine, S. Comerford, W.E. Lamar, J.J. Tallon Jr, J. Wain Hirschberg, J. Proszynski, G. Al Ghalith, K. Can Kurt, M.E. Sharkey, G.M. Church, G.S. Grills, H.M. Solo-Gabriele, and C.E. Mason, "Towards geospatially-resolved public-health surveillance *via* wastewater sequencing", *Nat. Commun.,* vol. 15, no. 1, p. 8386, 2024. [http://dx.doi.org/10.1038/s41467-024-52427-x] [PMID: 39333485]

[73] T. Zeng, X. Yu, and Z. Chen, "Applying artificial intelligence in the microbiome for gastrointestinal diseases: A review", *J. Gastroenterol. Hepatol.,* vol. 36, no. 4, pp. 832-840, 2021. [http://dx.doi.org/10.1111/jgh.15503] [PMID: 33880762]

[74] F.J. Colón-González, I.R. Lake, R.A. Morbey, A.J. Elliot, R. Pebody, and G.E. Smith, "A

methodological framework for the evaluation of syndromic surveillance systems: a case study of England", *BMC Public Health,* vol. 18, no. 1, p. 544, 2018.
[http://dx.doi.org/10.1186/s12889-018-5422-9] [PMID: 29699520]

[75] B. Zareie, J. Poorolajal, A. Roshani, A. Menbari, and M. Karami, "Outbreak detector: a web application to boost disease surveillance systems and timely detection of infectious disease epidemics", *BMC Res. Notes,* vol. 17, no. 1, p. 229, 2024.
[http://dx.doi.org/10.1186/s13104-024-06892-8] [PMID: 39164780]

[76] Varsha. P. S, "How can we manage biases in artificial intelligence systems – A systematic literature review," International Journal of Information Management Data Insights, vol. 3, no. 1, p. 100165, Apr. 2023.
[http://dx.doi.org/10.1016/J.JJIMEI.2023.100165]

[77] H. Yuan, K. Yu, F. Xie, M. Liu, and S. Sun, "Automated machine learning with interpretation: A systematic review of methodologies and applications in healthcare", *Medicine Advances,* vol. 2, no. 3, pp. 205-237, 2024.
[http://dx.doi.org/10.1002/med4.75]

[78] J. Waring, C. Lindvall, and R. Umeton, "Automated machine learning: Review of the state-of-the-art and opportunities for healthcare", *Artif. Intell. Med.,* vol. 104, 2020.101822
[http://dx.doi.org/10.1016/j.artmed.2020.101822] [PMID: 32499001]

CHAPTER 13

Advancements in Transformer-Based Models for NLP in Healthcare

Juhi Sharma[1], **Uzma Patel**[1], **Divyanshi Salundiya**[1], **Avantika Sharma**[1], **Kratika Pathak**[1] and **Sumit Govil**[1,*]

[1] *School of Life and Basic Sciences, Jaipur National University, Jaipur, Rajasthan, India*

Abstract: Transformer-based models have transformed the branch of Natural Language Processing (NLP), significantly developing healthcare applications. This abstract examines the advancements and effects of these models in healthcare, emphasizing their strengths, obstacles, and future possibilities. Notable transformer architectures such as BERT and GPT, along with their variants, have greatly improved the proficiency of NLP systems in comprehending and producing human language. These models are particularly effective for tasks like named entity recognition, relationship extraction, and clinical text generation, which are essential for managing and interpreting large volumes of healthcare information. Their ability to be pre-trained on extensive datasets and fine-tuned with specialized medical information has allowed transformers to attain cutting-edge performance in medical coding, Electronic Health Record (EHR) analysis, and patient sentiment evaluation. Implementing transformer-based models in the healthcare sector has enhanced diagnostic precision, provided more tailored treatment suggestions, and improved patient engagement through chatbots and virtual assistants. For instance, models like BioBERT and ClinicalBERT, specifically fine-tuned on biomedical and clinical literature, have demonstrated notable advancements in interpreting and predicting medical conditions based on clinical notes. Nevertheless, several challenges persist, including concerns about data privacy, the necessity for extensive and varied medical datasets, and the interpretability of complex model predictions. Tackling these issues requires ongoing research on model transparency, privacy-preserving methods, and strategies to address the imbalance and variability in healthcare data. Looking ahead, transformer-based models are set to further revolutionize healthcare by facilitating more accurate and scalable solutions. Improvement in model design, training approaches, and domain-specific customizations will be vital for realizing their full potential to enhance healthcare outcomes and operational efficiency.

Keywords: Diagnostic precision, Electronic health records, Healthcare, Model predictions, Patient engagement, Transformer architectures, Virtual assistants.

* **Corresponding author Sumit Govil:** School of Life and Basic Sciences, Jaipur National University, Jaipur, Rajasthan, India; E-mail: sumitgovil@jnujaipur.ac.in

A. Shankar, Saranya Jayapalan, & Basant. K. Tiwary (Eds.)

INTRODUCTION

Transformer models represent a significant advancement in deep learning architectures tailored for Natural Language Processing (NLP). They capture long-range dependencies, making them suitable for machine translation, text summarization, and question-answering [1]. The encoder-decoder framework is part of an architecture in which the encoder transforms the input into a compact summary while the decoder uses this summary to generate the output sequence. Both components are trained to minimize conditional log-likelihood, effectively allowing the model to handle input-output relationships [2].

The original transformer architecture features six identical layers in both the encoder and the decoder. Each encoder layer consists of two sublayers: a multi-head attention mechanism and a feed-forward network, enhanced with residual connections and layer normalization. The decoder adds a third attention layer that focuses on the encoder's output, with one layer masked to prevent future token visibility.

The transition to transformer models marks a pivotal shift from traditional sequential methods, like unidirectional RNNs and LSTMs, to attention-based architectures, thereby improving performance in NLP tasks [3]. Traditional models, including CNNs and RNNs, process data sequentially without revisiting previously processed tokens. While LSTMs improve RNNs by managing information flow through gating mechanisms, transformers leverage self-attention to capture dependencies more effectively [4].

Traditional deep learning models struggle with sequential reasoning, a capability enhanced by attention mechanisms. In human cognition, reasoning integrates and verifies facts through attention, effectively guiding the reasoning process by focusing on relevant information [5]. Similarly, in machine learning, tasks can be decomposed into specific subtasks that require concentrated attention on parts of the input or transformed data. This approach mimics the brain's neural processing, where attention helps manage information flow across multiple layers [6].

The Self-Attention Mechanism (SA) enables models to focus on important information while discarding less relevant details, which is particularly beneficial in computer vision by highlighting essential data for better outcomes. SA excels in establishing long-term dependencies within datasets, enhancing understanding of complex patterns. Multi-Head Self-Attention (MSA) processes multiple attention mechanisms simultaneously, capturing diverse data. This mechanism has notably improved neural machine translation through parallel computing, although the rise of large models often necessitates substantial computational resources [7]. In light of these developments, optimizing the sub-layers of transformer models can enhance their inference rates. This paper advocates tailoring language model architectures to specific languages, suggesting that parameter adjustments may benefit various machine translation applications [1].

Uses of Transformer Models in Healthcare

Initially created for NLP (Natural Language Processing), transformer models have been adapted across various fields, including speech processing, multimodal learning, time series analysis, and remote sensing (Fig. **1**). In healthcare, these models are employed across different data modalities, resulting in the development of modality-specific surveys focusing on areas such as medical imaging and biomedical language models. Large Language Models (LLMs) and

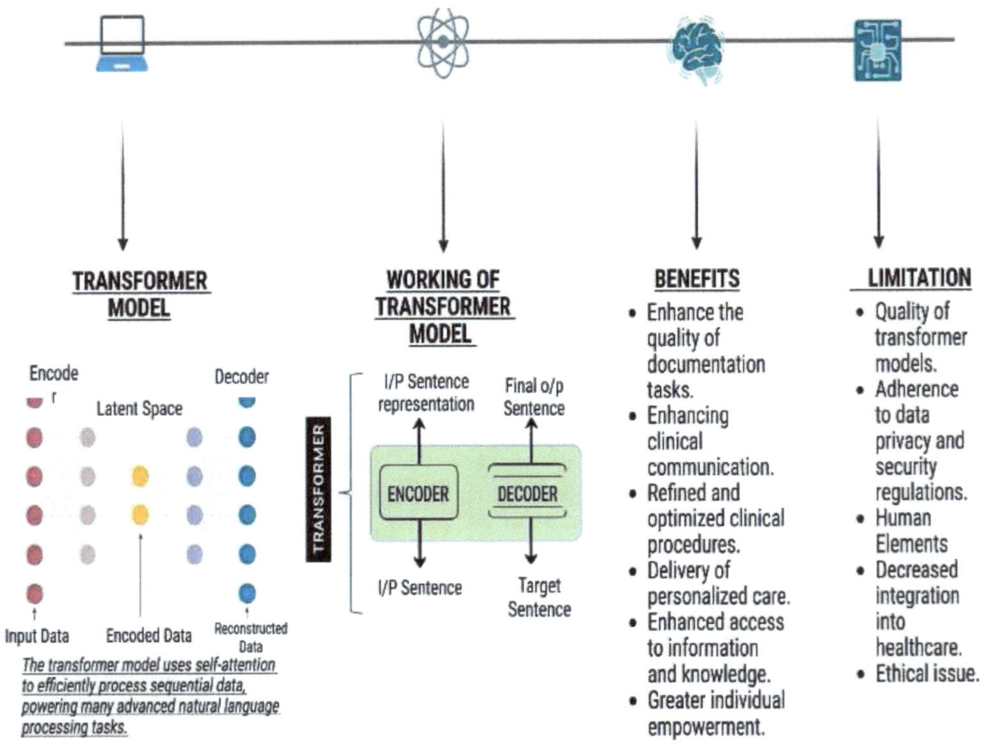

Fig. (1). Principles and architecture of transformer models.

transformers can revolutionize healthcare systems, significantly enhancing workflow management, clinical documentation, diagnosis, treatment, and communication. They facilitate personalized care, empower patients, and increase access to medical information. Despite this, their implementation comes with risks, including data-related issues, system impacts, quality and regulatory concerns, and economic implications requiring training programs to address shifts in the healthcare job landscape [6].

Key applications of transformer models in medicine include:

- ***Drug Discovery and Development***: Transformers analyze biological data to identify drug targets, support medication repurposing, and predict drug toxicity, thereby minimizing adverse side effects [8].
- ***GPT Model***: ChatGPT has potential in clinical diagnosis, medical education, and public health advice. Recent updates to the GPT-4 model have improved its clinical applicability, showcasing advancements in automation and AI in healthcare [9].

POTENTIAL CHALLENGES

Our study identifies substantial literature support for various applications of transformer models in healthcare:

- **Documentation and Clinical Coding (C1)**: AI has improved clinical documentation processes, particularly in radiation oncology [10].
- **Workflow and Healthcare Services (C2)**: Transformers have shown promise in optimizing triage processes.
- **Clinical Knowledge Management (C3)**: Effective clinical knowledge management, including diabetes care, has been reported.
- **Facilitating Healthcare Interactions (C4)**: Research indicates improved stakeholder interactions through speech-emotion recognition.
- **Education and Empowerment (C5)**: Positive patient empowerment outcomes have been observed.
- **Public Health (C7)**: Transformers can enhance public health initiatives like drug event monitoring and misinformation detection.
- **Decision-Making (C8)**: These models assist in computer-aided diagnosis and prediction of drug interactions [11].

DATA CHALLENGES IN HEALTH INDICATORS

- The WHO has defined over 750 indicators across various health domains, with 47 key indicators emphasized for evaluating health systems' progress. However, countries typically select between 15 and 30 core indicators, resulting in a large number of indicators across health programs that may operate independently.
- Integrating advanced NLP techniques and hybrid models represents a significant advancement in the collection and analysis of SDoH data, enhancing the ability to extract meaningful insights from EHRs. While challenges in data collection and health indicators persist, strategic data management and analysis approaches can improve public health outcomes and inform healthcare policies effectively [7].

Notably, the lack of concrete research on transformer systems in health management (C6) indicates an area for future exploration.

LIMITATION AND FUTURE WORK

One limitation of our study is the small sample size and varying levels of expertise among participants—32.1% had utilized ChatGPT without extensive technological expertise. The hiring process might have introduced bias by selectively choosing medical natural language processing experts. Additionally, the e-survey only offered a small amount of data, potentially leading to a misconception. Despite these challenges, our qualitative research identified eight potential applications of transformer models in healthcare. Upcoming research will focus on assessing the feasibility, significance, and results from the perspective of clinical specialists. We will also explore the risks and benefits of implementing transformer models in these contexts [12].

While transformer models are promising for various NLP tasks, their application in healthcare comes with unique challenges, particularly concerning accuracy and explainability:

- **Quantity and Quality of Data**

- ***Restricted and Biased Data***: The effectiveness of transformer models can be hampered by healthcare data that is noisy, biased, or limited in scale.
- ***Data Security and Privacy***: Handling sensitive patient information raises significant security and privacy concerns, necessitating robust protective measures.

- **Computational Resources**

- ***High Computational Costs***: Training and deploying large transformer models require substantial hardware resources, which can be expensive.
- ***Scalability***: Managing extensive healthcare databases may pose efficiency and scalability challenges [13].

- **Verifying Information**

- ***Data Quality***: Results from transformer models can be misleading if the underlying healthcare data is noisy or incomplete.
- ***Fact Verification***: Ensuring the integrity of data produced by these models is crucial, as inaccuracies can have profound implications.

- ***Data Sources***: Training data and evaluation must be precise and representative of the target population.

- **Handling Inaccuracies or Hallucinations**

- ***False Positives and Negatives:*** In diagnostic applications, transformer models may produce false results, which can mislead healthcare decisions.
- ***Hallucinations:*** These models can generate text that includes factually incorrect or nonsensical information, posing risks in clinical settings.
- ***Error Detection and Correction***: A significant challenge is developing methods to identify and rectify errors in transformer outputs.

- **Data Privacy Challenges**

- ***Data Exposure***: Using sensitive healthcare data for training can lead to unintended exposure of patient information.
- ***Data Breaches***: Patients face risks such as identity theft and financial loss from potential data breaches.
- ***Regulatory Compliance***: Healthcare organizations must comply with stringent data privacy laws, like GDPR and HIPAA.

- **Human Aspects**

- This concept highlights the medical experts who use transformer-based systems. Challenges include the need for human expertise to assess results, the risk of overreliance on technology, potential negligence, and the necessity for continuous skill development [14].

PRE-TRAINED TRANSFORMER MODELS

Transformer-Based Bidirectional Encoder Representations (BERT)

Overview of Transformer Models: BERT, T5, and GPT

BERT stands for Bidirectional Encoder Representations from Transformer, a type of transformer architecture tailored for encoding functions in Natural Language Processing (NLP). It generates comprehensive contextualized word and sentence embeddings by analyzing entire word sequences simultaneously, enhancing its understanding of context. To create context-sensitive embeddings, BERT utilizes self-supervised pretraining techniques like (MLM) Masked Language Modeling and (NSP) Sentence Prediction. MLM involves predicting masked tokens based on surrounding words, while NSP assesses sentence relationships. This approach allows BERT to develop deep bidirectional representations, making it suitable for language inference and question-answering [10].

Text-to-Text Transfer Transformer, or T5, is a flexible language model. The model presents different NLP assignments as text-to-text issues, facilitating its application across diverse challenges. Its encoder-decoder architecture allows it to process input text and generate output, effectively addressing tasks like text summarization and machine translation.

GPT stands for Generative Pre-trained Transformer models that employ a transformer-based architecture to process natural language text, utilizing unsupervised learning for pre-training on large text corpora. The training process includes pre-training to predict the next word, supervised fine-tuning on specific tasks, and reinforcement learning for performance enhancement. GPT generates text sequentially, predicting the next word based on prior context, which enables it to produce coherent and contextually relevant outputs [15].

IMPLICATION FOR HEALTHCARE

Both transformer models and Large Language Models (LLMs) provide significant ability to modify healthcare, enhancing areas such as diagnosis, treatment, clinical documentation, workflow management, therapy, clinical record keeping, and workflow management. They facilitate personalized care and make medical data more accessible. However, challenges exist, including data-related issues, system usage impacts, and concerns regarding quality and regulation. There is a pressing need for training programs and for adjustments to the employment landscape in healthcare.

Key considerations for the reliable application of these models in healthcare include:

- Implementing human oversight
- Ensuring openness in model interpretations.
- Maintaining high-quality data.
- Upholding system dependability and accuracy.
- Complying with regulations

The implementation of transformer models in healthcare provides substantial opportunities for invention, but it necessitates a careful approach to ensure safe and effective implementation [12].

COMPARATIVE STUDY OF TRANSFORMER MODELS IN TRANSLATION TECHNOLOGY

In the realm of Machine Translation (MT), transformer-based models like BERT, GPT, and T5 have significantly enhanced translation accuracy and efficiency, transforming how languages are understood and communicated [16].

- **GPT** excels at generating coherent translations and managing complex sentence structures effectively.
- **T5** frames all translation tasks as text generation challenges, showcasing versatility across various languages and translation domains.

Understanding the unique characteristics of BERT, GPT, and T5 is essential to understanding their advancements in translation technology, further illuminating their role in enhancing translation capabilities.

BERT, GPT, and T5 in Translation Technology

BERT, which stands for Bidirectional Encoder Representations from Transformers, is designed to understand the context of a sentence by reading text bidirectionally. This enables BERT to accurately capture the relationships between words, enhancing its ability to generate contextual embeddings crucial for translation tasks. Translators can leverage these embeddings to navigate complex sentence structures and ambiguous phrases, improving translation accuracy, especially for languages with nuanced meanings [10].

GPT stands for Generative Pre-trained Transformer, a class of models that generate fluent, contextually relevant translations. They use an autoregressive approach, predicting the next word from previous context. The sequential generation helps maintain coherence and meaning in translations. GPT's creative text generation capabilities allow translators to explore various expressions, making translations culturally appropriate and engaging.

Text-to-Text Transfer Transformer, or T5, approaches all natural language processing assignments, including translation, as challenges in the text-to-text tasks. This unified framework simplifies the translation process, treating source and target languages as text inputs. T5's ability to learn task-agnostic representations supports efficient transfer learning, allowing translators to fine-tune models for specific domains or styles, thus tailoring outputs to meet varying needs.

Understanding the unique features of BERT, GPT, and T5 enables translators to select the most appropriate model for improving the task, accuracy, fluency, and cultural relevance for translations. Staying informed about advancements in these NLP models is essential for improving translation technology and ensuring high-quality translations that resonate with target audiences [8].

Relevance of Transformer Models

BERT, GPT, and T5 significantly impact translation technology through various practical applications:

- ***BERT-based models*** enhance translation quality by generating contextual embeddings for both source and target language terms and expressions.
- ***GPT-based models*** can be trained for tasks involving translation, producing fluent translations from source texts.
- ***T5 models*** treat translation as a text-to-text problem, where the source-language prompt generates the translation in the target language.

In transformer models, the translation process starts with a sentence in the source language and ends with the target language output, involving encoder and decoder mechanisms, self-attention, and feed-forward layers to achieve the final translation.

Research Implications

The implications of BERT, GPT, and T5 in translation include:

- ***BERT's bidirectional nature*** excels at capturing contextual information, leading to accurate translations of ambiguous phrases.
- ***GPT's generative capabilities*** produce coherent translations, particularly effective for longer texts, preserving the natural flow and style.
- ***T5's text-to-text approach*** enhances versatility across various language pairs and domains, facilitating efficient translation.

These models demonstrate superior performance in understanding context and generating high-quality translations, capturing complex linguistic patterns.

GPT and T5 also excel in few-shot and zero-shot translation scenarios, allowing for flexibility in translation systems. These transformer models can be fine-tuned for multilingual applications, benefiting low-resource languages by leveraging insights from high-resource ones. Additionally, they can be customized for specific domains, improving accuracy in specialized fields like legal or medical translation.

Despite their advancements, challenges remain, including biases in training data and ethical concerns regarding content manipulation. Addressing these issues is crucial for responsible deployment in real-world applications.

In summary, BERT, GPT, and T5 have transformed translation technology by providing advanced solutions for various challenges. Their ability to understand context, generate fluent translations, manage multilingual tasks, and adapt to specific domains makes them essential for developing versatile translation systems. However, addressing ethical concerns and biases is critical for their responsible use in translation applications.

COLLECTING AND ANALYZING SOCIAL DETERMINANTS OF HEALTH (SDOH) DATA

A prevalent method for collecting SDoH data is through patient questionnaires administered during medical appointments. An advanced approach links Electronic Health Records (EHR) with SDoH data derived from state and county-level census analyses [17]. This method has been implemented by organizations like the Methodist Healthcare Ministries of South Texas and the statewide Health Information Exchange (HIE) for San Antonio. Given the absence of a standardized method for SDoH data collection, optimizing techniques for extracting relevant information is essential.

NLP techniques, especially BERT, are increasingly employed to extract information from text documents, including EHRs. BERT consists of encoder layers featuring a self-attention mechanism and feed-forward neural networks, having been pretrained on extensive datasets from Google's Book corpus. BioBERT extends the original BERT model by incorporating training on vast medical literature, which enhances its applicability in clinical contexts.

To fine-tune the Clinical BioBERT model for SDoH relevance, a dataset of paragraphs is labeled to indicate their relevance, followed by a binary classification process utilizing a cross-entropy loss function. This approach transforms embeddings of [CLS] tokens into classification outputs.

Hybrid Approaches to Relation Extraction

For Relation Extraction (RE), a hybrid method combining rule-based syntactic pattern matching with transformer-based techniques is employed. Initially, regex rules identify relations by extracting consecutive entities within sentences. Any remaining instances are processed using a transformer model, enhancing efficiency by reducing computational load.

Additionally, T5 is utilized to frame the RE problem as a natural language inference task, assessing whether a relationship exists between two entities. This method generates premise-hypothesis pairs to determine the validity of the relationship.

Indirect Sources of Health Information

Census Data

The census is a crucial indirect source of health information in India, conducted under the Union Ministry of Home Affairs. The latest census was conducted in 2001, following the Indian Census Act, 1948, which empowers the Central Government to carry out nationwide censuses. This act mandates truthfulness in responses and ensures the confidentiality of the data collected. The Indian Census serves as an authoritative source of demographic and geographic information, having begun systematic data collection in 1881, with regular updates every ten years.

Civil Registration System

The Civil Registration System (CRS) continuously records significant events, such as marriages, births, and deaths, which are crucial for evaluating socio-economic programs, including maternal and child healthcare. Established in 1969, the CRS has roots in British colonial administration but remains incomplete despite mandatory registration requirements. The system captures detailed information about births and deaths, including demographic details and medical care received, aiding in public health assessments.

Advancing Ubiquitous Healthcare: ALPH for Streamlined Applications and Transformer Models for Clinical Insights

Ubiquitous Healthcare

The field of ubiquitous healthcare combines advanced computing technologies to manage healthcare information effectively. However, the growth of healthcare applications has not kept pace with mobile and network advancements. A proposed domain-specific language (ALPH) simplifies the development of ubiquitous healthcare applications by using constructs that model healthcare tasks and entities. A case study application, MedHCP, demonstrated improved modularity and software quality through this approach [18].

Transformer Models in Healthcare

Transformer models, designed originally for NLP, are now applied in various healthcare domains. They excel at extracting information from EHRs, classifying medical images, and aiding drug discovery processes:

- **EHRs Synopsis:** Transformers summarize patient demographics and medical histories, enhancing clinical decision-making.
- **Medical Image Analysis**: These models accurately classify images (*e.g.*, CT scans, MRIs) and facilitate tasks like tumor segmentation [19].
- **Drug Development**: Transformers analyze biological data for potential drug targets, repurpose medications, and predict toxicity [8, 20].

Patient Education and Health Management

Transformer models can also improve patient education by powering virtual assistants that provide health information tailored to individual literacy levels. Additionally, they facilitate health management by analyzing data from sensors and questionnaires, offering personalized support for chronic conditions.

Public Health Monitoring with Transformer Models

Transformer-based models are increasingly being utilized in public health monitoring, particularly for tracking disease outbreaks and generating reports for epidemiological surveillance. These models streamline data collection and reporting processes, enhancing public health responses.

Document and Topic Classification

In NLP, document and topic classification are vital tasks for which transformer models have shown considerable effectiveness, particularly during the COVID-19 pandemic. The National Library of Medicine developed LitCovid, a search engine that categorizes COVID-19 literature into various topics, aiding researchers in accessing relevant information efficiently.

Named Entity Recognition and Linking

Named Entity Recognition (NER) and Named Entity Linking (NEL) are employed after identifying relevant documents, thus aiding in extracting significant biomedical hypotheses and further connecting them to biological databases. These tasks focus on identifying entities related to molecular biology and clinical domains, including genes, proteins, medications, and diseases [21].

Performance Metrics and Evaluation

Key Metrics

Performance in NLP and information retrieval systems is typically measured using metrics such as F1 score, precision, and recall. The F1 score combines these metrics to provide a balanced evaluation of a model's predictive accuracy. In healthcare applications, the F1 score is particularly useful for tasks like disease classification and clinical question answering [22].

ROC-AUC Analysis

The ROC-AUC (Receiver Operating Characteristic - Area Under the Curve) is an essential metric for analyzing the performance of binary classification models. It evaluates a model's ability to discriminate between positive and negative occurrences by mapping the True Positive Rate (TPR) against the False Positive Rate (FPR) across several thresholds [23]. AUC values range from 0.5, indicating random guessing, to 1.0, which represents perfect discrimination.

Transformer models offer significant advancements in public health monitoring through efficient data classification and the extraction of biomedical information. Performance evaluation using metrics like F1 score and ROC-AUC enables researchers and practitioners to assess model effectiveness comprehensively, ultimately enhancing healthcare outcomes.

Benchmark Datasets and Evaluation Standards for Healthcare NLP

Benchmark Datasets

Several key datasets are critical for advancing Natural Language Processing (NLP) in healthcare:

- **i2b2**: A prominent dataset for biomedical Named Entity Recognition (NER), featuring clinical notes annotated with entities like diseases and drugs.
- **CMeD**: Focuses on clinical concept extraction within the clinical text, aiding in identifying medical concepts.
- **MedMentions**: A large-scale dataset for NER in biomedical literature encompassing various medical entities.
- **BioCreative**: Comprises challenges and tasks for biomedical text mining, including relation extraction and question answering.
- **ClinicalTrials.gov**: A repository for clinical trial records useful for text classification and information extraction.

- **PubMed**: A vast corpus of biomedical literature suitable for tasks such as outlining text and question-answering [24].

Evaluation Standards

To assess the performance of healthcare NLP systems, various metrics are employed:

- **Precision**: Correct positive predictions: Total positive predictions.
- **Recall**: Actual positive prediction: Correct prediction.
- **F1-Score**: The harmonic mean of precision and recall.
- **Accuracy**: The overall proportion of correct predictions.
- **Macro-AveragedF1-Score**: The average F1-score across multiple classes.
- **Micro-AveragedF1-Score**: The overall F1-score considering all instances collectively.
- **AUC-ROC**: The area under the receiver operating characteristic curve, measuring the ability to differentiate between positive and negative occurrences [24].

Ethical and Privacy Considerations

The paper "Protecting Patient Information: Data Privacy Law and Its Challenges" discusses the landscape of data privacy regulations in India, emphasizing the importance of safeguarding patient information amid increasing digitization [25]. It highlights legislative frameworks like the Information Technology (IT) Rules and the proposed Personal Data Protection Bill, underscoring challenges in implementation and compliance among healthcare providers.

Addressing Biases in Transformer Models

This review focuses on gender bias in transformer models used in NLP, examining how biased training data can lead to skewed outputs. This study explores sources of bias and strategies for detection and mitigation, advocating interdisciplinary collaboration to develop fairer models and improved evaluation metrics [26].

Regulatory Considerations

The integration of IoT in healthcare raises concerns regarding patient data security. The need for compliance with privacy standards like HIPAA in the US and GDPR in the EU is critical to protect patient information [27, 28].

CHALLENGES AND LIMITATIONS

Challenges in developing transformer models for healthcare include biases in training data and the quality of outcomes generated. There is a need for high-quality, annotated data and rigorous testing to ensure reliability [29]. Ethical concerns also arise regarding health inequalities and the potential dehumanization of care due to increased automation [10].

This analysis underscores the need for diverse evaluation methods and a comprehensive understanding to effectively address the complexities of deploying transformer models in healthcare settings.

Scalability Issues and Computational Resources

Scalability encompasses a wide range of factors, and a system is only as scalable as its least scalable component—the one that becomes a bottleneck as the network expands. Research addressing Software-Defined Networking (SDN) scalability can be categorized into four main areas: data plane, control plane, applications, and cross-cutting issues [30].

- ***Varying Request and Resource Heterogeneity***

On the other hand, resource heterogeneity is characterized by the fact that the machines in a cluster are often built from commodity hardware rather than high-performance servers, resulting in significantly lower acquisition and operational costs. This configuration diversity among different machines leads to substantial variations within the cluster. These discrepancies can be described across magnitudes such as micro-architecture, chipset versions, CPU specifications, and reminiscence capacities [31].

- ***Workload Diversity and Resource Sharing***

Despite the advantages of these specialized systems, they often encounter challenges like low server utilization and inefficient data sharing. Many cloud facilities experience low resource utilization due to imbalances between busy and idle clusters, complicating data sharing across different frameworks. The necessity for data export and replication to permanent storage further exacerbates this inefficiency [32 - 35].

• *Increasing Request and Cluster Scale*

The expanding scale of payment and data processing systems is evident in the rising transaction volumes managed by significant platforms. For instance, Alipay surpassed Visa in 2015, achieving a peak of 85,900 transactions per second. As these systems grow, they must efficiently handle high request loads and minimize latency to ensure a seamless user experience. Larger cluster sizes, such as those operated by Yahoo, Alibaba, and Google, introduce management and scheduling complexities, resulting in challenges like message congestion and RPC call failures. Effective resource allocation and rapid scheduling are essential to meet the substantial scale and dynamic demands of modern systems [36 - 38]

INTEGRATING MODELS INTO CINICAL WORKFLOWS

Challenges in Integration: The study identifies several key challenges in incorporating ML systems into clinical workflows:

- ***Data Quality and Availability:*** Stakeholders pointed out issues related to the quality and accessibility of data necessary for training ML models. Inconsistent or incomplete data can significantly hinder the effectiveness of these systems.
- ***Integration with Existing Systems:*** Merging ML technologies with legacy EHR systems and supplementary clinical tools presents substantial technical and logistical challenges. Compatibility issues can disrupt workflows and reduce integration efficiency.
- ***Trust and Acceptance:*** Establishing trust among clinicians regarding the reliability and accuracy of ML systems is essential. There is a pressing need for transparent and interpretable models to ensure healthcare professionals feel comfortable relying on ML-generated recommendations.
- ***Training and Support:*** Comprehensive training and ongoing support are crucial for clinicians to adapt to new ML tools effectively. The study found that inadequate training can lead to resistance and underutilization of these technologies.

Opportunities for Improvement: Despite the challenges, the study highlights several opportunities to enhance the integration process [39 - 42].

FUTURE DIRECTIONS

Numerous challenges must be addressed to maximize the possibilities of transformer models. These include the extensive computational resources needed for training and deployment, the risk of bias in the training data, and the imperative to safeguard sensitive user information [43, 14, 44].

Transforming Healthcare Operations: Leveraging AI for Clinical Coding, Workflow Optimization, and Patient Empowerment

- ***Documentation and Clinical Coding:*** This involves automating transcription, summarizing clinical conversations, and structuring clinical data. For example, transformer models can generate patient-friendly discharge summaries and extract relevant details for healthcare professionals, streamlining the review of medical histories.
- ***Workflow and Healthcare Services***: Use cases in this category include patient triage and process guidance. Experts note that these systems can automate initial patient interactions, process reported symptoms, and identify urgent cases needing professional attention.
- ***Patient Education***: Transformer models can enhance patient education and ensure informed consent. Virtual assistants can answer patient inquiries, provide health information, and promote self-management skills.
- ***Health Management***: This encompasses monitoring patient health data to identify trends and implementing early warning systems to alert patients and providers about potential health issues.
- ***Enhanced Clinical Coding***: Automating the extraction of critical data from clinical notes and improving the accuracy of clinical coding processes can lead to more precise reimbursements.
- ***Scheduling Optimization***: Streamlining scheduling and resource allocation can minimize wait times and improve patient satisfaction.
- ***Decision Support***: Transformer models can offer personalized treatment recommendations based on patient data, predict outcomes, and assist in diagnosing complex diseases, enhancing overall healthcare delivery.

CONCLUSION

The application of transformer-based models has significantly influenced the development of NLP in the healthcare sector, particularly with named entity recognition, relationship extraction, and clinical text generation. Accuracy in diagnosis and personalized treatment recommendations, as well as patient engagement, is enhanced through pre-training and fine-tuning on big data and with specialized medical knowledge. However, concerns about data privacy, the volume of medical datasets, and the interpretability of predictions generated by these complex models remain. In the future, shifts in model architecture, training paradigms, and domain changes for applications must occur to improve healthcare outcomes and operational efficiency.

REFERENCES

[1] A. Vaswani, N. Shazeer, N. Parmar, J. Uszkoreit, L. Jones, A.N. Gomez, Ł. Kaiser, I. Polosukhin, I. Guyon, U.V. Luxburg, S. Bengio, H. Wallach, R. Fergus, S. Vishwanathan, and R. Garnett, "Advances

in neural information processing systems", In: *Curran Associates, Inc.* vol. 30. , 2017, pp. 5998-6008.

[2] K. Berahmand, F. Daneshfar, E.S. Salehi, Y. Li, and Y. Xu, "Autoencoders and their applications in machine learning: a survey", *Artif. Intell. Rev.*, vol. 57, no. 2, p. 28, 2024. [http://dx.doi.org/10.1007/s10462-023-10662-6]

[3] Y. Bengio, P. Simard, and P. Frasconi, "Learning long-term dependencies with gradient descent is difficult", *IEEE Trans. Neural Netw.*, vol. 5, no. 2, pp. 157-166, 1994. [http://dx.doi.org/10.1109/72.279181] [PMID: 18267787]

[4] R. S. Wadawadagi and V. Pagi, “Sentiment analysis with deep neural networks: Comparative study and performance assessment,” Artificial Intelligence Review, vol. 53, no. 5, Dec. 2020. [http://dx.doi.org/10.1007/s10462-020-09845-2]

[5] G.W. Lindsay, "Attention in psychology, neuroscience, and machine learning", *Front. Comput. Neurosci.*, vol. 14, no. 29, p. 29, 2020. [http://dx.doi.org/10.3389/fncom.2020.00029] [PMID: 32372937]

[6] A. Hernández, and J.M. Amigó, "Multilayer adaptive networks in neuronal processing", *Eur. Phys. J. Spec. Top.*, vol. 227, no. 10-11, pp. 1039-1049, 2018. [http://dx.doi.org/10.1140/epjst/e2018-800037-y]

[7] T. Lin, Y. Wang, X. Liu, and X. Qiu, “A survey of transformers,” AI Open, vol. 3, pp. 111–132, 2022. [Online]. Available: https://doi.org/10.1016/j.aiopen.2022.10.001

[8] X. Zeng, S. Zhu, W. Lu, Z. Liu, J. Huang, Y. Zhou, J. Fang, Y. Huang, H. Guo, L. Li, B.D. Trapp, R. Nussinov, C. Eng, J. Loscalzo, and F. Cheng, "Target identification among known drugs by deep learning from heterogeneous networks", *Chem. Sci. (Camb.)*, vol. 11, no. 7, pp. 1775-1797, 2020. [http://dx.doi.org/10.1039/C9SC04336E] [PMID: 34123272]

[9] R.I. Sifat, "ChatGPT and the future of health policy analysis: potential and pitfalls of using ChatGPT in policymaking", *Ann. Biomed. Eng.*, vol. 51, no. 7, pp. 1357-1359, 2023. [http://dx.doi.org/10.1007/s10439-023-03204-2] [PMID: 37061595]

[10] J.Y. Luh, R.F. Thompson, and S. Lin, "Clinical documentation and patient care using artificial intelligence in radiation oncology", *J. Am. Coll. Radiol.*, vol. 16, no. 9, pp. 1343-1346, 2019. [http://dx.doi.org/10.1016/j.jacr.2019.05.044] [PMID: 31238022]

[11] A. Howard, W. Hope, and A. Gerada, "ChatGPT and antimicrobial advice: the end of the consulting infection doctor?", *Lancet Infect. Dis.*, vol. 23, no. 4, pp. 405-406, 2023. [http://dx.doi.org/10.1016/S1473-3099(23)00113-5] [PMID: 36822213]

[12] K. Denecke, R. May, and O. Rivera-Romero, "Transformer models in healthcare: a survey and thematic analysis of potentials, shortcomings and risks", *J. Med. Syst.*, vol. 48, no. 1, p. 23, 2024. [http://dx.doi.org/10.1007/s10916-024-02043-5] [PMID: 38367119]

[13] V. Braun, and V. Clarke, "Using thematic analysis in psychology", *Qual. Res. Psychol.*, vol. 3, no. 2, pp. 77-101, 2006. [http://dx.doi.org/10.1191/1478088706qp063oa]

[14] G. Eysenbach, "The role of ChatGPT, generative language models, and artificial intelligence in medical education: A conversation with ChatGPT and a call for papers", *JMIR Med. Educ.*, vol. 9, p. e46885, 2023. [http://dx.doi.org/10.2196/46885] [PMID: 36863937]

[15] A. Onan, H. A. Alhumyani, DeepExtract: Semantic-driven extractive text summarization framework using LLMs and hierarchical positional encoding, Journal of King Saud University - Computer and Information Sciences, Volume 36, Issue 8, 2024, 102178, ISSN 1319-1578, https://doi.org/10.1016/j.jksuci.2024.102178. (https://www.sciencedirect.com/science/article/pii/S1319157824002672)

[16] N. Sabharwal and A. Agrawal, “BERT model applications: Other tasks,” in Hands-on Question Answering Systems with BERT. Berkeley, CA, USA: Apress, 2021. [Online]. Available:

https://doi.org/10.1007/978-1-4842-6664-9_6

[17] M. Chen, X. Tan, and R. Padman, "Social determinants of health in electronic health records and their impact on analysis and risk prediction: A systematic review", *J. Am. Med. Inform. Assoc.,* vol. 27, no. 11, pp. 1764-1773, 2020. [http://dx.doi.org/10.1093/jamia/ocaa143] [PMID: 33202021]

[18] X. Yang, A. Chen, N. PourNejatian, H.C. Shin, K.E. Smith, C. Parisien, C. Compas, C. Martin, A.B. Costa, M.G. Flores, Y. Zhang, T. Magoc, C.A. Harle, G. Lipori, D.A. Mitchell, W.R. Hogan, E.A. Shenkman, J. Bian, and Y. Wu, "A large language model for electronic health records", *NPJ Digit. Med.,* vol. 5, no. 1, p. 194, 2022. [http://dx.doi.org/10.1038/s41746-022-00742-2] [PMID: 36572766]

[19] M. Wornow, Y. Xu, R. Thapa, B. Patel, E. Steinberg, S. Fleming, M.A. Pfeffer, J. Fries, and N.H. Shah, "The shaky foundations of large language models and foundation models for electronic health records", *NPJ Digit. Med.,* vol. 6, no. 1, p. 135, 2023. [http://dx.doi.org/10.1038/s41746-023-00879-8] [PMID: 37516790]

[20] L. Chen, Z. Fan, J. Chang, R. Yang, H. Hou, H. Guo, Y. Zhang, T. Yang, C. Zhou, Q. Sui, Z. Chen, C. Zheng, X. Hao, K. Zhang, R. Cui, Z. Zhang, H. Ma, Y. Ding, N. Zhang, X. Lu, X. Luo, H. Jiang, S. Zhang, and M. Zheng, "Sequence-based drug design as a concept in computational drug design", *Nat. Commun.,* vol. 14, no. 1, p. 4217, 2023. [http://dx.doi.org/10.1038/s41467-023-39856-w] [PMID: 37452028]

[21] A. Nentidis, A. Krithara, K. Bougiatiotis, and G. Paliouras, “Overview of BioASQ 8a and 8b: Results of the eighth edition of the BioASQ tasks a and b,” in Proceedings of the BioASQ Workshop, CEUR Workshop Proceedings, vol. 2696, 2020. [Online]. Available: https://ceur-ws.org/Vo--2696/paper_164.pdf

[22] C. Sun, Z. Yang, L. Wang, Y. Zhang, H. Lin, and J. Wang, "Biomedical named entity recognition using BERT in the machine reading comprehension framework", *J. Biomed. Inform.,* vol. 118, p. 103799, 2021. [http://dx.doi.org/10.1016/j.jbi.2021.103799] [PMID: 33965638]

[23] R. You, Y. Liu, H. Mamitsuka, and S. Zhu, "BERTMeSH: deep contextual representation learning for large-scale high-performance MeSH indexing with full text", *Bioinformatics,* vol. 37, no. 5, pp. 684-692, 2021. [http://dx.doi.org/10.1093/bioinformatics/btaa837] [PMID: 32976559]

[24] K. Järvelin, and J. Kekäläinen, "Cumulated gain-based evaluation of IR techniques", *ACM Trans. Inf. Syst.,* vol. 20, no. 4, pp. 422-446, 2002. [http://dx.doi.org/10.1145/582415.582418]

[25] S. Gupta, "Challenges in implementing data privacy laws in India’s healthcare sector", *Int. J. Health Care Qual. Assur.,* vol. 34, no. 5, pp. 456-469, 2021.

[26] P. Nemani, Y.D. Joel, P. Vijay, and F.F. Liza, "Gender bias in transformer models: A comprehensive survey", *J. Artif. Intell. Res.,* vol. 72, pp. 1-30, 2024.

[27] A. Riahi Sfar, E. Natalizio, S. Mazlout, Y. Challal, and Z. Chtourou, “Privacy preservation using game theory in e-health applications,” Journal of Information Security and Applications, vol. 66, Art. no. 103158, 2022, doi: 10.1016/j.jisa.2022.103158.

[28] T.F. Lee, I.P. Chang, and G.J. Su, "Compliance with HIPAA and GDPR in certificate-less based authenticated key agreement using extended chaotic maps", *Electronics (Basel),* vol. 12, no. 5, p. 1108, 2023. [http://dx.doi.org/10.3390/electronics12051108]

[29] F. Eggmann, R. Weiger, N.U. Zitzmann, and M.B. Blatz, "Implications of large language models such as ChatGPT for dental medicine", *J. Esthet. Restor. Dent.,* vol. 35, no. 7, pp. 1098-1102, 2023. [http://dx.doi.org/10.1111/jerd.13046] [PMID: 37017291]

[30] S.H. Yeganeh, A. Tootoonchian, and Y. Ganjali, "On scalability of software-defined networking", *IEEE Commun. Mag.,* vol. 51, no. 2, pp. 136-141, 2013. [http://dx.doi.org/10.1109/MCOM.2013.6461198]

[31] B. Sharma, V. Chudnovsky, J.L. Hellerstein, R. Rifaat, and C.R. Das, "Modeling and synthesizing task placement constraints in Google compute clusters", *Proceedings of the ACM Symposium on Cloud Computing,* 2011pp. 1-10 [http://dx.doi.org/10.1145/2038916.2038919]

[32] M. Isard, M. Budiu, Y. Yu, A. Birrell, and D. Fetterly, "Dryad", *Oper. Syst. Rev.,* vol. 41, no. 3, pp. 59-72, 2007. [http://dx.doi.org/10.1145/1272998.1273005]

[33] J. Dean, and S. Ghemawat, "MapReduce", *Commun. ACM,* vol. 51, no. 1, pp. 107-113, 2008. [http://dx.doi.org/10.1145/1327452.1327492]

[34] M. Zaharia, M. Chowdhury, T. Das, A. Dave, J. Ma, M.J. McCauley, M.J. Franklin, S. Shenker, and I. Stoica, "Resilient distributed datasets: A fault-tolerant abstraction for in-memory cluster computing", *Proceedings of the USENIX Symposium on Networked Systems Design and Implementation,* 2012pp. 15-28

[35] B. Saha, H. Shah, S. Seth, G. Vijayaraghavan, A. Murthy, and C. Curino, "Apache Tez: A unifying framework for modeling and building data processing applications", *Proceedings of the ACM SIGMOD International Conference on Management of Data,* 2015pp. 1357-1368 [http://dx.doi.org/10.1145/2723372.2742790]

[36] A. Verma, L. Pedrosa, M. Korupolu, D. Oppenheimer, E. Tune, and J. Wilkes, "Large-scale cluster management at Google with Borg", *Proceedings of the ACM EuroSys,* 2015pp. 1-12 [http://dx.doi.org/10.1145/2741948.2741964]

[37] V.K. Vavilapalli, A.C. Murthy, C. Douglas, S. Agarwal, M. Konar, R. Evans, T. Graves, J. Lowe, H. Shah, and S. Seth, "Apache Hadoop YARN: Yet another resource negotiator", *Proceedings of the ACM Symposium on Cloud Computing,* 2013pp. 1-10 [http://dx.doi.org/10.1145/2523616.2523633]

[38] Z. Zhang, C. Li, Y. Tao, R. Yang, H. Tang, and J. Xu, "Fuxi", *Proceedings VLDB Endowment---,* vol. 7, no. 13, pp. 1393-1404, 2014. [http://dx.doi.org/10.14778/2733004.2733012]

[39] M.R. Endsley, "Toward a theory of situation awareness in dynamic systems", *Hum. Factors,* vol. 37, no. 1, pp. 32-64, 1995. [http://dx.doi.org/10.1518/001872095779049543]

[40] B. Saunders, J. Sim, T. Kingstone, S. Baker, J. Waterfield, B. Bartlam, H. Burroughs, and C. Jinks, "Saturation in qualitative research: exploring its conceptualization and operationalization", *Qual. Quant.,* vol. 52, no. 4, pp. 1893-1907, 2018. [http://dx.doi.org/10.1007/s11135-017-0574-8] [PMID: 29937585]

[41] R.J. Holden, and B.T. Karsh, "The Technology Acceptance Model: Its past and its future in health care", *J. Biomed. Inform.,* vol. 43, no. 1, pp. 159-172, 2010. [http://dx.doi.org/10.1016/j.jbi.2009.07.002] [PMID: 19615467]

[42] O. Asan, A.E. Bayrak, and A. Choudhury, "Artificial intelligence and human trust in healthcare: Focus on clinicians", *J. Med. Internet Res.,* vol. 22, no. 6, p. e15154, 2020. [http://dx.doi.org/10.2196/15154] [PMID: 32558657]

[43] R. Seetharaman, "Revolutionizing medical education: Can ChatGPT boost subjective learning and expression?", *J. Med. Syst.,* vol. 47, no. 1, p. 61, 2023. [http://dx.doi.org/10.1007/s10916-023-01957-w] [PMID: 37160568]

[44] J. Homolak, "Opportunities and risks of ChatGPT in medicine, science, and academic publishing: a modern Promethean dilemma", *Croat. Med. J.,* vol. 64, no. 1, pp. 1-3, 2023. [http://dx.doi.org/10.3325/cmj.2023.64.1] [PMID: 36864812]

CHAPTER 14

Revolutionizing Mental Health Care with AI-Driven NLP Chatbots: Innovations, Applications, and Future Directions

Maharaja Muthuvairam Subbulakshmi[1], **Manikandan Jayaraman**[1], **Pradeep Kumar Sriram**[1] and **Jeyaraman Jeyakanthan**[1,*]

[1] *Structural Biology and Biocomputing Lab, Department of Bioinformatics, Alagappa University, Karaikudi-630003, Tamil Nadu, India*

Abstract: The advent of modern technologies has revolutionized healthcare, introducing innovative solutions through Artificial Intelligence (AI), Deep Learning (DL), Machine Learning (ML), and the Internet of Things (IoT). These technologies have been leveraged to significantly enhance the quality of medical care. AI, particularly through ML and DL, automatically utilizes models derived from medical and biological data to improve decision-making and generate recommendations. For high-performance statistical tasks and input classification, Natural Language Processing (NLP) has been effectively employed to manage the healthcare sector. In natural language processing, chatbots have been utilized to implement NLP for various purposes, such as generating timely suggestions and alerts for patients in critical scenarios, particularly in mental health care. Traditional NLP chatbots, like Bidirectional Encoder Representations from Transformers (BERT), have been adapted for mental health applications, achieving an accuracy rate of approximately 98% with specialized terminology and personalized suggestions. The advancement of NLP techniques through AI-driven chatbots is expected to improve response generation for mental health issues and aid in developing technical solutions to reduce mental health problems within social populations. This chapter provides detailed insights into the development, advancement, and framework of NLP-associated chatbots in mental health. It covers technical aspects, performance metrics, implemented methodologies, case studies, real-time applications, drawbacks, and future perspectives. This chapter offers transformative information on NLP-driven technology for improving mental health care.

Keywords: Artificial Intelligence (AI), Deep Learning (DL), Machine Learning (ML), Medical chatbots, Mental health care, Natural Language Processing (NLP).

* **Corresponding author Jeyaraman Jeyakanthan:** Structural Biology and Biocomputing Lab, Department of Bioinformatics, Alagappa University, Karaikudi-630003, Tamil Nadu, India; E-mail: jjbioinformatics@gmail.com

A. Shankar, Saranya Jayapalan, & Basant. K. Tiwary (Eds.)

INTRODUCTION

Incorporating futuristic technology, AI-ML (Artificial Intelligence and Machine Learning) has advanced healthcare informatics, paving the way for innovations in healthcare records, diagnosis, and treatment strategies. Implementing Machine Learning (ML) and Deep Learning (DL) algorithms has enabled AI models to process vast amounts of medical data and generate insights through an automated process, allowing AI to think and react like humans based on specific dependencies. This computerized task is decision-making, where AI assists healthcare professionals in reducing errors, improving accuracy, and providing personalized support. Furthermore, real-time monitoring of patients, which captures vital signs and parameters through connected devices, ensures that these data are continuously recorded and utilized to generate AI models for decision-making [1]. This synergy ensures that healthcare informatics is proactive rather than reactive, making it more predictive. Among its various impacts on healthcare, AI powers Natural Language Processing (NLP), a prominent area that allows machine models to interpret and understand human language patterns. NLP acts as a layer between humans and machine models, managing and understanding patients' queries, feedback, and clinical reports. With AI, NLP can analyze medical interventions and generate suggestions based on patient communication. One significant application of NLP is in medical chatbots, where users can chat or talk to the chatbot and obtain solutions to their queries around the clock. These conversational agents can seamlessly interact with users in natural language, assisting with diagnosis, scheduling appointments, and generating recommendations [2]. NLP medical chatbots have become a critical tool in mental healthcare, providing alerts with immediate responses and therapeutic interventions. Through meaningful conversations, these chatbots support users' queries on mental health conditions and offer instant guidance during critical moments. In mental health diagnosis, speech and text can be analyzed by NLP models, utilizing data from Electronic Health Records (EHRs) to detect conditions such as anxiety, depression, and schizophrenia. Emotion detection and sentiment analysis techniques are applied in conversations by extracting emotional cues that may signal mental health risks. Speech and voice patterns, such as tone, pitch, and prosody, are detected using NLP models combined with acoustic analysis, indicating cognitive decline [3].

NLP algorithms are built on a transformer model called BERT (Bidirectional Encoder Representations from Transformers), which constructs models in both forward and backward directions. This model is highly effective in recognizing linguistic markers of anxiety or depression using extensive datasets, enabling proactive interventions. The structured framework of BERT allows it to reach at-risk clients before their health conditions escalate [4]. This chapter explores mental healthcare interventions through AI-powered NLP medical chatbots modeled with BERT, discussing innovations, applications, and future perspectives (Fig. **1**).

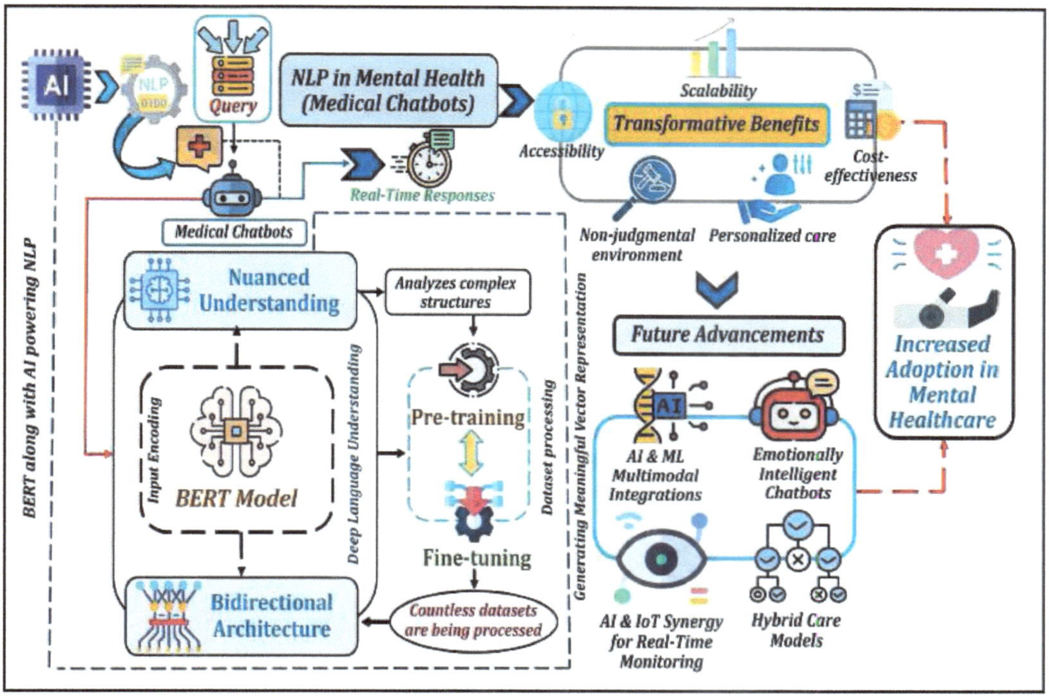

Fig. (1). Pictorial representation illustrating the workflow of AI-driven Natural Language Processing (NLP) medical chatbots.

ARCHITECTURAL FRAMEWORK OF NLP MEDICAL CHATBOTS

The Bidirectional Encoder Representations from Transformers (BERT) is an advanced model for sentence context analysis, revolutionizing NLP medical chatbots (Fig. **2**). Through deep analysis, BERT captures words and their surrounding context in both left and right directions, making it exceptionally effective for language understanding tasks. This capability has been widely adopted in healthcare, enabling the development of medical chatbots with nuanced awareness [5]. BERT-based NLP medical chatbots demonstrate remarkable performance in comprehending the intricacies of mental healthcare terminology and conversations in a more informed and empathetic manner. BERT's latent ability to handle complex sentence structures and recognize the intent behind a client's query ensures accurate solutions, making these medical chatbots highly reliable in mental healthcare. This architecture processes input by encoding it into meaningful vector representations, generating contextually relevant solutions that are both medically appropriate and conversationally engaging in a human-like manner [6]. The model is pre-trained on a vast dataset and fine-tuned on mental health-specific datasets to effectively address nuances and provide guidance on sensitive issues such as anxiety and depression. In addition, this BERT-NLP architecture enables real-time interactions with immediate interventions, offering scalability to handle countless conversations simultaneously. This scalability makes the framework a viable tool, acting as a virtual therapist for mental healthcare interventions [7].

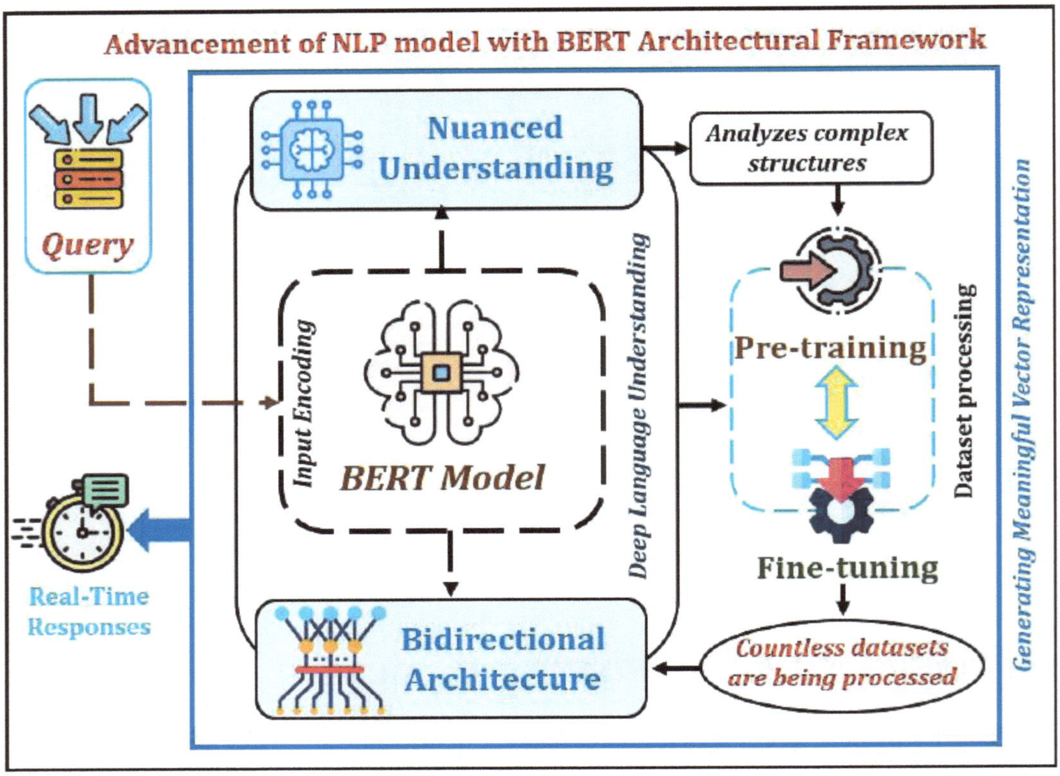

Fig. (2). Graphical model depicting the architectural framework of Bidirectional Encoder Representations from Transformers (BERT).

NLP MEDICAL CHATBOTS IN MENTAL HEALTH DISORDERS

Mental health disorders are a global concern, with the World Health Organization (WHO) estimating that 12–13% of the population worldwide faces mental illnesses, including conditions such as schizophrenia, anxiety, depression, and bipolar disorder. The COVID-19 pandemic exacerbated mental health issues that increased stress-related disorders globally. Despite the pressing need for accessible mental healthcare services, NLP medical chatbots offer an innovative platform that delivers scalable and wide-ranging mental healthcare support [8]. These chatbots provide impactful therapeutic interventions, often based on

Cognitive Behavioral Therapy (CBT), to offer confidential and personalized support. Chatbots such as Wysa and Woebot utilize CBT techniques to deliver therapy exercises, helping users identify negative thought patterns and reframe them with positive strategies. CBT models leverage queries to generate empathetic and contextually appropriate solutions. With access to extensive longitudinal conversational data, these chatbots can track user progress over time and adjust therapeutic approaches accordingly. Mental health chatbots also serve as early detection tools, identifying signs of mental health concerns from user inputs and offering self-care tips [9]. In critical cases, alerts are generated, or conversations are escalated to professional psychiatrists to ensure timely intervention. NLP medical chatbots reduce the burden on healthcare systems, enabling more efficient management of mental health issues and leading to improved long-term outcomes.

TECHNICAL STANDPOINTS OF MEDICAL CHATBOTS IN MENTAL HEALTHCARE INTERVENTIONS

NLP medical chatbots are built on sophisticated language models integrated with Deep Learning (DL) strategies to generate responses in a human-like manner. Across multiple interactions, mental health chatbots retain contextual understanding, maintaining conversation continuity by referencing the context from previous exchanges. By incorporating sentiment analysis algorithms, these chatbots can detect emotional tones and generate tailored responses, offering empathetic support [10]. To create meaningful and coherent responses, chatbots automatically craft replies that mimic human interactions rather than relying on scripted or robotic responses. Advances in multimodal input processing enable medical chatbots to support dynamic interactions, including visual input analysis. For example, facial expressions captured through camera integration can be analyzed to gauge emotional states [11]. Natural Language Understanding (NLU) is enhanced by algorithms such as BERT and Support Vector Machines (SVM), enabling the extraction of deeper meanings from inputs [12]. Entities and relevant information are extracted using NER (Named Entity Recognition) and modeled with CRF (Conditional Random Fields) [13]. Appropriate responses are then generated using Natural Language Generation (NLG) algorithms, such as LSTM (Long Short-Term Memory) networks, which provide template-based responses. Additionally, sequence-to-sequence models dynamically constructed by Recurrent Neural Networks (RNN) ensure coherent responses [14, 15]. Dialogue management algorithms further contribute to maintaining the flow of communication, learning optimal strategies through Reinforcement Learning (RL) based on the Deep Q-learning algorithm (Table **1**) [16]. Emotional and sentiment detection is categorized into neutral, positive, and negative tones using BERT-based sentiment classifiers, enhancing the chatbot's ability to provide nuanced and supportive mental healthcare interventions.

Table. 1. A comprehensive process flow for multimodal chatbot response generation.

S No	Stage	Step	Description	Techniques/Algorithms
1.	Input	Client's Input	The user provides text, voice, or visual input	The multimodal inputs are processed with dynamic interactions to gauge emotional states.
2.	Initial Processing	Natural Language Understanding (NLU)	Processing the input to understand the intent of the context	BERT (Bidirectional Encoder Representations from Transformers) and SVM (Support Vector Machine)
3.	First Processing	Entity Extraction	Extracts relevant entity from the keywords or emotional inputs	Named Entity Recognition (NER) and Conditional Random Fields (CRF)
4.	Second Processing	Response Generation	Human-like responses are generated based on the extracted entities	LSTM (Long Short-Term Memory) and RNN (Recurrent Neural Networks) (sequence-to-sequence models)
5.	Initial Output	The initial response of the Chatbot	Generates the first response based on the initial NLU processing	Based on the template or dynamic responses
6.	Multimodal Processing	The multimodal inputs are processed	Processing the additional inputs	Camera integration or visual analysis techniques
7.	Initial Multimodal Processing	Emotion detection	Emotions are detected from the flow of communication	Strategy processed by BERT and Deep Learning
8.	First Multimodal Processing	Sentiment analysis	The sentiment categories are detected as positive, neutral, and negative	BERT-based sentiment classifiers
9.	Second Multimodal Processing	Dialogue management	The flow of conversation is managed, and coherent responses are optimized.	Reinforcement Learning (RL) from the Deep Q-Learning
10.	Final Output	Chatbot response	Refined responses are provided considering the multimodal data	The Dynamic response technique, Context-aware output

REAL-TIME AI-POWERED MEDICAL CHATBOTS IN MENTAL HEALTH CARE

Wysa, Woebot, and Replika are AI-powered medical chatbots that provide real-time assistance around the clock (Fig. **3**). The Wysa chatbot addresses anxiety, depression, and sleep problems by combining NLP and CBT-based self-care exercises. It also recommends specialized psychiatrists for critical cases [17]. The clinically evaluated Woebot chatbot uses NLP-CBT strategies to manage mental health conditions. It offers mood-tracking and self-care advice, making it a valuable tool for timely assistance [18]. Replika is a companion chatbot that creates a safe platform for users to convey their emotions and thoughts. This chatbot is particularly effective in helping users cope with loneliness and promoting emotional well-being [19]. These chatbots have successfully paved the way for scalable mental healthcare solutions, reaching a wide range of populations that might otherwise lack access to traditional therapies due to geographical disparities and financial constraints.

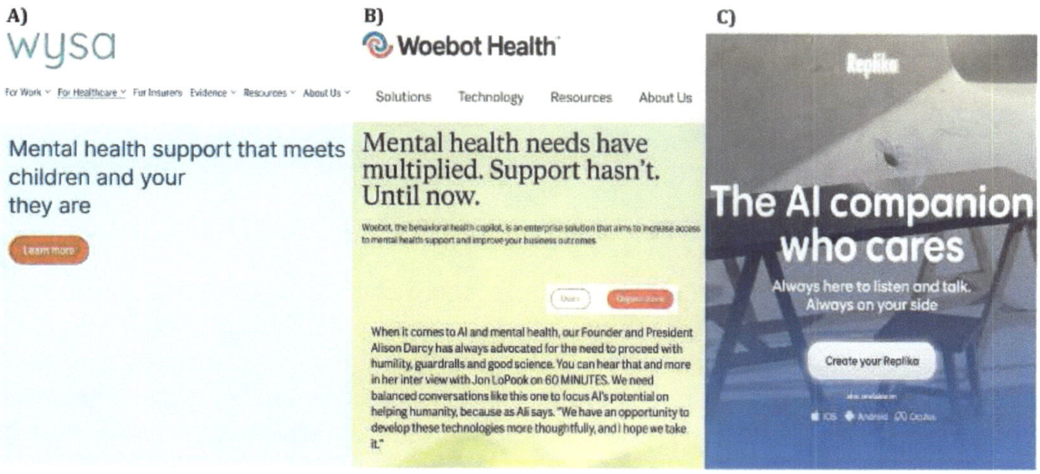

Fig. (3). Real-time AI-powered medical chatbots in mental health care. (**A**) Wysa, (**B**) Woebot, and (**C**) Replika.

TRANSFORMATIVE BENEFITS OF NLP MEDICAL CHATBOTS IN MENTAL HEALTHCARE INTERVENTIONS

Accessibility is a significant advantage of NLP medical chatbots, as they provide continuous assistance around the clock without the need for human intervention. These chatbots are highly scalable and capable of handling multiple tasks for numerous clients simultaneously while delivering high-quality healthcare services. Medical chatbots are designed to offer personalized suggestions by recognizing past consultations and providing accurate solutions based on clients' queries. Another key benefit is that these chatbots create a secure and non-judgmental environment where clients can express their emotions freely, without fear or judgment (Table **2**) [20]. Additionally, NLP medical chatbots offer cost-effective services compared to traditional therapy, making mental health care more accessible to a broader population and providing transformative benefits to those in need.

Table. 2. Characteristics of AI-driven NLP medical chatbots for enhanced mental healthcare.

S. No	Category	Description
1.	Accessibility	Providing round-the-clock assistance without human intervention, making healthcare support always available.
2.	Scalability	Capable of managing multiple tasks from multiple users, delivering efficient and scalable healthcare assistance to a large-scale population.
3.	Personalized care	Personalized recommendations are delivered based on past interactions, ensuring tailored solutions for unique needs and concerns.
4.	Non-judgmental environment	Providing a non-judgmental space to express all emotions openly without fear of stigma or criticism.
5.	Cost-effectiveness	Alternative to traditional therapy offers assistance with affordability, expanding access to mental healthcare, especially in under-resourced areas.

LIMITATIONS OF NLP CHATBOTS IN MENTAL HEALTH CARE

Despite their benefits, medical chatbots face several limitations in mental healthcare. While they are capable of multilingual understanding, NLP chatbots often lack the emotional depth and nuanced intelligence of psychiatrists, making it challenging for them to comprehend complex emotions and generate the same level of empathy. Concerns about security and privacy also arise, as patient data fed into chatbots often includes highly sensitive medical information. It is essential to ensure that these platforms comply with data protection regulations, such as the GDPR (General Data Protection Regulation), to protect patient confidentiality (Table **3**) [21]. A significant risk lies in the lack of critical thinking, which could lead clients to over-rely on chatbot interactions while potentially forgoing access to professional mental healthcare. Although chatbots can offer valuable insights into severe mental health conditions, they cannot substitute for a human therapist.

Table 3. Overview of the limitations of NLP medical chatbots in mental healthcare interventions.

S. No	Category	Description
1.	Emotional Limitations	The lack of emotional depth and empathy in human therapists makes it challenging for them to understand and fully respond to complex emotional states.
2.	Security and Privacy concerns	Handling patients' sensitive data raises privacy risks, and compliance with regulations like GDPR is critical to protect confidential information.
3.	Over-Reliance on Technology	Regular users may become too dependent on the chatbots, potentially reducing engagement with professional mental healthcare services.
4.	Lack of Critical Thinking	The chatbots do not possess the capacity for critical thinking, which limits their ability to handle nuanced or severe mental healthcare issues.
5.	Not a Complete Replacement	Although chatbots are helpful, they cannot fully replace the expertise and empathy provided by human therapists, especially in critical mental health disorders.

CHALLENGES OF AI AND NLP IN MENTAL HEALTH CARE

The heterogeneity of numerous mental health cases makes it critically challenging to apply generalized models. While AI and NLP-generated models can categorize large volumes of clinical data, they may not accurately represent clinical realities. Although these models provide multiple perspectives, they tend to conform to existing clinical hypotheses in complex cases, limiting their ability to generate novel responses. This challenge extends to ethical considerations, where patients might become overly dependent on the NLP chatbot. In non-English contexts, language complexity may lead to misunderstandings of the query, affecting NLP performance and making global applicability more difficult. Although NLP provides crucial support, it cannot evaluate some clinical terms, as the algorithms are based on existing data. Therefore, the responses generated by NLP should ensure proper query evaluation, with ethical considerations integrated into mental healthcare chatbots [22].

THE FUTURE OF NLP MEDICAL CHATBOTS IN MENTAL HEALTHCARE: OPPORTUNITIES AND INNOVATIONS

The ongoing advancements in AI and ML, particularly in BERT-Natural Language Processing, expand the capabilities of NLP medical chatbots, with exciting developments on the horizon. Integrating multimodal AI systems and NLP medical chatbots can drive speech, language, facial expression, and gesture detection advancements. These advancements allow chatbots to provide more comprehensive assistance, not only from user input but also by detecting how and in what way the query is being communicated, including tone and expressions [23]. Futuristic chatbots, with a continuous focus on AI, will become emotionally intelligent and better equipped to address the emotional needs of clients, leading to more empathetic interactions. Real-time mental health monitoring *via* the AI-IoT (Artificial Intelligence-Internet of Things) synergy facilitates the creation of a powerful framework using gadgets such as wearable smartwatches or biosensors. This will enable the monitoring of not only mental health conditions like anxiety and depression but also heart rate changes, sleep patterns, and physiological indicators, allowing for personalized alerts and live relaxation techniques. Combining the strengths of NLP chatbots and psychiatrists, hybrid care models will emerge to address critical cases requiring in-depth interventions. In the future, NLP medical chatbots will become more widely recognized, leading to increased adoption in healthcare sectors and making them widely accessible alongside traditional therapy.

CONCLUSION

In addressing the emerging mental health crisis, the significant innovation of NLP-based medical chatbots in mental health care represents scalable, accessible, effective, and personalized care, making it a valuable AI technology. With the assistance of the architectural framework of BERT, unprecedented accuracy and performance are achieved, with the potential to revolutionize mental health care. Moreover, combining AI-driven BERT-NLP and neuroscience in cross-disciplinary research leads to breakthroughs in supportive cognitive underpinnings of mental illnesses, providing effective and accurate treatment. The mental health care ecosystem's interventions in the future will be more personalized, reliably accessible, and data-driven, leading to improved outcomes that empower patients to maintain their mental well-being.

CONSENT FOR PUBLICATION

None Declared

CONFLICT OF INTEREST

The authors declare no competing financial interest.

Figs. (**1** and **2**) have been designed using free resources from www.flaticon.com.

ACKNOWLEDGEMENT

This book chapter was supported by the Department of Biotechnology- National Network Project (DBT-NNP) [Grant No. BT/PR40156/BTIS/137/54/2023];

Department of Biotechnology -Bioinformatics Centre (DBT-BIC): [Grant No. (BIC)-No.BT/PR40154/BTIS/137/34/2021] and MoE-STARS [No.MoE-STARS/STARS-2/2023-0966 dt: 29-05-2024].

REFERENCES

[1] A. Barragán-Montero, U. Javaid, G. Valdés, D. Nguyen, P. Desbordes, B. Macq, S. Willems, L. Vandewinckele, M. Holmström, F. Löfman, S. Michiels, K. Souris, E. Sterpin, and J.A. Lee, "Artificial intelligence and machine learning for medical imaging: A technology review", *Phys. Med.,* vol. 83, pp. 242-256, 2021. [http://dx.doi.org/10.1016/j.ejmp.2021.04.016] [PMID: 33979715]

[2] Z. Wei, Y. Chen, Q. Zhao, P. Zhang, L. Zhou, J. Ren, Y. Piao, B. Qiu, X. Xie, S. Wang, J. Liu, D. Zhang, R.C. Kadosh, and X. Zhang, "Implicit perception of differences between NLP-produced and human-produced language in the mentalizing network", *Adv. Sci. (Weinh.),* vol. 10, no. 12, 2023.2203990 [http://dx.doi.org/10.1002/advs.202203990] [PMID: 36748300]

[3] M.L. Graber, C. Byrne, and D. Johnston, "The impact of electronic health records on diagnosis", *Diagnosis (Berl.),* vol. 4, no. 4, pp. 211-223, 2017. [http://dx.doi.org/10.1515/dx-2017-0012] [PMID: 29536944]

[4] N.Q.K. Le, Q.T. Ho, T.T.D. Nguyen, and Y.Y. Ou, "A transformer architecture based on BERT and 2D convolutional neural network to identify DNA enhancers from sequence information", *Brief. Bioinform.,* vol. 22, no. 5, 2021.bbab005 [http://dx.doi.org/10.1093/bib/bbab005] [PMID: 33539511]

[5] J. Lee, W. Yoon, S. Kim, D. Kim, S. Kim, C.H. So, and J. Kang, "BioBERT: a pre-trained biomedical language representation model for biomedical text mining", *Bioinformatics,* vol. 36, no. 4, pp. 1234-1240, 2020. [http://dx.doi.org/10.1093/bioinformatics/btz682] [PMID: 31501885]

[6] S. Kula, R. Kozik, and M. Choraś, "Implementation of the BERT-derived architectures to tackle disinformation challenges", *Neural Comput. Appl.,* vol. 34, no. 23, pp. 20449-20461, 2022. [http://dx.doi.org/10.1007/s00521-021-06276-0] [PMID: 34316097]

[7] D. Xu, M. Gopale, J. Zhang, K. Brown, E. Begoli, and S. Bethard, "Unified Medical Language System resources improve sieve-based generation and Bidirectional Encoder Representations from Transformers (BERT)–based ranking for concept normalization", *J. Am. Med. Inform. Assoc.,* vol. 27, no. 10, pp. 1510-1519, 2020. [http://dx.doi.org/10.1093/jamia/ocaa080] [PMID: 32719838]

[8] F. Shah-Mohammadi, I. Parvanova, and J. Finkelstein, "NLP-assisted pipeline for COVID-19 core outcome set identification using ClinicalTrials.gov", *Stud. Health Technol. Inform.,* vol. 290, pp. 622-626, 2022. [http://dx.doi.org/10.3233/SHTI220152] [PMID: 35673091]

[9] D. Gifu, and E. Pop, "Smart solutions to keep your mental balance", *Procedia Comput. Sci.,* vol. 214, pp. 503-510, 2022. [http://dx.doi.org/10.1016/j.procs.2022.11.205] [PMID: 36514712]

[10] M. Alawad, H.J. Yoon, S. Gao, B. Mumphrey, X.C. Wu, E.B. Durbin, J.C. Jeong, I. Hands, D. Rust, L. Coyle, L. Penberthy, and G. Tourassi, "Privacy-preserving deep learning NLP models for cancer registries", *IEEE Trans. Emerg. Top. Comput.,* vol. 9, no. 3, pp. 1219-1230, 2021. [http://dx.doi.org/10.1109/TETC.2020.2983404] [PMID: 36117774]

[11] A. Aggarwal, C.C. Tam, D. Wu, X. Li, and S. Qiao, "Artificial intelligence-based chatbots for promoting health behavioral changes: Systematic review", *J. Med. Internet Res.,* vol. 25, 2023.e40789 [http://dx.doi.org/10.2196/40789] [PMID: 36826990]

[12] Y. Wei, J. Zhou, Y. Wang, Y. Liu, Q. Liu, J. Luo, C. Wang, F. Ren, and L. Huang, "A review of algorithms and hardware design for AI-based biomedical applications", *IEEE Trans. Biomed. Circuits Syst.,* vol. 14, no. 2, pp. 145-163, 2020. [http://dx.doi.org/10.1109/TBCAS.2020.2974154] [PMID: 32078560]

[13] E. Munzone, A. Marra, F. Comotto, L. Guercio, C.A. Sangalli, M. Lo Cascio, E. Pagan, D. Sangalli, I. Bigoni, F.M. Porta, M. D'Ercole, F. Ritorti, V. Bagnardi, N. Fusco, and G. Curigliano, "Development and validation of a natural language processing algorithm for extracting clinical and pathological features of breast cancer from pathology reports", *JCO Clin. Cancer Inform.,* vol. 8, no. 8, 2024.e2400034 [http://dx.doi.org/10.1200/CCI.24.00034] [PMID: 39137368]

[14] A. Roux, S. Changey, J. Weber, and J.P. Lauffenburger, "LSTM-based projectile trajectory estimation in a GNSS-denied environment", *Sensors (Basel),* vol. 23, no. 6, p. 3025, 2023. [http://dx.doi.org/10.3390/s23063025] [PMID: 36991737]

[15] T. Casy, A. Grasseau, A. Charras, B. Rouvière, J.O. Pers, N. Foulquier, and A. Saraux, "Assessing the robustness of clinical trials by estimating Jadad's score using artificial intelligence approaches", *Comput. Biol. Med.,* vol. 148, 2022.105851 [http://dx.doi.org/10.1016/j.compbiomed.2022.105851] [PMID: 35947929]

[16] D. Niraula, J. Jamaluddin, M.M. Matuszak, R.K.T. Haken, and I.E. Naqa, "Quantum deep reinforcement learning for clinical decision support in oncology: application to adaptive radiotherapy", *Sci. Rep.,* vol. 11, no. 1, p. 23545, 2021. [http://dx.doi.org/10.1038/s41598-021-02910-y] [PMID: 34876609]

[17] C. Beatty, T. Malik, M. Saha, and C. Sinha, "Evaluating the therapeutic alliance with a free-text CBT conversational agent (Wysa): A mixed-methods study," Frontiers in Digital Health, vol. 4, 2022. [Online]. Available: https://doi.org/10.3389/fdgth.2022.847991

[18] K.K. Fitzpatrick, A. Darcy, and M. Vierhile, "Delivering cognitive behavior therapy to young adults with symptoms of depression and anxiety using a fully automated conversational agent (Woebot): A randomized controlled trial", *JMIR Ment. Health,* vol. 4, no. 2, 2017.e19 [http://dx.doi.org/10.2196/mental.7785] [PMID: 28588005]

[19] R. Meadows, C. Hine, and E. Suddaby, "Conversational agents and the making of mental health recovery", *Digit. Health,* vol. 6, 2020.2055207620966170 [http://dx.doi.org/10.1177/2055207620966170] [PMID: 33282335]

[20] E. M. Boucher, N. R. Harake, H. E. Ward, S. E. Stoeckl, J. Vargas, J. Minkel, … R. Zilca, "Artificially intelligent chatbots in digital mental health interventions: A review," Expert Review of Medical Devices, vol. 18, sup. 1, pp. 37–49, 2021. [Online]. Available: https://doi.org/10.1080/17434440.2021.2013200

[21] R. Hussein, D. Wurhofer, E.M. Strumegger, A. Stainer-Hochgatterer, S.T. Kulnik, R. Crutzen, and J. Niebauer, "General Data Protection Regulation (GDPR) toolkit for digital health", *Stud. Health Technol. Inform.,* vol. 290, pp. 222-226, 2022. [http://dx.doi.org/10.3233/SHTI220066] [PMID: 35673005]

[22] A. Le Glaz, Y. Haralambous, D.H. Kim-Dufor, P. Lenca, R. Billot, T.C. Ryan, J. Marsh, J. DeVylder, M. Walter, S. Berrouiguet, and C. Lemey, "Machine learning and natural language processing in mental health: Systematic review", *J. Med. Internet Res.,* vol. 23, no. 5, 2021.e15708 [http://dx.doi.org/10.2196/15708] [PMID: 33944788]

[23] P. Rajpurkar, and M.P. Lungren, "The current and future state of AI interpretation of medical images", *N. Engl. J. Med.,* vol. 388, no. 21, pp. 1981-1990, 2023. [http://dx.doi.org/10.1056/NEJMra2301725] [PMID: 37224199]

CHAPTER 15

Emerging Technologies in NLP for Healthcare

R. Sofia[1,*] and **S. Yazhinian**[2]

[1] *Department of Electronics and Communication Engineering, Manakula Vinayagar Institute of Technology, Puducherry, India.*

[2] *Department of Computer Science, Vel Tech Rangarajan Dr. Sagunthala R&D Institute of Science & Technology, Chennai, India*

Abstract: Emerging technologies in Natural Language Processing (NLP) are generating substantial breakthroughs across different sectors, notably in healthcare, where they are transforming patient care, diagnostics, and medical research. By utilizing the power of transformers and Large Language Models (LLMs) like GPT-3/4 and BERT, NLP is improving text production, contextual comprehension, and the interpretation of complex medical jargon. These technologies also evolve into multimodal applications, merging text with visuals and audio for thorough data processing. In banking and customer service, conversational AI leads to the development of sophisticated chatbots and emotion-sensitive systems. At the same time, explainable and ethical NLP provides openness and fairness in decision-making processes. Domain-specific models are being adapted to address the particular demands of specialized domains, and the combination of NLP with edge computing allows real-time processing for mobile and IoT devices. Moreover, NLP is breaking down language barriers with cross-lingual models, supporting low-resource languages, and encouraging inclusion. As these technologies continue to grow, they are establishing new norms in human-machine interaction, with substantial implications for tailored care, efficient operations, and new paths of discovery across numerous industries.

Keywords: BERT, GPT-3/4, Healthcare, Transformers, Large Language Models (LLMs), Natural Language Processing (NLP).

INTRODUCTION

From electronic health records to medical research publications, the healthcare sector faces a paradox in a time when digital information generation is unparalleled. While data has never been more plentiful, extracting actionable insights from this great ocean of information has never been more challenging. Emerging as a revolutionary branch of artificial intelligence, Natural Language Processing (NLP) is a critical tool for bridging this gap by giving sophisticated

* **Corresponding author R. Sofia:** Department of Electronics and Communication Engineering, Manakula Vinayagar Institute of Technology, Puducherry, India; E-mail: sofiaece@mvit.edu.in

A. Shankar, Saranya Jayapalan, & Basant. K. Tiwary (Eds.)

solutions to negotiate, assess, and exploit the complexity of medical information in inconceivable ways [1, 2].

In a contemporary hospital, a usual day comprises doctors dictating patient notes, radiologists writing thorough reports, nurses recording treatment events, and researchers reporting new clinical outcomes. Each of these endeavors provides valid but unstructured textual data. Designed for structured information, conventional data processing tools find it challenging to retrieve the intricacies, context, and linkages buried in these natural language descriptions [3 - 5]. This is where NLP technologies have become essential, as they are the intelligent link between computational analysis and human communication.

NLP has had an impact on healthcare in ways beyond simple text processing. NLP technologies radically alter healthcare delivery's critical components by enabling robots to perceive, interpret, and generate human language. From automating fundamental administrative tasks to recognizing tiny patterns in patient histories that may escape human observation, these technologies are increasing the efficiency and quality of healthcare services. Furthermore, in global health catastrophes like the COVID-19 pandemic, NLP's ability to swiftly scan and analyze enormous amounts of medical literature and clinical data has become increasingly crucial for hastening research and improving patient treatment choices.

As we stand at the intersection of artificial intelligence and healthcare, new NLP technologies are pushing the limits of what is attainable in medical practice. Advanced language models, driven by deep learning architectures, can now understand challenging medical tales with near-human accuracy. These computers can continually analyze several languages, adapt to expert medical jargon, and even recognize the contextual factors necessary for practical medical interpretation.

This chapter reviews developing NLP technologies in healthcare, examining their current uses and future potential. The progress of NLP from basic text processing to strong AI-driven systems capable of complex medical reasoning.

- Examines how cutting-edge NLP technologies are being applied to various parts of healthcare delivery, from clinical decision support to individualized patient care
- Investigates the problems and potential of adopting NLP technologies within healthcare settings
- Considers the ethical implications and privacy issues surrounding the employment of these technologies

- Explores new trends and future directions that promise to impact healthcare delivery radically

The impact of this technological discovery cannot be overstated. As healthcare systems worldwide face expanding demand, resource constraints, and a desire for improved patient outcomes, NLP technologies offer powerful tools to enhance the efficiency, accuracy, and accessibility of medical services. Understanding the use and implications of these evolving technologies is crucial for healthcare professionals, technologists, and legislators [6 - 10].

This chapter presents a detailed evaluation of the current state of NLP in healthcare and a forward-looking examination of developing trends and future potential. By evaluating these technologies' theoretical underpinnings and practical implementations, we aim to equip readers with a thorough knowledge of how NLP is revolutionizing healthcare and what we anticipate in the years ahead.

Historical Context: The Evolution of NLP in Healthcare

The route of natural language processing in healthcare reflects one of the most significant technical changes in medical informatics, moving from simple text processing systems to today's powerful artificial intelligence technology. This trend spans several decades, each distinguished by new technologies that profoundly modified how we handle and interpret medical information.

The narrative began in the 1960s, during what we now call the Rule-Based Era. This epoch witnessed the emergence of vital medical terminology standards with the invention of SNOMED (Systematized Nomenclature of Medicine). Early NLP systems mainly focused on pattern-matching algorithms and manually built rules to comprehend medical language. These basic systems employed regular expressions and Boolean logic to recognize medical terms and parse simple texts. The invention of MYCIN in the 1970s was a crucial milestone as one of the early medical expert systems, including rudimentary NLP capabilities. The Linguistic String Project (LSP) followed, pioneering systematic ways of medical language processing. While rigid rule-based architectures restricted these systems, they laid the fundamental basis for future developments.

The 1990s introduced the Statistical Revolution, signaling a paradigm shift in medical NLP. This period featured probabilistic models that could learn from data rather than depending only on predetermined rules. Hidden Markov Models have been developed as potent tools for medical entity recognition, whilst Maximum Entropy models have changed text categorization skills. The discovery of Conditional Random Fields enhanced sequence labeling skills, enabling more accurate processing of medical narratives. This decade also saw the integration of the Unified Medical Language System (UMLS), which provided a comprehensive foundation for standardized medical vocabularies and proved a helpful resource for NLP systems.

Machine learning techniques gained prominence as processing power expanded and medical data became more available. Support vector machines performed remarkably in medical document categorization, whereas decision trees produced interpretable models for symptom analysis. Adopting n-gram models provided greater comprehension of medical language patterns, enabling more complicated text processing capabilities. These statistical techniques marked a significant improvement over rule-based systems, offering greater flexibility and better management of the inherent diversity in medical literature.

The beginning of the 2010s saw the beginning of the deep learning transformation, altering medical NLP with neural networks of remarkable sophistication. Recurrent Neural networks, particularly LSTM networks, introduced new capabilities for understanding temporal medical data and recognizing long-term relationships in clinical narratives. The emergence of word embeddings through Word2Vec in 2012 altered how computers express and understand medical concepts, enabling a more advanced understanding of medical language and linkages.

Today's NLP systems reflect the conclusion of this rich historical growth, combining the precision of rule-based procedures with the flexibility of statistical methods and the strength of deep learning. Modern algorithms can parse intricate medical narratives with near-human accuracy, identifying the words and the subtle contextual distinctions required for medical interpretation. They thrive at tasks ranging from automated medical coding to real-time clinical decision support, exhibiting skills that would have appeared unfeasible during the early days of rule-based systems.

The technology has complex features such as zero-shot and few-shot learning, enabling systems to adapt to novel medical conditions and language without considerable training. Multimodal processing capabilities allow the integration of numerous kinds of data, from clinical notes to medical imaging reports, delivering comprehensive analytical tools for healthcare practitioners. These systems can translate medical acronyms, comprehend temporal correlations, and produce structured data from unstructured text while maintaining high accuracy and dependability.

The improvement continues with expanding capabilities in predictive modeling, outcome analysis, and population health management. Modern NLP systems serve as crucial tools for clinical trial matching, risk prediction, and therapy recommendations, fundamentally altering how healthcare practitioners access and utilize medical information. This progression from simple pattern matching to complicated AI-driven solutions demonstrates technology innovation and a fundamental shift in how we approach medical information processing and healthcare delivery.

As we move into the future, the foundation laid by this historical pattern promises even more revolutionary developments. Integrating quantum computing, enhanced privacy-preserving techniques, and more sophisticated multi-modal processing capabilities promises to further revolutionize how we process and utilize medical information, continuing the remarkable journey that began with thefirst rule-based systems decades ago.

Significance in Modern Healthcare: Technical Implementation and Architecture

The exponential expansion of digital health data has created significant technological issues in healthcare informatics. Modern healthcare systems create vast amounts of unstructured data - over 80% of medical data is in unstructured format, with hospitals generating an average of 50 petabytes of data yearly. This technology landscape demands powerful NLP frameworks to analyze, assess, and draw relevant insights from this complex medical information ecosystem.

At the architectural level, contemporary healthcare NLP systems feature multi-layered processing pipelines developed to handle the complexity of medical language. The foundation begins with specialized medical tokenization systems that must account for complicated medical vocabulary, acronyms, and domain-specific language patterns. These systems employ strong tokenization algorithms incorporating medical ontologies like SNOMED-CT and RxNorm, enabling accurate segmentation of medical words and phrases. Contemporary versions employ transformer-based architectures such as Clinical BERT variants, which have been pre-trained on vast corpora of medical literature to comprehend context-specific medical language and linkages.

The technological development of modern healthcare NLP systems follows a sophisticated processing hierarchy, including three basic tiers. The pre-processing layer forms the basis, incorporating Unicode normalization for managing various character sets in medical documents, medical-specific text segmentation algorithms, and specialized medical abbreviation extension tools. This layer also offers context-aware sentence boundary detection suited for clinical notes and better noise reduction algorithms for tackling clinical artifacts. These preparatory processing phases assure the quality and homogeneity of input data for future analysis.

Building upon this premise, the language processing layer employs complicated analytic algorithms. This covers medical-domain Part-of-Speech (POS) tagging using particular medical tagsets and deep learning-based medical Named Entity Recognition (NER) employing BiLSTM-CRF architectures. The layer also supports dependency parsing optimized for clinical narrative structures, temporal expression detection using hybrid rule-based and machine-learning techniques, and medical concept normalization using the UMLS meta-thesaurus. These components operate in unison to extract ordered linguistic information from medical texts.

The semantic analysis layer delivers maximum processing sophistication, leveraging medical concept embeddings using domain-adapted word2vec and BERT models. This layer enables relation extraction using attention-based transformer topologies and features, particularly components such as negation detection *via* clinical NegEx techniques. Uncertainty detection leverages probabilistic deep learning models, whereas medical temporal reasoning is handled utilizing temporal graph networks. This advanced semantic processing allows thorough comprehension of medical information and linkages.

The technical design incorporates critical components that interact synergistically to manage medical information. Enhanced vector representations comprise a significant component, with newer systems adding domain-specific word embeddings acquired on medical corpora. These include BioWord2Vec, specialized for biological language; Clinical BERT embeddings for contextualized representations; Med2Vec, for patient and visit embeddings; and graph embeddings for medical knowledge representation. Advanced neural architectures complement these representations by employing BERT variants optimized for the medical domain, specialized attention mechanisms for clinical text, hierarchical attention networks for processing long clinical documents, and graph neural networks for medical knowledge integration.

Information extraction systems represent another significant component, implementing Named Entity Recognition using CRF-BiLSTM structures and relation extraction leveraging dependency parsing and attention approaches. Event extraction utilizes temporal convolutional networks, whereas attribute extraction involves multi-task learning approaches. Knowledge integration is crucial, combining UMLS for medical concept normalization, RxNorm for drug standardization, SNOMED-CT for clinical terminology, and ICD-10 coding, leveraging hierarchical categorization models.

The technological implementation addresses different domain-specific issues necessary for healthcare applications. Privacy and security challenges are tackled *via* differential privacy techniques, federated learning methodologies for distributed model training, secure multi-party computing for collaborative learning, and homomorphic encryption for privacy-preserving analysis. Scalability and performance needs are satisfied by distributed processing architectures, in-memory processing for real-time applications, GPU acceleration for complex computations, and optimization strategies for managing vast clinical records. Model interpretability, a core necessity in healthcare, is addressed by utilizing attention visualization techniques, layer-wise relevance propagation, LIME, and SHAP implementations for local interpretability, and hierarchical attention mechanisms for document-level explanation.

This sophisticated technical infrastructure extends to specific healthcare applications, enabling advanced clinical decision support through real-time processing of clinical narratives, integration with FHIR-based EHR systems, complex event processing for clinical alerts, and dynamic knowledge graph updates. Research and analytics skills are enhanced by automated literature review utilizing transformer-based models, clinical trial matching, cohort identification, and outcome prediction using temporal convolutional networks. Population health management benefits from distributed processing of population-level health data, real-time epidemic monitoring, risk stratification through multi-modal data integration, and social determinants analysis utilizing text mining methods.

The value of these technical solutions continues to rise as healthcare data volumes expand and new applications develop. Future developments will likely focus on more vigorous privacy-preserving techniques, improved model interpretability, and more complicated multi-modal integration capabilities, further increasing the impact of NLP in healthcare services and research.

This evolving technical landscape enables healthcare organizations to process and analyze unstructured medical text in real time, extract and normalize medical concepts across diverse data sources, identify complex patterns and relationships in clinical data, and support evidence-based decision-making through automated analysis, ultimately advancing the frontier of healthcare informatics and patient care.

The papers explore the growing role of Natural Language Processing (NLP) and multimodal AI across various sectors, particularly healthcare. Z. Liu *et al.* 2019 discussed the transformative impact of NLP on healthcare, enhancing diagnostics, patient care, and medical research [11]. A. Holzinger *et al.* 2019 focused on multimodal explainable AI and reviewed its applications in healthcare and beyond [12]. F. Doshi-Velez & B. Kim, 2017 delved into the development of explainable and interpretable large language models, which are gaining traction across industries [13]. K. Huang *et al.* 2019 examined the integration of explainable AI with multimodal and longitudinal healthcare data to improve clinical decision support [14]. S. J. R. Meystre *et al.* 2008 specifically explored the direct clinical applications of NLP in neurology, showcasing its role in diagnosis and patient care [3]. A. Radford *et al.*, 2021 introduced Gemini AI, a breakthrough in multimodal AI that is changing the landscape of healthcare and other fields [15]. Y. Wang *et al.* 2018 reviewed the use of NLP in clinical decision support systems and electronic health records, which help improve patient outcomes [2]. J. Lee *et al.* 2020 highlighted how large language models are evolving to handle multimodal data, enhancing their capabilities in medical imaging and text analysis tasks [7]. M. T. Ribeiro *et al.* 2016 analyzed NLP applications in healthcare, focusing on both clinical and administrative settings [16]. D. T. Nguyen *et al.* 2022 a comprehensive survey of explainable and interpretable multimodal large language models, exploring their potential across various domains [17].

CORE NLP CONCEPTS IN MEDICAL CONTEXT

Text Preprocessing and Normalization in Medical Documents

Medical text preprocessing provides unique issues that go well beyond essential text normalization. When I worked on developing preprocessing pipelines for a large hospital system, we learned that medical texts contain an intricate mix of standard English, medical vocabulary, acronyms, and numeric values that require specialized handling.

The procedure begins with basic cleaning – deleting extraneous characters and standardizing forms. However, medical text requires additional specific measures. Consider a typical clinical note: "Pt c/o SOB & CP x2d, hx of MI." This seemingly simple text requires numerous normalization processes. Medical abbreviation expansion translates this into "Patient complains of shortness of breath and chest pain for 2 days, history of myocardial infarction." This extension is not straightforward — context matters significantly. "MI" either implies "myocardial infarction" or "mental illness," depending on the context.

Time phrases in medical texts need specific consideration. Phrases like "bid" (twice daily) or "q4h" (every 4 hours) require unique parsing rules. We have discovered that integrating rule-based systems with machine-learning approaches works well for handling these medical-specific temporal expressions.

Medical Entity Recognition

Healthcare entity identification involves recognizing and categorizing clinical concepts in literature. Despite a general-purpose named entity recognition, medical NER works with complex, overlapping entities and requires substantial domain knowledge. For instance, in the sentence "patient presents with acute anterior wall myocardial infarction," we need to distinguish both the entire ailment "acute anterior wall myocardial infarction" and its anatomical component "anterior wall."

Modern medical NER systems often feature mixed architectures. The foundation usually comprises a BiLSTM-CRF network, reinforced with attention mechanisms and pre-trained on medical corpora. These models are then enhanced with domain knowledge from medical ontologies like UMLS and SNOMED-CT. This combination helps capture both contextual patterns and known medical knowledge.

Relation Extraction in Clinical Text

Relation extraction in medical settings focuses on discovering links between medical phenomena. This work is especially tough because of the intricate structure of medical interactions. Consider a clinical note: "Patient's father died of lung cancer at age 45. Mother has a history of breast cancer." Here, we must identify the illnesses, familial links, and temporal features.

Modern techniques employ graph-based neural networks paired with attention processes. These systems may capture both local syntactic links and more significant document-level contexts. One incredibly successful strategy includes developing medical knowledge graphs that connect extracted links with existing medical knowledge bases, allowing more complex reasoning about medical interactions.

Semantic Analysis in Healthcare

Medical semantic analysis goes beyond mere word definitions to explore the intricate interaction of medical ideas. A significant problem is addressing denial and uncertainty. In medical textbooks, "no evidence of pneumonia" or "possible early signs of diabetes" convey essential therapeutic importance.

Implementation often includes numerous levels of investigation. At the basic level, we apply contextual embeddings learned on medical corpora. These are augmented with medical ontologies to capture domain-specific interactions. Negation detection needs specialized algorithms — the conventional NegEx technique provides a baseline, while contemporary solutions employ neural networks trained on clinical literature to handle complicated scenarios.

Medical Document Classification

Medical document categorization includes organizing clinical records into appropriate groupings. This process is exacerbated by the highly technical nature of medical records and their different forms. A single patient record could comprise progress notes, discharge summaries, radiological reports, and pathology reports, each needing separate categorization techniques.

Current best practices use hierarchical attention networks that can analyze documents at various levels - word, phrase, and document. These networks are often trained on massive medical corpora and fine-tuned for particular classification tasks. We have observed that integrating document structural information (headers, sections) considerably increases categorization accuracy.

Medical Information Extraction

Medical information extraction links all the aforementioned elements to produce organized data from unstructured medical material. This method includes finding and retrieving relevant clinical information, such as diagnoses, drugs, treatments, test results, and their properties and relationships.

Modern systems employ pipeline topologies that incorporate numerous specialized components. For example, we need to identify the medicine name, dose, frequency, route, and duration while retrieving prescription information. Each element needs specialist processing — a medical NER module may handle medicine names, while dose information would require a separate numeric expression parser.

The key to good medical information extraction lies in managing context and temporality. A medicine stated in a patient's history has different ramifications than one in the current medications section. Similarly, differentiating between active and stopped drugs involves recognizing temporal linkages in the text. Implementation often comprises a mix of deep learning models for entity and connection extraction, rule-based systems for managing structured inputs like lab data, and knowledge-based techniques for validating against medical ontologies. The retrieved information is then standardized to standard medical vocabularies (RxNorm for drugs, LOINC for lab testing, *etc.*) to facilitate interoperability.

This comprehensive approach to medical text processing has altered how we manage clinical documentation, allowing applications ranging from automated coding to clinical decision support. We witness more sophisticated capabilities in analyzing and exploiting medical text data as these technologies advance.

UNIQUE CHALLENGES IN MEDICAL TEXT PROCESSING

Medical text processing is complicated and varies from conventional text processing owing to specific terminology, frequent use of abbreviations, context-dependency, linguistic variety, and system integration needs. Here is a summary of each difficulty in a simplified, technical overview:

Domain-Specific Terminology

Medical Vocabulary Complexity: Medical literature includes a wide variety of specialized terminology that is infrequently used in general English. These include anatomical words (like "dorsolateral prefrontal cortex"), illness names (such as "keratoconjunctivitis"), pharmaceutical names (both generic and brand), and specialized medical procedures.

Rooted in Greek and Latin: Much of medical terminology combines Greek and Latin origins. This structure makes it hard for automated systems to correctly read and process the material.

For instance, "pneumonoultramicroscopicsilicovolcanoconiosis" is a single name for a lung illness but incorporates numerous roots that hold particular meanings related to lung health and sickness.

Variability in Naming: Some illnesses and ailments have many names or synonyms. For example, "heart attack" might alternatively be referred to as "myocardial infarction." This heterogeneity needs processing systems to comprehend that these phrases may signify the same thing even if they are stated differently.

Abbreviations and Acronyms

Frequent and Overloaded Usage: Medical documentation widely employs acronyms, which might indicate multiple things, depending on the context. "HR," for instance, might refer to "heart rate" in one context or "hormone receptor" in another. Similarly, "PT" may signify "patient," "physical therapy," or "prothrombin time."

Specialty and Institutional Variations: Different specializations (such as cardiology, oncology, or physical therapy) may use the same acronym differently. Furthermore, individual hospitals or healthcare organizations may use abbreviations, making uniformity problematic across contexts.

Rapidly Evolving: With medical developments, new acronyms indicate new illnesses, treatments, or approaches. This fast vocabulary growth demands ongoing changes to medical text processing systems to remain current.

Context-Dependent Interpretation

Patient Context: The interpretation of medical language may differ depending on patient-specific circumstances such as age, gender, and medical history. For instance, some symptoms or pharmaceutical effects may change depending on age, while a patient's past diagnosis may influence the interpretation of new data. Medication interactions also need contextual expertise to determine contraindications effectively.

Clinical Setting Context: The context in which documentation occurs influences language and concentration. Notes from an emergency department setting may vary in tone and substance from those of routine check-ups. Similarly, documentation techniques varied across specialists, primary care providers, and inpatient and outpatient settings, with each context contributing a distinct layer of meaning.

Workflow Context: Medical literature also depends on comprehending workflows, such as diagnostic orders, treatment plans, or current health conditions. Systems need to evaluate phrases in connection with past entries, enabling healthcare providers to analyze changes or improvements appropriately.

Multiple Languages and Writing Styles

Language Variability: Medical paperwork might contain terminology in several languages, including Greek, Latin, and local languages. International spelling variants add another layer; for instance, "haematology" in British English is spelled "hematology" in American English. Consequently, multilingual medical records need complex translation and normalization techniques to standardize information.

Differences in Writing Styles: Medical writing spans from serious research publications to quick clinical notes. Research publications may have organized, technical language, but clinical notes are generally in free-text style, which might include shorthand and fragmentary sentences. Specialty-specific documentation patterns provide extra diversity since terminology or phrases may be more prevalent in certain professions than others.

Structured *vs.* Unstructured Data: Some data, like test findings, are structured and standardized, while others, like patient notes, are unstructured. Medical text processing systems must be prepared to handle both kinds and combine them usefully.

Integration with Existing Medical Systems

Compatibility with EHR Systems: Medical text processing typically has to function within Electronic Health Record (EHR) systems. EHRs vary considerably in design, data formats, and standards, such as HL7 and FHIR. Effective medical text processing needs interoperability with various platforms to seamlessly access, interpret, and analyze data.

Legacy System Challenges: Many healthcare institutions still utilize outdated systems that may not be compatible with newer processing tools, making integration problematic. Updating these systems or establishing middleware solutions is frequently essential to ensure effective data interchange.

Data Security and Privacy Compliance: Medical text processing must meet stringent privacy standards like HIPAA in the United States, ensuring patient information is secured. Security requirements are critical for protecting data security and integrity, particularly when patient data is transferred across several departments or locations.

Workflow Integration: For practical application, medical text processing systems should integrate into healthcare workflows, enabling real-time or near-real-time processing. This can require connecting with clinical decision support tools, simplifying paperwork, and ensuring data flow seamlessly to maximize patient care.

By addressing unique challenges involving specific medical nuances, context requirements, and integration standards, medical text processing can contribute significantly to more accurate, efficient, and meaningful healthcare insights.

CURRENT STATE OF NLP TECHNOLOGIES IN HEALTHCARE

NLP (Natural Language Processing) technology alters healthcare by helping extract, organize, and analyze vast volumes of medical information. Here is a simple overview of how NLP is utilized in clinical documentation, Electronic Health Records (EHR), and clinical research.

Clinical Documentation

NLP systems are highly effective at managing the intricacies of clinical documentation, which includes clinical notes, discharge summaries, and numerous medical reports. These systems aid in the following ways:

Extracting Relevant Medical Information: NLP can filter through unstructured language in medical data to extract relevant information, such as symptoms, diagnoses, prescriptions, and treatments. This enables professionals to immediately obtain vital patient facts without going through lengthy reports.

Identifying Key Clinical Findings: NLP systems may identify key clinical insights (such as vital signs, test results, and health changes) and highlight them in the record. This decreases the danger of losing essential information in patient notes.

Standardizing Medical Terminology: Medical terminologies vary significantly, and NLP systems may standardize terminology by mapping synonyms to a single preferred phrase (*e.g.*, converting both "heart attack" and "myocardial infarction" to a standard term). This provides for more consistent recordkeeping and more straightforward data analysis.

Generating Structured Data from Free Text: Most clinical notes are written as free text, which may be challenging for computers to evaluate. NLP translates this text into structured data (*e.g.*, tables or fields in a database), making it more straightforward to search, analyze, and exchange across systems.

Supporting Clinical Coding and Billing: NLP may aid with assigning codes (*e.g.*, ICD-10 or CPT) used for medical billing. By automatically recognizing phrases linked to certain illnesses or treatments, NLP helps decrease human workload and increase coding accuracy.

Electronic Health Records (EHR)

NLP is crucial to strengthening EHR systems, making it easier to organize and retrieve patient information and speed up healthcare operations. Key NLP applications in EHRs include:

Automated Data Input and Validation: NLP may assist in eliminating manual data input by automatically extracting information from clinical notes and entering it into the relevant EHR fields. This avoids mistakes, saves time, and assures data correctness by checking submitted information.

Real-Time Clinical Decision Support: NLP systems deliver real-time warnings and suggestions based on patient data. For example, if a patient's record contains particular symptoms and test findings, the NLP system might propose probable diagnoses or highlight pharmaceutical interactions.

Patient Cohort Identification: NLP can identify groups of patients with similar features for targeted therapies or clinical trials. This entails evaluating unstructured data, including medical notes, to categorize patients based on diagnosis, demographics, or treatment response.

Quality Metrics Monitoring: NLP helps hospitals monitor quality metrics (such as readmission rates and infection control measures) by recognizing essential data in patient records. This allows healthcare providers to satisfy regulatory obligations and enhance care standards.

Compliance Checking: NLP systems check paperwork for compliance with healthcare laws (like HIPAA) and hospital rules. By recognizing missing information or inconsistent entries, NLP helps guarantee that patient records are complete and fulfill legal criteria.

Clinical Research Support

In clinical research, NLP aids researchers by offering efficient techniques to collect and evaluate data from multiple sources. Key ways NLP assists clinical research include:

Analyzing Scientific Literature: NLP helps researchers analyze vast scientific papers and clinical trials. By extracting essential information, such as results, methodology, and statistical outcomes, NLP helps researchers remain informed with the newest knowledge and make data-driven choices.

Identifying Potential Study Participants: NLP can swiftly scan patient data to locate people who satisfy specific criteria for clinical trials or research projects. This reduces time compared to manual searches and enables faster recruitment of qualified individuals.

Extracting Data from Published Studies: NLP systems extract data points (such as sample sizes, results, and side effects) from existing studies, making it more easier researchers to conduct meta-analyses or compare findings across studies.

Supporting Systematic Reviews: Systematic reviews must collect and assess several papers on a particular issue. NLP automates elements of this process, locating relevant articles, extracting crucial facts, and helping arrange data for more straightforward analysis.

Monitoring Adverse Events: NLP may assist in monitoring reported adverse events (such as pharmaceutical side effects or unexpected symptoms) from patient records or clinical research reports. This is especially valuable in pharmacovigilance, where researchers must discover and follow safety risks across massive databases.

EMERGING NLP APPLICATIONS IN CLINICAL SETTINGS

Emerging NLP applications in healthcare are transforming clinical settings by delivering improved help in decision-making, patient communication, and even integration with medical imaging. Here is a breakdown of each section in simple, technical terms:

Clinical Decision Support Systems

NLP-based Clinical Decision Support Systems (CDSS) are meant to aid healthcare practitioners by evaluating patient data and offering appropriate actions:

Analyzing Patient Symptoms and Medical History: NLP systems may scan patient records and present symptoms, comparing them to vast medical databases. Doing so helps detect trends and aids healthcare practitioners in rapidly determining a patient's health state.

Suggesting probable Diagnoses: Based on symptoms, medical history, and risk factors, NLP systems may recommend probable diagnoses. For example, if a patient appears to have chest discomfort, the system might suggest conditions such as heart disease or anxiety, enabling the clinician to evaluate these options.

Recommending Treatment Options: Using treatment recommendations and historical case data, NLP systems may offer acceptable therapies for specific diagnoses. For instance, for a diagnosis of hypertension, the system can prescribe lifestyle adjustments combined with conventional drugs.

Alerting Healthcare Providers to Potential Risks: NLP systems may discover high-risk scenarios by evaluating patient data for warning indicators. For example, if a patient's test results reveal abnormal kidney function while on certain drugs, the system may notify clinicians of a probable risk of kidney damage.

Monitoring Treatment Effectiveness: NLP monitors symptom changes, test data, and drug reactions reported in patient records. By evaluating these patterns, NLP systems may assist therapists in assessing whether a therapy is working or whether changes are required.

Patient Engagement and Communication

NLP is boosting patient engagement by delivering services that make healthcare more accessible and personalized:

Automated Appointment Scheduling: NLP can read patient appointment requests *via* text or speech, match their demands with available time slots, and automatically book appointments. This lessens the strain on administrative personnel and enhances convenience for patients.

Patient Query Handling: NLP chatbots and virtual assistants can answer patient queries regarding symptoms, drugs, or general health information. This provides patients with quick help, particularly for frequent queries that do not need a doctor's urgent response.

Symptom Checking: NLP-powered symptom checkers enable patients to enter symptoms and obtain information on probable disorders. These systems employ medical information databases to deliver appropriate counsel, typically advising people on whether to seek medical assistance.

Treatment Adherence Monitoring: NLP may evaluate text messages, app entries, or other patient input to monitor whether patients are taking prescriptions as recommended. If a patient shows they are missing medications or encountering adverse effects, the system may warn clinicians or offer solutions.

Health Education Delivery: NLP-based systems may offer health education materials suited to a patient's condition. For instance, following a diabetes diagnosis, the system may deliver instructional information on controlling blood sugar, nutritional suggestions, and exercise instructions.

Medical Image Analysis Integration

Integrating NLP with medical imaging is a breakthrough strategy that combines textual data with visual information, boosting diagnostic and reporting capabilities:

Report Generation from Medical pictures: NLP can generate summaries or reports based on radiological images, such as X-rays, MRIs, or CT scans. The technology analyzes the data and converts them into structured language, which helps radiologists write observations quickly.

Cross-Modal Information Extraction: NLP may combine information from text (*e.g.*, clinical notes) with data from pictures. For instance, if an MRI indicates a lung anomaly, the NLP system may correlate this discovery with earlier text notes on respiratory symptoms, offering a comprehensive picture of the patient's health.

Automated Annotation of Medical Images: NLP can aid in labeling or annotating regions of interest in medical images. For example, it may identify a tumor in an MRI or a fracture in an X-ray based on keywords or patterns found in linked text, supporting radiologists in speedier analysis.

Clinical Finding Correlation: NLP systems can connect image findings with textual patient data, such as symptoms and test results, to increase diagnosis accuracy. If an X-ray reveals indications of pneumonia and notes indicate a cough, NLP may integrate these ideas for a more thorough diagnosis.

Multi-Modal Diagnosis: Combining NLP with picture data enables systems to provide multi-modal diagnostics, which requires synthesizing information from text (like patient symptoms) and images (like scans). This integrated perspective may increase diagnostic accuracy by combining data from diverse sources.

ADVANCED LANGUAGE MODELS IN HEALTHCARE

Advanced language models transform how medical information is handled, boosting accuracy in clinical decision-making and facilitating adaptation to varied healthcare situations. This section addresses transformer-based models, few-shot and zero-shot learning, and multilingual capabilities in medical NLP.

Transformer-Based Models

Transformer-based architectures have significantly increased NLP capabilities, with healthcare-specific modifications increasing their efficacy in medical settings:

BERT-Based Medical Models: BERT (Bidirectional Encoder Representations from Transformers) is a core NLP model, and specific medical versions have been trained on medical data to comprehend the intricacies of healthcare language. These models excel at understanding context and ambiguity in medical texts.

BioClinicalBERT: BioClinicalBERT is a variant of BERT that is trained particularly on clinical notes and biological literature. It assists in tasks like extracting information from patient data, recognizing medical words, and processing complicated clinical paperwork more accurately than general-purpose models.

PubMedBERT: PubMedBERT has been trained on biomedical literature from PubMed, making it especially effective at interpreting research papers and scientific language. It is essential for clinical research, systematic reviews, and literature analysis in healthcare.

Clinical XLNet: Based on the XLNet architecture, Clinical XLNet is geared for clinical workloads and delivers solid performance on longer documents. This paradigm increases contextual comprehension in medical records and is effective for processing extensive patient histories or discharge summaries.

Domain-Specific GPT Variants: Generative models like GPT, modified for healthcare, aid in activities that involve text production, such as summarizing clinical notes, preparing patient reports, or composing replies to patient questions. Domain-specific GPT variations may be trained on healthcare data to deliver relevant and accurate medical replies.

These transformer-based models boost NLP tasks by enhancing contextual comprehension, minimizing mistakes in terminology, and aiding structured data extraction from unstructured medical literature.

Few-Shot and Zero-Shot Learning

Few-shot and zero-shot learning models benefit medical NLP for applications with insufficient data. These strategies enable models to generalize from minimum instances or adapt without any previous data on the given task:

Rare Disease Identification: Few-shot learning allows models to detect rare illnesses by training on a limited number of instances. This is particularly effective in rare diseases when significant data is not accessible, enabling the model to learn from a few cases.

Novel Symptom Pattern Recognition: Zero-shot learning allows models to recognize novel symptom patterns without previous training data on the individual symptoms. This may be critical for recognizing developing illnesses or identifying atypical symptom clusters that might suggest an epidemic.

Adaptation to New Medical Terminology: With new illnesses and therapies continually developing, few-shot learning enables models to swiftly absorb new terminology with minimal emerging data, minimizing the need for significant retraining on novel words.

Cross-profession Knowledge transmits: These models may transmit knowledge from one medical profession to another. For example, a model trained on cardiology data might apply information to other disciplines, like pulmonology, if they have related symptoms or treatment regimens.

Emergency Response Scenarios: In emergency response, zero-shot models can swiftly adapt to novel scenarios by relying on basic medical knowledge, especially in crisis situations when instant decision-making is essential. Providing flexible learning with less input, few-shot and zero-shot learning models give adaptable solutions to growing medical demands.

Multilingual Medical NLP

Multilingual capabilities in NLP enable models to analyze healthcare data in many languages, which is vital for global health initiatives and cross-cultural medical collaboration:

Cross-Lingual Medical Information Extraction: Multilingual models can extract and analyze medical data across languages, vital for international research and global health monitoring. This permits studying health data from varied populations and languages, offering insights into larger health patterns.

Multilingual Clinical Documentation: Multilingual NLP helps translate and standardize medical data in locations with varied language populations. This guarantees that health practitioners have consistent access to patient information regardless of language barriers, which enhances patient care.

Global Health Monitoring: Multilingual NLP models can follow and analyze health data globally, revealing trends in disease distribution, outbreak causes, and cross-border health concerns. This is especially crucial for pandemic response and global disease control activities.

Worldwide Research Cooperation: By overcoming language barriers, multilingual NLP improves cooperation on research initiatives, clinical trials, and medical studies worldwide. It permits research results to be shared and interpreted internationally, supporting collective medical progress.

Cultural Context Adaptation: Multilingual models may also adapt medical information to varied cultural settings, helping healthcare personnel to interact more effectively with patients from diverse backgrounds. This helps ensure that health advice is culturally appropriate and accessible.

These sophisticated NLP models—transformers, few-shot learning, and multilingual models—are boosting the capacity of healthcare systems to offer accurate, timely, and accessible information. They enable various healthcare applications, from clinical decision-making to multinational cooperation.

CHALLENGES AND ETHICAL CONSIDERATIONS

While NLP technologies have achieved tremendous improvements in healthcare, they also raise technological, privacy, and ethical difficulties. Addressing these concerns is critical for the responsible and successful deployment of NLP in therapeutic contexts.

Technical Challenges

Implementing NLP in healthcare comes with specific technological barriers that need to be solved for dependable and scalable systems:

Data Quality and Standardization: Medical data varies in quality and format across sources, making it challenging to ensure consistency. NLP models need standardized data to work effectively, and inconsistencies in medical language, acronyms, or record structure might affect model performance.

System Integration: It may be complicated to integrate NLP systems with current healthcare systems, such as Electronic Health Records (EHRs) and other health IT infrastructure. Compatibility with standards like HL7 or FHIR is needed to allow smooth data transmission.

Scale and Performance: NLP systems need to manage massive amounts of data, frequently in real-time, for activities like monitoring health trends or notifying physicians. Scaling NLP systems to work consistently under heavy loads without sacrificing accuracy or speed is a major challenge.

Model Interpretability: Healthcare professionals must comprehend how NLP models reach confident conclusions to accept their suggestions. Many NLP models, intense learning-based ones, act as "black boxes," meaning their decision-making processes are not interpretable.

Continuous Learning and Adaptation: Medical knowledge and procedures develop swiftly. NLP models must adapt to new knowledge, medical words, and standards. Establishing strategies for continual learning without jeopardizing model performance is critical.

PRIVACY AND SECURITY

Privacy and security are crucial when working with sensitive health data since NLP models routinely analyze vast volumes of patient information:

Patient Data Protection: Patient data must be safeguarded against illegal access and possible breaches. Encryption, anonymization, and other data security measures are necessary to ensure patient confidentiality.

HIPAA Compliance: NLP systems in the United States must comply with the Health Insurance Portability and Accountability Act (HIPAA) to safeguard patient data privacy. Ensuring compliance is a legal and technological concern that NLP systems must handle.

Secure Data Sharing: In healthcare, data sharing across institutions is generally essential for cooperation and continuity of service. NLP systems must guarantee that shared data stays safe, employing secure routes and effective encryption technologies.

Access Control: Controlling who may access patient data inside the NLP system is critical. Role-Based Access Control (RBAC) and related strategies guarantee that only authorized individuals can access sensitive information.

Audit Trails: NLP systems must preserve thorough records of who accessed or edited data, maintaining accountability and allowing audits to identify and prevent improper access or abuse of patient information.

Ethical Considerations

Ethics play a key part in using NLP in healthcare since the technology directly affects patient care and well-being:

Bias in Medical NLP Systems: NLP models might accidentally convey biases if trained on datasets that lack diversity. This might lead to disproportionate treatment recommendations or misinterpretations of data for particular patient groups, possibly leading to healthcare inequities.

Algorithmic Fairness: NLP systems must deliver fair and equitable results for all patients, regardless of age, gender, ethnicity, or other demographic characteristics. Ensuring algorithmic fairness demands careful dataset selection and frequent reviews of model performance across diverse groups.

Transparency in Decision-Making: Patients and doctors should know how NLP systems generate recommendations or judgments, mainly when the NLP model's input affects patient treatment plans. Transparent systems create trust and allow better-informed decision-making.

Medical agreement: Using NLP on medical data must be done with explicit patient agreement. Patients should be notified about how their data will be used, kept, and shared, enabling them to opt out if desired.

Professional Responsibility: Clinicians must still monitor and evaluate NLP results, since depending only on automated systems might lead to mistakes. Medical NLP should aid healthcare practitioners rather than replace human judgment, keeping the physician's role in decision-making.

Addressing these problems and ethical issues is vital for the appropriate and successful use of NLP in healthcare, ensuring that patient data is secured, systems are fair and trustworthy, and healthcare personnel remain integral to patient care.

FUTURE DIRECTIONS

Breakthroughs in new technologies, integration with other systems, and specific research activities will likely define the future of NLP in healthcare. These initiatives seek to make NLP more accurate, accessible, and secure, eventually boosting patient care and medical discoveries.

Emerging Technologies

Innovations in technology promise to expand the frontiers of what medical NLP can achieve:

Quantum Computing Applications in NLP: Quantum computing offers promise for expediting complicated NLP calculations, enabling quicker and more efficient analysis of big medical datasets. Quantum algorithms might boost pattern detection in vast datasets, providing speedier insights in real-time applications.

Edge Computing for Medical NLP: Edge computing enables data processing closer to the data source, such as wearable devices or local healthcare systems. This minimizes latency, allowing real-time language processing for applications like remote monitoring and diagnostics in rural or resource-limited areas.

Federated Learning Approaches: Federated learning enables NLP models to learn from decentralized data sources without exchanging patient data between regions. This privacy-preserving strategy promotes cooperation across institutions, making it feasible to increase model performance without compromising patient confidentiality.

Automated Medical Knowledge Graph Construction: Knowledge graphs organize medical information in a manner that computers can comprehend, linking concepts like symptoms, diagnoses, and therapies. Automated knowledge graph creation helps NLP models grasp links between medical concepts, enhancing accuracy in applications like clinical decision support.

Real-Time Language Understanding Systems: Real-time NLP systems can quickly analyze and interpret patient-provider communications or clinical documents. This technology might support physicians during patient contacts by delivering real-time information and minimizing paperwork time.

Integration with Other Technologies

Integrating NLP with other cutting-edge technologies allows new applications and increases data security, usability, and clinical support:

IoT and Medical Devices: NLP combined with Internet of Things (IoT) devices can evaluate real-time data from wearables, home health monitoring, and hospital equipment. This connectivity may offer fast alarms for arrhythmias, blood sugar changes, or breathing concerns, boosting patient safety.

Blockchain for Secure Data Sharing: Blockchain provides a decentralized and tamper-proof mechanism to communicate patient data securely. Integrating blockchain with NLP guarantees that sensitive medical information stays safe throughout exchanges among institutions, increasing trust and openness in patient data management.

Augmented Reality (AR) Applications: AR paired with NLP may enhance medical training and surgical operations. NLP may parse spoken instructions or contextual information, directing physicians through procedures or delivering real-time diagnostic help *via* an AR interface.

Robots and Autonomous Systems: NLP-enhanced robots may improve patient care in hospitals and rural areas. Robots equipped with NLP may aid in triaging, issuing treatment reminders, monitoring patient health, and enhancing access to care when human resources are limited.

Individualized Medicine Platforms: NLP systems paired with genetic and clinical data may produce individualized treatment strategies for patients. By knowing individual risk factors and reactions to therapy, NLP may aid physicians in offering precision medicine suited to each patient's requirements.

Research Priorities

Research in NLP for healthcare is focused on resolving present constraints and laying the way for future innovations:

Improved Model Interpretability: Research aims to make NLP models more interpretable, enabling physicians to comprehend and trust model outputs. Efforts concentrate on building transparent models that clearly explain their decision-making process, particularly for healthcare contexts where human monitoring is vital.

Enhanced Privacy-Preserving methods: Privacy is a key problem in healthcare, and research is undertaken to create more effective privacy-preserving methods, such as differential privacy, homomorphic encryption, and secure multi-party computing, guaranteeing patient data stays secret.

Better Handling of Medical Uncertainty: Healthcare is inherently unpredictable, with symptoms and results changing among people. NLP models are being created to accommodate this ambiguity, boosting their dependability in clinical applications where accuracy is critical.

Cross-Modal Learning Advancement: Cross-modal learning integrates text, visual, and other data sources for a more holistic understanding. For instance, connecting text from medical notes with images from scans helps NLP algorithms generate more accurate diagnoses by using different data sources.

Robust Evaluation procedures: Developing standardized and rigorous evaluation procedures is crucial to analyzing NLP model performance and dependability in clinical settings. Research is focused on developing benchmarks that represent real-world applications to guarantee models are safe, trustworthy, and therapeutically useful.

The future of NLP in healthcare is optimistic, with rising technology, integrated applications, and targeted research driving progress. These advances offer the potential to make healthcare more customized, secure, and responsive to patient requirements.

CONCLUSION

The field of NLP in healthcare is expanding at an unprecedented rate, fueled by technical innovation and the rising need for efficient, data-driven healthcare solutions. This advancement offers greater patient care, more efficient clinical operations, and transformational discoveries in medical research. Future work in NLP for healthcare is anticipated to concentrate on increasing model accuracy, assuring interpretability, and sustaining ethical norms, with a strong emphasis on safeguarding privacy and data security. As NLP continues to interact with new technology, it offers great promise to transform healthcare, making it more accessible, tailored, and sensitive to the intricacies of individual patient demands.

REFERENCES

[1] K. Kreimeyer, M. Foster, A. Pandey, N. Arya, G. Halford, S. F. Jones, R. Forshee, M. Walderhaug, and T. Botsis, "Natural language processing systems for capturing and standardizing unstructured clinical information: A systematic review", *J. Biomed. Informat.*, vol. 73, pp. 14-29, 2017. [http://dx.doi.org/10.1016/j.jbi.2017.07.012]

[2] Y. Wang, L. Wang, M. Rastegar-Mojarad, S. Liu, F. Shen, R. Wang, and H. Liu, "Clinical information extraction applications: A literature review", *J. Biomed. Informat.*, vol. 77, pp. 34-49, 2018. [http://dx.doi.org/10.1016/j.jbi.2018.10.007]

[3] S. M. Meystre, G. K. Savova, K. C. Kipper-Schuler, and J. F. Hurdle, "Extracting information from textual documents in the electronic health record: A review", *J. Biomed. Informat.,* vol. 41, no. 5, pp. 807-817, 2008.
[http://dx.doi.org/10.1016/j.jbi.2008.10.005]

[4] P. B. Jensen, L. J. Jensen, and S. Brunak, "Mining electronic health records: Towards better research applications and clinical care", *Nat. Rev. Genet.,* vol. 13, no. 6, pp. 395-405, 2012.
[http://dx.doi.org/10.1038/nrg3208]

[5] C. Friedman, and N. Elhadad, "Natural language processing in health care and biomedicine", In: *Biomedical Informatics,* E. H. Shortliffe, J. J. Cimino, Eds., Springer: New York, NY, USA, 2014, pp. 255-284.
[http://dx.doi.org/10.1007/978-1-84628-754-1_10]

[6] L. L. Wang, K. Lo, Y. Chandrasekhar, R. Reas, J. Yang, D. Burdick, D. Eide, K. Funk, Y. Kinney, Z. Liu, W. Merrill, P. Mooney, D. A. Murdick, D. Rishi, J. Sheehan, Z. Shen, B. Stilson, A. D. Wade, K. Wang, N. Xie, D. Raymond, S. Weld, O. Etzioni, and S. Kohlmeier, "CORD-19: The COVID-19 Open Research Dataset", *arXiv preprint arXiv:2004.10706,* 2020.
[http://dx.doi.org/10.48550/arXiv.2004.10706]

[7] J. Lee, W. Yoon, S. Kim, D. Kim, S. Kim, C. H. So, and J. Kang, "BioBERT: A pre-trained biomedical language representation model for biomedical text mining", *Bioinformatics,* vol. 36, no. 4, pp. 1234-1240, 2020.
[http://dx.doi.org/10.1093/bioinformatics/btz682]

[8] E. Alsentzer, J. Murphy, W. Boag, W. Weng, D. Jindi, T. Naumann, and M. McDermott, "Publicly available clinical BERT embeddings", In: *Proceedings of the 2nd Clinical Natural Language Processing Workshop*, 2019, pp. 72-78.
[http://dx.doi.org/10.18653/v1/W19-1909]

[9] H. J. Murff, V. F. FitzHenry, M. Matheny, J. Gentry, K. L. Kotter, K. Crimin, R. S. Dittus, and H. Xu, "Automated identification of postoperative complications within an electronic medical record using natural language processing", *JAMA,* vol. 306, no. 8, pp. 848-855, 2011.
[http://dx.doi.org/10.1001/jama.2009.1191]

[10] W. Nicholson Price II, and I. G. Cohen, "Privacy in the age of medical big data", *Nat. Genet.,* vol. 48, no. 1, pp. 37-43, 2016.
[http://dx.doi.org/10.1038/ng.3702]

[11] Z. Liu, Y. Chen, B. Tang, X. Wang, Q. Qen, H. Li, and B. Wang, "Clinical natural language processing in China: Systematic review", *JMIR Med. Informat.,* vol. 7, no. 2, p. e12239, 2019.
[http://dx.doi.org/10.2196/12239]

[12] A. Holzinger, G. Langs, H. Denk, K. Zatloukal, and H. Müller, "Causability and explainability of artificial intelligence in medicine", *Wiley Interdiscip. Rev. Data Min. Knowl. Discov.,* vol. 9, no. 4, p. e1312, 2019.
[http://dx.doi.org/10.1002/widm.1312]

[13] F. Doshi-Velez, and B. Kim, "Towards a rigorous science of interpretable machine learning", *arXiv preprint arXiv:1702.08608,* 2017.
[http://dx.doi.org/10.48550/arXiv.1702.08608]

[14] K. Huang, J. Altosaar, and R. Ranganath, "ClinicalBERT: Modeling clinical notes and predicting hospital readmission", *arXiv preprint arXiv:1904.05342,* 2019.
[http://dx.doi.org/10.48550/arXiv.1904.05342]

[15] A. Radford, J. Wu, R. Child, D. Luan, D. Amodei, and I. Sutskever, "Learning Transferable Visual Models From Natural Language Supervision", In: *Proceedings of the 38th International Conference on Machine Learning (ICML)*. PMLR, 2021, pp. 8748-8763.
[http://dx.doi.org/10.5555/3504035.3505536]

[16] M. T. Ribeiro, S. Singh, and C. Guestrin, "Why should I trust you? Explaining the predictions of any classifier", In: *Proceedings of the 22nd ACM SIGKDD International Conference on Knowledge Discovery and Data Mining*, 2016, pp. 1135-1144. [http://dx.doi.org/10.1145/2939672.2939778]

[17] D. T. Nguyen, S. R. Joty, S. M. Hasan, and M. Mohiuddin, "Multimodal machine learning: A survey and taxonomy", *IEEE Trans. Pattern Anal. Mach. Intell.,* 2022. [http://dx.doi.org/10.1109/TPAMI.2021.3086807]

CHAPTER 16

Navigating the Future of Healthcare: Exploring the Next Phase in NLP

M. K. Bhanuja[1] and **K. Suresh Joseph**[1,*]

[1] *Department of Computer Science, Pondicherry University, Puducherry, India*

Abstract: Natural Language Processing (NLP) uses modern machine learning techniques to help machines study human-understandable language. Innovations in NLP help change healthcare by being implemented in various domains of the healthcare sector. NLP can be used in domains such as making clinical decisions, enhancing patient care, and performing administrative tasks. Advances in deep learning methods, improved transformer models, and modern diverse datasets will open new horizons in the medical sector. However, challenges such as ethics and data privacy still remain. Exploring new areas that can be used in the healthcare sector, along with NLP, will give new ideas for research. This chapter examines the prospective utilization of NLP within the healthcare sector, elucidating its potential benefits for patients and healthcare providers. The discourse encompasses the foundational relevance of NLP, current implementation landscapes, key contemporary applications, anticipated future trends, inherent implementation challenges, the role of NLP in facilitating personalized medicine, and a prospective outlook for the technology's integration into healthcare systems.

Keywords: Clinical decision-making, Data privacy, Healthcare, Natural Language Processing (NLP), Transformer models.

INTRODUCTION

Natural Language Processing (NLP), a subset of Artificial Intelligence (AI), focuses on the interaction between computers and human languages. NLP enables machines to read, interpret, and derive meaning from unstructured data such as spoken conversations, handwritten notes, emails, and textual reports. Unlike structured data such as spreadsheets or coded data, which is easy for computers to analyze, unstructured data like clinical notes, discharge summaries, or pathology reports presents challenges due to its variability and ambiguity [1].

* **Corresponding author K. Suresh Joseph:** Department of Computer Science, Pondicherry University, Puducherry, India; E-mail: ksjdeptofcs@gmail.com

A. Shankar, Saranya Jayapalan, & Basant. K. Tiwary (Eds.)

The primary objective of NLP is to enable machines to understand language like humans, including understanding grammar, syntax, context, semantics, and intent. Various techniques, such as tokenization, part-of-speech tagging, named entity recognition (NER), sentiment analysis, and semantic parsing, are employed to understand and analyze language data. Recent advancements in NLP have been driven by complex machine learning models, like Bidirectional Encoder Representations from Transformers (BERT) and Generative Pre-trained Transformer (GPT), which are good at processing and generating natural text with perfect accuracy.

The new application of NLP in healthcare will bring significant changes using advanced AI techniques, mainly deep learning and transformer models. These technologies can be used to solve complex problems in healthcare. NLP can be used in multilingual patient communication, ensuring that all patients are cared for and understood correctly. However, as we adopt these technologies, we must address the important concerns that can come with this. Data privacy is a significant concern that should be taken care of. Sensitive patient information should be protected from unauthorized access, and ethical considerations should be considered. This chapter will explore how NLP is changing healthcare delivery and management. We will look at various new applications and discuss the current limitations of NLP technologies, including challenges in understanding context and the need for diverse training datasets. To move forward, we aim to show how NLP can become a key part of a more brilliant healthcare system. This will improve health outcomes, ensure that care is accessible and tailored to each patient's needs, and make a better tomorrow.

Relevance of NLP in Healthcare

The healthcare sector generates a significant amount of unstructured data daily. It can be a doctor's note, lab results, radiology reports, patient discharge summaries, or research articles. Early on, about 80% of these data lacked structure, which challenged analytics and decision-making. NLP can address this issue by uncovering unseen insights from this data, providing clinicians, administrators, and patients with better and more accurate information.

Below are some key areas where NLP plays an essential role in healthcare:

Clinical Documentation and Physician Burnout Reduction

Healthcare providers spend much time documenting patient information in Electronic Health Records (EHRs). NLP systems can automatically extract relevant details from voice recordings or clinical notes. This helps workers reduce documentation burden, prevent burnout, and enhance the quality of care [2].

Enhanced Clinical Decision Support (CDS)

NLP is pivotal in analyzing and interpreting a patient's comprehensive health history alongside their current medical condition. By leveraging advanced algorithms, NLP systems can sift through vast amounts of medical literature, extracting relevant insights to provide tailored recommendations for each patient. For instance, these systems can propose individualized treatment plans or highlight potential drug interactions, enabling healthcare professionals to make more informed, real-time decisions. This capability not only aids clinicians in delivering personalized care but also enhances the overall quality of patient outcomes by ensuring that all relevant information is considered [3].

Improved Patient Outcomes and Experience

NLP improves patient outcomes by automating appointment scheduling, medication reminders, and mental health assessments. Additionally, sentiment analysis of patient feedback can help identify areas for improvement in care delivery, ultimately leading to higher patient satisfaction [4].

Public Health Surveillance

NLP algorithms play a crucial role in analyzing a wide range of data sources, including news articles, social media platforms, and other publicly available information, to effectively monitor disease outbreaks and discern trends in public health. A notable application of these tools emerged during the COVID-19 pandemic, where NLP was employed to sift through diverse datasets [5]. By identifying clusters of symptoms reported in various contexts, these algorithms significantly assisted health authorities in detecting potential outbreaks early and formulating timely responses. This proactive approach illustrates the power of NLP in enhancing public health surveillance and response strategies.

Automation of Administrative Workflows

NLP significantly enhances administrative workflows, particularly in insurance claims processing, denial management, and billing. By automatically extracting pertinent information from various documents, NLP minimizes the likelihood of errors, boosts operational efficiency, and speeds up the reimbursement processes.

This technology not only streamlines the handling of complex data but also allows for quicker decision-making and improved accuracy in financial transactions, ultimately leading to a smoother experience for providers and patients.

Sentiment and Emotion Analysis in Mental Health

NLP applications can evaluate patients' emotional states by meticulously examining language patterns found in various forms of communication, such as text messages, therapy notes, and conversations with chatbots. By analyzing the nuances of these interactions, like word choice, tone, and sentiment, NLP can uncover valuable insights that facilitate the early detection of mental health issues, including conditions like anxiety and depression [6]. This innovative technology enhances understanding of a patient's emotional well-being and supports timely intervention and personalized care.

Current Landscape of NLP in Healthcare

The adoption of NLP in healthcare has seen remarkable growth over the past few years. This surge is primarily attributed to advancements in machine learning algorithms, the proliferation of cloud computing resources, and the digitization of healthcare data, which has transformed how information is recorded and analyzed [7].

Today, the landscape of NLP in healthcare is characterized by various innovative technologies and models. Machine learning techniques, intense learning, and transformer models have enhanced the ability to process and understand complex medical texts [8]. These advancements allow for more accurate interpretation of clinical notes, patient records, and research articles, improving patient care and outcomes.

Furthermore, applications of NLP in healthcare are becoming increasingly diverse. They range from automated transcription services for healthcare providers to more sophisticated systems that can analyze patient sentiment from feedback forms. Other applications include clinical decision support systems, predictive analytics for patient outcomes, and personalized treatment recommendations based on patient data. The convergence of various technologies transforms how healthcare professionals interact with data, leading to more efficient workflows and improved patient care through data-driven insights. Early NLP systems relied on rule-based algorithms that followed predefined patterns to identify and extract relevant terms. While these systems were adequate for specific tasks, such as extracting diagnosis codes or identifying adverse events in clinical notes, their performance was limited by their inability to adapt to complex language variations [9].

Modern NLP systems utilize supervised and unsupervised machine learning models trained on large datasets to recognize patterns in text, allowing for more accurate information extraction. Standard algorithms used for NLP tasks in healthcare include Support Vector Machines (SVMs), random forests, and Recurrent Neural Networks (RNNs) [10]. The advent of transformer-based models, such as BERT and GPT, has revolutionized NLP by enabling the learning of contextual relationships in text [11]. These models process language bi-directionally, understanding the meanings of individual words and their contextual usage. Specialized models like ClinicalBERT have been fine-tuned for medical texts, making them particularly effective for healthcare applications [12]. Cloud computing platforms such as the Google Cloud Healthcare Application Programming Interface (API), Microsoft Azure Healthcare Bot, and Amazon Web Services (AWS) Comprehend Medical offer NLP services that facilitate large-scale deployment [13, 14]. These platforms provide APIs for extracting clinical entities, summarizing medical notes, and identifying key trends from patient data.

Key Applications of NLP in Healthcare Today

NLP addresses healthcare's most pressing challenges by transforming unstructured data into actionable insights. Its ability to extract meaning from clinical notes, patient records, and other medical data helps streamline workflows, improve care delivery, and support decision-making. Below are some of the key applications of NLP in healthcare today. Many healthcare providers are increasingly leveraging advanced Natural Language Processing (NLP)-based transcription tools to convert spoken dictations into structured, easily accessible text for EHRs [15]. These innovative tools transcribe and analyze clinical notes' content to suggest appropriate billing codes. Streamlining documentation processes significantly reduces the time healthcare professionals spend on paperwork while improving the accuracy and quality of data entered into patient records [16]. NLP technology has also paved the way for developing sophisticated voice-enabled virtual assistants. These assistants support physicians by accurately transcribing conversations during patient consultations, generating comprehensive summaries of those interactions, and setting timely reminders for follow-up actions. This automation allows physicians to concentrate more on direct patient care than on administrative tasks, ultimately enhancing patient experience.

In addition, NLP empowers clinicians to retrieve specific information quickly and efficiently from EHRs by understanding and processing natural language queries. Pharmaceutical companies are also harnessing the power of NLP to analyze extensive datasets, including research papers, clinical trial results, and patient reports. This analysis helps identify promising new drug candidates while facilitating the early detection of adverse events. NLP is crucial in advancing healthcare innovation by accelerating the drug development process and ensuring comprehensive patient safety measures.

Furthermore, healthcare providers are deploying NLP-powered chatbots to enhance patient engagement. These chatbots are programmed to respond to patient inquiries, provide self-care advice, and facilitate appointment scheduling. They are essential in chronic disease management and mental health support, offering patients 24/7 assistance and guidance [17]. By fostering continuous communication, these chatbots contribute significantly to patient well-being and adherence to treatment plans.

One of the most labor-intensive and time-consuming responsibilities for healthcare providers is the process of documentation. Physicians often dedicate considerable time entering various information into EHRs. This extensive documentation requirement can contribute to professional burnout, negatively impacting efficiency and reducing the time available for direct patient care.

NLP systems have emerged as a powerful solution to mitigate this challenge by automating the extraction and organization of pertinent information from clinical notes and spoken interactions. These advanced systems employ sophisticated algorithms to transcribe physicians' conversations with patients during visits into structured textual formats, which can then be seamlessly integrated into EHR systems with minimal manual intervention [18]. In addition to transcription, many NLP solutions can generate concise summaries of patient interactions, effectively highlighting critical details such as presenting symptoms, diagnoses, and prescribed treatments. This capability streamlines the documentation process and ensures that all relevant information is accurately captured and easily accessible. Furthermore, NLP tools can automatically extract diagnosis and procedure codes from clinical notes, such as International Classification of Diseases (ICD) or Current Procedural Terminology (CPT) codes. This functionality simplifies the often complex billing and reimbursement processes, reducing errors and ensuring that providers receive timely service payments.

By automating administrative tasks, NLP systems greatly reduce the workload of healthcare providers, ultimately leading to enhanced accuracy in medical records. This efficiency enables physicians to devote more time and energy to patient care, improving the overall quality of care. Tools such as Nuance Dragon Medical One and Suki AI are already making significant advancements in transforming clinical documentation practices, paving the way for a more efficient and patient-centered healthcare system [19]. NLP also markedly enhances Clinical Decision Support (CDS) by providing healthcare professionals with pertinent information extracted from unstructured data sources. These tools analyze patient histories, lab results, and clinical notes to generate personalized treatment recommendations and alerts. NLP-powered CDS tools can identify critical insights from EHRs, including allergies, medications, and past diagnoses, ensuring that clinicians make well-informed decisions [20].

Additionally, NLP systems can detect potential drug interactions by cross-referencing a patient's medications with clinical literature, helping to prevent adverse events. They can also analyze clinical research papers, guidelines, and case studies to suggest optimal treatment options tailored to the individual patient. Overall, NLP-powered CDS systems enhance care outcomes and minimize medical errors by providing clinicians with timely, data-driven insights [21].

Healthcare providers increasingly recognize the importance of patient feedback in enhancing their services. This transformation is primarily supported by advanced NLP tools, which facilitate the efficient and effective analysis of extensive feedback data. A key aspect of NLP is sentiment analysis, which aims to comprehend the emotions and opinions conveyed in written text. This technique enables hospitals and clinics to gather significant insights into patient experiences [22].

NLP systems can navigate various types of patient feedback, including online reviews, survey responses, and social media interactions. Healthcare organizations can better understand the factors influencing these sentiments by systematically identifying patient satisfaction and dissatisfaction patterns. For example, recurring challenges such as long wait times, insufficient communication from staff, or the quality of care received can be identified through this analysis, allowing organizations to address these concerns before they escalate. Furthermore, sentiment analysis can extend to patient messages, therapy notes, and other communication forms. By monitoring the emotional tone and content of these interactions, healthcare providers can detect subtle shifts that may signal deteriorating mental health conditions, such as depression or anxiety. This continuous monitoring fosters an environment of engagement, enabling providers to make timely adjustments to their services based on real-time feedback. Ultimately, leveraging sentiment analysis not only enhances patient satisfaction but also contributes to improved health outcomes by allowing healthcare providers to respond effectively to the needs and concerns of their patients. This approach signifies a substantial advancement in how healthcare organizations can utilize technology to enhance the overall patient care experience [23].

NLP-powered chatbots and virtual assistants transform patient engagement by providing 24/7 access to healthcare information. These tools assist with various tasks, from triaging symptoms to sending reminders for medication and managing chronic conditions. Patients can describe their symptoms in natural language, allowing the chatbot to offer essential guidance or direct them to the appropriate care provider. Virtual assistants also automate administrative tasks, such as scheduling appointments and reminding patients to take their medications. Additionally, chatbots can provide mental health support by engaging users in conversations that help identify emotional distress and suggest coping strategies. Examples of such chatbots include Wysa and Woebot, which facilitate empathetic interactions. These conversational agents enhance healthcare accessibility, reduce waiting times, and offer personalized care, particularly for patients with chronic diseases or mental health conditions [24].

Healthcare professionals often find themselves in the challenging position of needing rapid access to crucial patient information embedded within vast and complex EHR systems. Navigating these extensive databases can be cumbersome and time-consuming. NLP is a powerful technology that significantly enhances information retrieval by seamlessly interpreting and understanding intricate natural language queries. For instance, clinicians are empowered to articulate specific inquiries such as, "Can you show me all patients diagnosed with diabetes in the last year?" In response, NLP tools swiftly sift through the data, efficiently providing the information needed to aid clinical decision-making.

Moreover, NLP systems go beyond mere retrieval; they delve into the depths of clinical data to uncover significant trends and patterns. This analytical capability enables healthcare organizations to make informed, data-driven decisions that can improve operational efficiency and patient outcomes. Additionally, researchers benefit immensely from NLP-powered systems, which allow them to quickly extract valuable insights from thousands of medical papers [25]. This functionality accelerates the research process and enriches clinical efficiency by ensuring healthcare providers have timely access to critical information. Ultimately, this innovative approach contributes to enhanced patient care and better health outcomes, marking a significant advancement in healthcare and technology.

NLP plays a pivotal role in pharmacovigilance, which focuses on detecting, assessing, understanding, and preventing adverse effects or any other drug-related problems. Given the enormous amount of unstructured data generated from various sources, including patient medical records, clinical notes, research publications, and post-marketing surveillance, NLP tools have become indispensable for pharmaceutical companies and healthcare practitioners. One of the primary applications of NLP in pharmacovigilance is its ability to sift through extensive patient records to uncover previously unreported adverse events [26, 27]. These events may not be documented in structured fields, leading to significant gaps in safety data. By employing advanced algorithms, NLP systems can automatically identify patterns or mentions of adverse effects in narrative forms, which are often overlooked in traditional data collection methods.

Moreover, NLP is equipped to analyze social media interactions, online forums, and consumer reviews, uncovering public discourse around medications. By monitoring these platforms to discuss side effects, drug recalls, or other safety concerns, NLP can provide early warnings and insights into user experiences that might not otherwise be captured through formal channels. In addition to monitoring and detection, NLP streamlines the reporting process by automating the generation of adverse event reports to be submitted to regulatory authorities, such as the Food and Drug Administration (FDA) in the United States [28]. This automation enhances report generation efficiency and helps ensure compliance with regulatory standards, thus reinforcing patient safety. Integrating NLP into pharmacovigilance systems significantly improves the speed and accuracy of identifying drug-related risks while fostering a safety culture in the healthcare landscape. This innovative approach ultimately contributes to better medication management and informed decision-making among healthcare providers.

NLP is crucial in helping health authorities monitor public health trends and identify potential disease outbreaks by analyzing diverse text-based data sources. NLP systems evaluate news articles, blogs, and social media platforms to detect early indicators of epidemics. Additionally, NLP tools extract pertinent information from epidemiological reports, assisting health officials in tracking the spread of infectious diseases. During the COVID-19 pandemic, these tools were instrumental in monitoring case trends, patient symptoms, and vaccine distribution, enabling governments to respond effectively. This real-time surveillance facilitates quicker responses to health crises, ultimately improving outcomes and reducing public health risks. Precision medicine customizes treatment based on a patient's genetic, clinical, and lifestyle information. NLP is essential in this process, as it extracts valuable insights from various data sources to support personalized care [29]. NLP tools connect relevant clinical data with genomic information to recommend tailored treatments.

Additionally, NLP systems analyze patient-generated health data, such as information from wearable devices, to provide early warnings or interventions. By examining patient histories, NLP can also predict the risk of future complications, allowing clinicians to intervene proactively. Ultimately, by facilitating personalized care, NLP improves patient outcomes, leading to more effective treatments.

Future Trends in NLP for Healthcare

NLP has significantly impacted healthcare by enhancing clinical documentation, decision-making, and patient engagement. However, the rapid evolution of NLP technologies promises even greater potential for improving healthcare outcomes and delivery. Emerging trends, such as conversational agents, multimodal NLP, real-time clinical analytics, and privacy-aware NLP federated learning, can potentially change the future of healthcare. This section looks closely at these trends.

Conversational agents and chatbots powered by NLP are becoming essential components of patient care. These systems provide 24/7 support and can perform various functions, ranging from symptom triage to mental health assistance and answering Frequently Asked Questions (FAQs). As patients increasingly seek convenience and immediate access to healthcare information, chatbots present a scalable solution for patient engagement and the self-management of chronic diseases. By analyzing symptoms, chatbots can guide patients and recommend appropriate actions, such as self-care measures or visiting a physician. This capability is particularly beneficial in alleviating the strain on emergency departments.

Furthermore, chatbots aid patients with chronic conditions, such as diabetes, by reminding them to take their medications, track symptoms, and adhere to lifestyle guidelines. Overall, conversational agents enhance accessibility and continuity of care, especially for populations facing barriers to in-person healthcare services. They also encourage self-management and early intervention, thereby reducing the burden on healthcare providers.

The future of healthcare is evolving toward an integrative approach known as multimodal analysis, where NLP is seamlessly blended with diverse data types. This includes not just textual information but also images, lab reports, and genomic data, all aimed at delivering highly personalized, precise care. In this interconnected framework, advanced NLP tools play a vital role by analyzing unstructured clinical data, like physician notes, alongside structured numerical and visual data from various sources, such as X-rays, MRI scans, and genetic sequences [30]. This powerful combination allows healthcare professionals to gain a comprehensive and nuanced understanding of an individual patient's health status. These NLP systems are adept at extracting valuable insights from narrative radiology reports and imaging studies, providing doctors with a broader and more holistic perspective on patient well-being.

Moreover, by considering a variety of data sources, including patient histories, genetic profiles, and extensive medical records, these tools can recommend highly personalized treatment plans that are fine-tuned to meet each patient's unique needs. Furthermore, data gathered from wearable technology, such as heart rate monitors and sleep trackers, can be integrated with clinical notes to create timely and contextual alerts and predictive insights. By merging various types of information, multimodal NLP significantly enhances the development of targeted care pathways and improves diagnostic accuracy [31]. This innovative approach aligns seamlessly with the principles of precision medicine, ensuring that healthcare interventions are specifically tailored to individual patients' distinct biology and health histories [32].

The capacity to process real-time clinical data revolutionizes how healthcare providers respond to emergencies and monitor patient conditions [33]. NLP systems can analyze streaming data from ICUs, operating rooms, and other clinical environments to identify patterns and generate alerts. This real-time insight empowers providers to take proactive measures before conditions deteriorate, improving patient outcomes. NLP systems examine unstructured data from ICU devices and clinical notes to detect early signs of complications, such as sepsis or respiratory failure. By analyzing lab results, nursing observations, and vital signs, NLP can predict potential emergencies (*e.g.*, cardiac arrests) and alert healthcare teams accordingly. Additionally, NLP tools scrutinize patient records and triage notes to forecast bottlenecks in emergency care, enabling hospitals to allocate resources more efficiently. Real-time clinical analytics enhances patient safety by facilitating early interventions and aiding hospitals in streamlining workflows, ensuring patients receive appropriate care promptly. As these systems advance, they will become increasingly vital in managing high-risk and critical-care patients.

One of the most promising trends in healthcare NLP is federated learning, which enables models to be trained across multiple institutions while safeguarding sensitive patient data. This approach guarantees compliance with healthcare regulations like HIPAA and facilitates collaboration among institutions in AI model development histories. In federated learning, the NLP model is trained locally at each participating institution, with only the model parameters (not the raw patient data) shared with a central server that aggregates updates from all institutions. This decentralized method maintains data privacy, as patient records never leave their host institution. Hospitals can work together to train models on larger datasets without compromising patient privacy, ultimately enhancing model performance. Federated learning allows for creating NLP tools that securely analyze patient data across various healthcare settings, including clinics and telehealth platforms. Federated learning aligns with data privacy regulations like HIPAA and GDPR by ensuring that patient data remains within its originating institution. It unlocks significant potential for large-scale collaboration in healthcare AI without sacrificing patient privacy. It promotes data security while ensuring that NLP tools are trained on diverse datasets, improving their fairness and generalizability.

Challenges in Implementing NLP in Healthcare

NLP has revolutionized healthcare by enabling the analysis of unstructured data, improving patient outcomes, and optimizing workflows. However, implementing NLP in healthcare is not without challenges. These challenges can affect the accuracy, scalability, and adoption of NLP solutions across the healthcare ecosystem. Below is an in-depth discussion of four critical barriers: data privacy and security, interoperability, bias and fairness in models, and domain-specific customization.

The intricate nature of healthcare data presents significant challenges regarding privacy and security, particularly when deploying NLP solutions. Healthcare data encompasses many personal patient information, including detailed medical histories, diagnostic reports, treatment plans, and medication lists. Protecting this sensitive information is critical, as it is governed by stringent regulations such as the Health Insurance Portability and Accountability Act (HIPAA) in the United States and the General Data Protection Regulation (GDPR) in Europe. NLP systems rely on vast datasets drawn from EHRs, clinical notes, and various other medical documents. This reliance on large-scale data introduces multiple potential vulnerabilities. A breach can lead to the exposure of sensitive patient information, which has legal ramifications resulting in hefty fines and penalties, and can also severely undermine patient trust. Healthcare providers often must collaborate with third-party NLP vendors to enhance their data processing capabilities. This collaboration typically necessitates sharing patient data across different platforms and systems, which inherently increases the risk of unauthorized access or data mismanagement. To minimize risks while utilizing NLP, these systems must comply with existing regulations by implementing robust methods for anonymizing patient data before data processing occurs. However, the inherent complexity of clinical language poses challenges in fully de-identifying sensitive information. Unique medical conditions, rare diseases, and specific patient identifiers can sometimes inadvertently remain traceable, risking the re-identification of individuals. One innovative approach to address these privacy concerns is federated learning [34]. This technique allows NLP models to be trained on decentralized data without transferring data to a central server. Keeping the data local to its source reduces the risk of data breaches.

Additionally, employing strong encryption methods for data, both at rest and in transit, further safeguards against potential interception. Encryption ensures that the information remains unreadable and secure if data is intercepted during transfer. Furthermore, establishing role-based access control is essential in managing who can access sensitive patient data [35]. By strictly limiting access to authorized personnel, healthcare organizations can significantly reduce vulnerability exposure and protect patient privacy more effectively. This multi-layered approach to security, comprising regulatory compliance, advanced technologies, and strict access controls, forms a comprehensive strategy to mitigate risks associated with NLP deployments in healthcare settings.

The fragmented nature of healthcare systems poses significant interoperability challenges for implementing NLP. Hospitals, clinics, and healthcare providers utilize various EHR systems, often lacking compatibility. This diversity complicates and prolongs the integration of NLP tools across these systems. EHR systems frequently store information in multiple formats, including free text, coded data, and scanned documents, making it challenging for NLP tools to retrieve and analyze data consistently. NLP solutions must be compatible with various healthcare data standards, such as HL7, Fast Healthcare Interoperability Resources (FHIR), and ICD coding. Ensuring alignment with these standards necessitates customization, which can increase development time and costs.

Additionally, many healthcare providers rely on outdated or legacy EHR systems incompatible with contemporary NLP solutions, limiting their ability to adopt new technologies. Global initiatives to promote standards like FHIR can enhance data consistency across various systems, simplifying the implementation of NLP tools. Application Programming Interfaces (APIs) facilitate interactions between NLP systems and multiple EHR platforms, improving interoperability. Moreover, middleware solutions serve as intermediaries between different healthcare systems, enabling seamless integration of NLP tools with existing infrastructures.

Bias in NLP models poses a significant challenge, particularly within the healthcare sector, where biased algorithms can lead to disparities in treatment outcomes. Often, NLP models are trained on datasets that reflect existing societal or systemic biases, which can disproportionately impact specific patient populations. For instance, a model trained predominantly on English-language data may struggle with non-English-speaking patients or individuals from marginalized communities. Additionally, NLP systems frequently underperform across various demographic groups, resulting in inequities in healthcare. For example, mental health chatbots designed using Western data may find it challenging to interpret the language patterns of users from non-Western backgrounds, potentially leading to misdiagnoses or overlooked interventions. These systems may also miss medical terminology, idioms, or expressions common among non-English speakers or specific ethnic groups, leading to inaccurate analyses. If NLP tools rely on biased medical literature, they may further reflect and perpetuate inequalities within healthcare. Medical research often underrepresents women and minority groups, thereby limiting the effectiveness of NLP models for these populations. NLP models should be developed using datasets encompassing a wide range of languages, dialects, and demographic groups to minimize bias. Furthermore, implementing algorithms to detect and mitigate bias during the model development phase can enhance fairness. Regular performance evaluations of NLP models across diverse patient populations will help identify and address potential biases over time.

Unlike general NLP models designed for typical language tasks, healthcare NLP systems necessitate fine-tuning to comprehend the specific terminology, context, and nuances inherent in clinical data. General-purpose NLP tools may struggle to accurately interpret specialized medical language, including abbreviations, jargon, and diagnostic codes. Clinical notes frequently contain abbreviations (such as "HTN" for hypertension) and specialized terminology that general NLP models often misinterpret. In healthcare, words or phrases can carry different meanings based on context. For instance, the term "discharge" might refer to either a fluid discharge or the release of a patient from a hospital.

Moreover, medical science evolves rapidly, compelling NLP models to be routinely updated with new terminologies, research findings, and clinical guidelines. These models must be trained and refined using domain-specific corpora like clinical notes, EHRs, and medical journals. Models such as ClinicalBERT and BioBERT have been developed for this precise purpose. NLP developers must collaborate closely with healthcare professionals to ensure that these models accurately capture the subtleties of clinical language. Continuous retraining of NLP models with the latest medical knowledge is essential to maintain their relevance and accuracy.

The Role of NLP in Shaping Personalized Medicine

Personalized medicine aims to tailor healthcare interventions to individual patients based on their unique genetic, clinical, and lifestyle data. NLP enables personalized care by extracting insights from vast amounts of unstructured data, such as clinical notes, research articles, and patient-generated data from wearables. By facilitating predictive analytics and integrating with IoT devices,

NLP allows for timely interventions, improved disease management, and precision in treatment. This section explores how NLP shapes personalized medicine through its applications in predictive analytics and the integration of wearables and IoT.

Predictive analytics employs statistical techniques and machine learning models to forecast patient outcomes, identify risks, and suggest personalized treatment options. NLP enhances predictive analytics by extracting valuable insights from unstructured clinical data, such as physician notes and lab reports, as well as from genetic information [36]. This helps healthcare providers deliver more precise and tailored treatments. NLP can analyze genetic data, including information from genome sequencing, to pinpoint biomarkers associated with specific diseases. It also aids in matching patients with targeted therapies based on their molecular profiles.

Additionally, NLP-enabled systems can examine clinical notes, family histories, and research data to predict an individual's risk of developing chronic conditions like diabetes or cardiovascular diseases. This enables healthcare providers to intervene early and implement preventive measures. NLP tools assist in identifying patient cohorts that would benefit most from specific treatments. By analyzing data from clinical trials and medical literature, NLP supports the creation of evidence-based care protocols that align with each patient's unique health profile. Enhanced by NLP, predictive analytics promotes precision medicine, ensuring patients receive the proper treatment at the right time. By recognizing patterns across various datasets, NLP helps healthcare providers predict outcomes more accurately, reducing the trial-and-error approach commonly associated with treatment planning.

The rapid advancement and widespread adoption of wearable devices, alongside the growth of the Internet of Things (IoT) in the healthcare sector, present unprecedented opportunities for delivering personalized patient care. Devices such as smartwatches, continuous glucose monitors, and advanced heart rate sensors continuously generate vast amounts of health-related data. NLP systems can effectively analyze this data stream, allowing healthcare professionals to monitor patient health conditions in real time. The integration of NLP with wearable technology facilitates timely and targeted interventions, particularly for the management of chronic diseases such as diabetes, hypertension, and cardiovascular disorders. These NLP tools can efficiently process and interpret diverse data sets gathered from wearables, including activity logs, sleep patterns, heart rate variability, and glucose levels. By analyzing this data, healthcare providers gain a holistic understanding of an individual’s health status, enabling them to observe trends over time and identify potential areas of concern. For instance, NLP-powered systems can automatically generate alerts in case of abnormal readings, such as an unusually elevated heart rate or irregular glucose levels. These alerts promptly notify healthcare teams, ensuring necessary interventions occur before situations escalate. This proactive approach to health management enhances patient safety and optimizes treatment plans based on real-time data feedback. Moreover, remotely monitoring patients reduces the requirement for frequent in-person visits, thereby increasing patient convenience and allowing healthcare providers to allocate resources more efficiently. Insights drawn from wearable data can be invaluable during virtual consultations, as doctors can offer tailored advice based on empirical evidence rather than relying solely on patient-reported experiences. The seamless integration of NLP with wearables and IoT devices enhances the speed and quality of healthcare interventions and encourages patients to take proactive measures in managing their health. This empowerment leads to more engaged patients likely to adhere to treatment protocols and make lifestyle changes that contribute to improved health outcomes.

In summary, healthcare providers benefit from a richer, more complete picture of each patient's health status, which translates to better disease management, reduced hospital admissions, and improved overall patient care. This innovative convergence of technology heralds a new era in healthcare, where personalized attention and timely interventions become the standard.

The Road Ahead for NLP in Healthcare

The future of NLP in healthcare is poised to bring about transformative changes that can significantly enhance patient care, streamline clinical workflows, and drive advancements in precision medicine. As NLP technologies evolve and mature, their potential to revolutionize various aspects of healthcare becomes increasingly evident. These technologies promise to bolster diagnostic accuracy, improve patient outcomes, and increase operational efficiency across healthcare settings. However, continuous innovation is essential to fully realize NLP's potential in this sector. It will require collaborative efforts across multiple domains, including technology development, clinical practice, and regulatory frameworks. NLP is already vital in key areas such as clinical decision support systems, documentation automation, and initiatives to enhance patient engagement. Looking ahead, we can expect to see the emergence of more sophisticated conversational agents designed to facilitate seamless interactions between patients and healthcare providers, as well as real-time monitoring tools that enable proactive responses to patient needs.

Furthermore, future applications may incorporate multimodal systems that integrate various data types, such as clinical texts with imaging and genomics, producing a more comprehensive view of patient health. The capability of NLP to analyze vast amounts of unstructured data will empower healthcare professionals with actionable insights, enabling quicker diagnoses and more personalized treatment plans tailored to individual patient needs. Despite its promising potential, applying NLP in healthcare is not without challenges. Issues related to bias, data privacy, and interoperability pose significant obstacles to its widespread adoption. Models developed using limited or biased datasets can lead to inaccurate or inequitable healthcare outcomes, particularly affecting underrepresented populations who may not have been adequately included in training data. This raises the urgent need to ensure that data privacy and security measures are robust, given that NLP systems often handle highly sensitive patient information. To address these challenges, ongoing research and innovation are crucial. There is a pressing need for reliable solutions that enhance the accuracy and fairness of NLP systems and protect patient information. Advances in federated learning and privacy-preserving artificial intelligence will be critical for mitigating privacy concerns while allowing for effective data utilization. Building a sustainable future for NLP in the healthcare sector necessitates strong collaboration among various stakeholders, including technology firms, healthcare providers, researchers, and regulatory bodies. These partnerships are vital for aligning AI innovations with healthcare practices' real-world needs and ensuring compliance with regulatory requirements. Developers must work closely with clinicians to design user-friendly tools that cater to their requirements. At the same time, regulators must ensure that the deployment of NLP systems adheres to ethical standards and complies with legal frameworks such as HIPAA and GDPR. Through concerted, collaborative efforts, we can accelerate the adoption of NLP technologies in healthcare, ensuring they serve the best interests of both patients and providers, ultimately leading to a more efficient, equitable, and effective healthcare system.

CONCLUSION

NLP is changing the healthcare sector by using various applications. This technology improves different healthcare areas, such as diagnosis and patient care, and makes the workflow of clinics efficient. As healthcare systems adopt new AI techniques such as transformer models, deep learning, *etc*, they are becoming more capable of providing personalized solutions to patients. However, implementing these new ideas using NLP will also come with challenges. It is important to address data privacy, ethical concerns, bias, *etc*. These problems should be addressed to ensure that the output of these suggested methods will be accurate and valid. Healthcare professionals need to thoroughly understand the changes that can occur when implementing these ideas in the healthcare sector, and they should work together to encourage and enhance innovations. This suggests that the next phase of NLP in healthcare will have a significant impact. It can create a more innovative, patient-focused approach that simplifies complex tasks. This change can lead to an improved and effective healthcare system.

REFERENCES

[1] T. Beaney, S. Jha, A. Alaa, A. Smith, J. Clarke, T. Woodcock, A. Majeed, P. Aylin, and M. Barahona, "Comparing natural language processing representations of coded disease sequences for prediction in electronic health records", *J. Am. Med. Inform. Assoc.,* vol. 31, no. 7, pp. 1451-1462, 2024. [http://dx.doi.org/10.1093/jamia/ocae091] [PMID: 38719204]

[2] V. Digumarthi, T. Amin, S. Kanu, J. Mathew, B. Edwards, L.A. Peterson, M.E. Lundy, and K.E. Hegarty, "Preoperative prediction model for risk of readmission after total joint replacement surgery: a random forest approach leveraging NLP and unfairness mitigation for improved patient care and cost-effectiveness", *J. Orthop. Surg. Res.,* vol. 19, no. 1, p. 287, 2024. [http://dx.doi.org/10.1186/s13018-024-04774-0] [PMID: 38725085]

[3] Y. A. Ali, P. Pathak, N. Dogra, A. M. Potshangbam, S. Tuteja, D. P. Katare, S. D. Bhattacharjee, M. A. Hussain, and R. J. Mani, "Exploring the role of natural learning processing in Alzheimer's disease research and prediction", In: *AI-Driven Alzheimer's Disease Detection and Prediction* 1st. , 2024, pp. 1-14. [http://dx.doi.org/10.1016/B978-0-443-13233-9.00001-4]

[4] S.Y.J. Lee, M. Alzeen, and A. Ahmed, "Estimation of racial and language disparities in pediatric emergency department triage using statistical modeling and natural language processing", *J. Am. Med. Inform. Assoc.,* vol. 31, no. 4, pp. 958-967, 2024. [http://dx.doi.org/10.1093/jamia/ocae018] [PMID: 38349846]

[5] J. Bambi, H. Sadri, K. Moselle, E. Chang, Y. Santoso, J. Howie, A. Rudnick, L.T. Elliott, and A. Kuo, "Approaches to extracting patterns of service utilization for patients with complex conditions: graph community detection *vs.* natural language processing clustering", *BioMedInformatics,* vol. 4, no. 3, pp. 1884-1900, 2024. [http://dx.doi.org/10.3390/biomedinformatics4030103]

[6] A.Y. Landau, Harnessing the power of machine learning and electronic health records to support child abuse and neglect identification in emergency department settings.*Studies in Health Technology and Informatics.,* J. Mantas, A. Hasman, G. Demiris, K. Saranto, M. Marschollek, T.N. Arvanitis, I. Ognjanović, A. Benis, P. Gallos, E. Zoulias, E. Andrikopoulou, Eds., IOS Press, 2024. [http://dx.doi.org/10.3233/SHTI240740]

[7] N. Nazyrova, S. Chahed, T. Chausalet, and M. Dwek, "Leveraging large language models for medical text classification: a hospital readmission prediction case", [http://dx.doi.org/10.1109/ICPRS62101.2024.10677826]

[8] T. Fang, Y. Yang, and L. Zhou, "Enhanced precision in chinese medical text mining using the ALBERT+Bi-LSTM+CRF model", *Appl. Sci. (Basel),* vol. 14, no. 17, p. 7999, 2024. [http://dx.doi.org/10.3390/app14177999]

[9] B. Fonferko-Shadrach, H. Strafford, C. Jones, R.A. Khan, S. Brown, J. Edwards, J. Hawken, L.E. Shrimpton, C.P. White, R. Powell, I.M.S. Sawhney, W.O. Pickrell, and A.S. Lacey, "Annotation of epilepsy clinic letters for natural language processing", *J. Biomed. Semantics,* vol. 15, no. 1, p. 17, 2024. [http://dx.doi.org/10.1186/s13326-024-00316-z] [PMID: 39277770]

[10] T. Manaka, T.V. Zyl, D. Kar, and A. Wade, "Multi-step transfer learning in natural language processing for the health domain", *Neural Process. Lett.,* vol. 56, no. 3, p. 177, 2024.

[http://dx.doi.org/10.1007/s11063-024-11526-y]

[11] S. Chopra, P. Agarwal, J. Ahmed, S.S. Biswas, and A.J. Obaid, "Roberta and BERT: revolutionizing mental healthcare through natural language", *SN Comput. Sci.,* vol. 5, no. 7, p. 889, 2024. [http://dx.doi.org/10.1007/s42979-024-03202-8]

[12] A. Babu, and S.B. Boddu, "BERT-based medical chatbot: enhancing healthcare communication through natural language understanding", *Explor. Res. Clin. Soc. Pharm.,* vol. 13, 2024.100419 [http://dx.doi.org/10.1016/j.rcsop.2024.100419] [PMID: 38495953]

[13] C. Crema, F. Verde, P. Tiraboschi, C. Marra, A. Arighi, S. Fostinelli, G.M. Giuffré, V.P.D. Maschio, F. L'Abbate, F. Solca, B. Poletti, V. Silani, E. Rotondo, V. Borracci, R. Vimercati, V. Crepaldi, E. Inguscio, M. Filippi, F. Caso, A.M. Rosati, D. Quaranta, G. Binetti, I. Pagnoni, M. Morreale, F. Burgio, M. Stanzani-Maserati, S. Capellari, M. Pardini, N. Girtler, F. Piras, F. Piras, S. Lalli, E. Perdixi, G. Lombardi, S.D. Tella, A. Costa, M. Capelli, C. Fundarò, M. Manera, C. Muscio, E. Pellencin, R. Lodi, F. Tagliavini, and A. Redolfi, "Medical information extraction with NLP-powered QABots: a real-world scenario", *IEEE J. Biomed. Health Inform.,* vol. 28, no. 11, pp. 6906-6917, 2024. [http://dx.doi.org/10.1109/JBHI.2024.3450118] [PMID: 39190519]

[14] S. Alghnam, M. Bosaeed, A. Aljouie, S.M. Alshahrani, O. Alshenqeety, R. Atun, and S. Alqahtani, "Estimating the prevalence of select non-communicable diseases in Saudi Arabia using a population-based sample: econometric analysis with natural language processing", *Ann. Saudi Med.,* vol. 44, no. 5, pp. 329-338, 2024. [http://dx.doi.org/10.5144/0256-4947.2024.329] [PMID: 39368120]

[15] M.E. Azzouzi, G. Coatrieux, R. Bellafqira, D. Delamarre, C. Riou, N. Oubenali, S. Cabon, M. Cuggia, and G. Bouzillé, "Automatic de-identification of French electronic health records: a cost-effective approach exploiting distant supervision and deep learning models", *BMC Med. Inform. Decis. Mak.,* vol. 24, no. 1, p. 54, 2024. [http://dx.doi.org/10.1186/s12911-024-02422-5] [PMID: 38365677]

[16] J. Margetta, and A. Sale, "Distinguishing cardiac catheter ablation energy modalities by applying natural language processing to electronic health records", *J. Comp. Eff. Res.,* vol. 13, no. 3, 2024.e230053 [http://dx.doi.org/10.57264/cer-2023-0053] [PMID: 38261335]

[17] E.D. Oikonomou, P. Karvelis, N. Giannakeas, A. Vrachatis, E. Glavas, and A.T. Tzallas, "How natural language processing derived techniques are used on biological data: a systematic review", *Netw. Model. Anal. Health Inform. Bioinform.,* vol. 13, no. 1, p. 23, 2024. [http://dx.doi.org/10.1007/s13721-024-00458-1]

[18] M. Cascella, F. Semeraro, J. Montomoli, V. Bellini, O. Piazza, and E. Bignami, "The breakthrough of large language models release for medical applications: 1-year timeline and perspectives", *J. Med. Syst.,* vol. 48, no. 1, p. 22, 2024. [http://dx.doi.org/10.1007/s10916-024-02045-3] [PMID: 38366043]

[19] F. Sigona, D.P. Radicioni, B. Gili Fivela, D. Colla, M. Delsanto, E. Mensa, A. Bolioli, and P. Vigorelli, "A computational analysis of transcribed speech of people living with dementia: The Anchise 2022 Corpus", *Comput. Speech Lang.,* vol. 89, 2025.101691 [http://dx.doi.org/10.1016/j.csl.2024.101691]

[20] K. Klug, K. Beckh, D. Antweiler, N. Chakraborty, G. Baldini, K. Laue, R. Hosch, F. Nensa, M. Schuler, and S. Giesselbach, "From admission to discharge: a systematic review of clinical natural language processing along the patient journey", *BMC Med. Inform. Decis. Mak.,* vol. 24, no. 1, p. 238, 2024. [http://dx.doi.org/10.1186/s12911-024-02641-w] [PMID: 39210370]

[21] M.T. Mefford, A.P. Ambrosy, R. Wei, C. Zheng, R.V. Parikh, T.N. Harrison, M.S. Lee, A.S. Go, and K. Reynolds, "Rule-based natural language processing to examine variation in worsening heart failure hospitalizations by age, sex, race and ethnicity, and left ventricular ejection fraction", *Am. Heart J.,*

vol. 278, pp. 117-126, 2024.
[http://dx.doi.org/10.1016/j.ahj.2024.09.001] [PMID: 39251103]

[22] G. Huang, Y. Li, S. Jameel, Y. Long, and G. Papanastasiou, "From explainable to interpretable deep learning for natural language processing in healthcare: How far from reality?", *Comput. Struct. Biotechnol. J.,* vol. 24, pp. 362-373, 2024.
[http://dx.doi.org/10.1016/j.csbj.2024.05.004] [PMID: 38800693]

[23] V. Torri, M. Ercolanoni, F. Bortolan, O. Leoni, and F. Ieva, "A NLP-based semi-automatic identification system for delays in follow-up examinations: an Italian case study on clinical referrals", *BMC Med. Inform. Decis. Mak.,* vol. 24, no. 1, p. 107, 2024.
[http://dx.doi.org/10.1186/s12911-024-02506-2] [PMID: 38654295]

[24] Y. Liu, H. Wang, H. Zhou, M. Li, Y. Hou, S. Zhou, F. Wang, R. Hoetzlein, and R. Zhang, "A review of reinforcement learning for natural language processing and applications in healthcare", *J. Am. Med. Inform. Assoc.,* vol. 31, no. 10, pp. 2379-2393, 2024.
[http://dx.doi.org/10.1093/jamia/ocae215] [PMID: 39208319]

[25] X. Ye, X. Wang, and H. Lin, "Global research on pandemics or epidemics and mental health: a natural language processing study", *J. Epidemiol. Glob. Health,* vol. 14, no. 3, pp. 1268-1280, 2024.
[http://dx.doi.org/10.1007/s44197-024-00284-8] [PMID: 39117794]

[26] J.B. Oehm, O. Wenning, M. Storck, X. Jiang, and J. Varghese, "Automatic extraction of medication data from semi-structured prescriptions", In: *Studies in Health Technology and Informatics.,* J. Mantas, A. Hasman, G. Demiris, K. Saranto, M. Marschollek, T.N. Arvanitis, I. Ognjanović, A. Benis, P. Gallos, E. Zoulias, E. Andrikopoulou, Eds., IOS Press, 2024.
[http://dx.doi.org/10.3233/SHTI240749]

[27] B. Probierz and A. Straś, "Automation of the analysis of medical interviews to improve diagnoses using NLP for medicine," in Intelligent Information and Database Systems, N. T. Nguyen et al., Eds., Lecture Notes in Computer Science, vol. 14795. Singapore: Springer, 2024. [Online]. Available: http://dx.doi.org/10.1007/978-981-97-4982-9_10

[28] A. Nayak, and K.S. Raghatate, "Health policy reforms and their effect on healthcare delivery: utilizing Natural Language Processing (NLP) to analyze public sentiment and policy feedback", *S. East. Eur. J. Public Health,* no. Aug, pp. 359-367, 2024.
[http://dx.doi.org/10.70135/seejph.vi.713]

[29] R.F. Xiang, "Use of n-grams and K-means clustering to classify data from free text bone marrow reports", *J. Pathol. Inform.,* vol. 15, 2024.100358
[http://dx.doi.org/10.1016/j.jpi.2023.100358] [PMID: 38292072]

[30] A. Turkmen and O. Can, "Natural language processing for ontology development in IoT-enabled smart healthcare," in Studies on the Semantic Web, A. Carbonaro, S. Tiwari, F. Ortiz-Rodriguez, and V. Janev, Eds. Amsterdam, Netherlands: IOS Press, 2024.
[http://dx.doi.org/10.3233/SSW230027]

[31] J. Hotchkiss, E. Ridderman, and W. Buftin, "Overall US hospice quality according to decedent caregivers—natural language processing and sentiment analysis of 3389 online caregiver reviews", *Am. J. Hosp. Palliat. Care,* vol. 41, no. 5, pp. 527-544, 2024.
[http://dx.doi.org/10.1177/10499091231185593] [PMID: 37338245]

[32] M. Lal, and S. Neduncheliyan, "Enhanced V-Net approach for the emotion recognition and sentiment analysis in the healthcare data", *Multimedia Tools Appl.,* vol. 83, no. 29, pp. 72765-72787, 2024.
[http://dx.doi.org/10.1007/s11042-024-18364-z]

[33] S.D. Goryachev, C. Yildirim, C. DuMontier, J. La, M. Dharne, J.M. Gaziano, M.T. Brophy, N.C. Munshi, J.A. Driver, N.V. Do, and N.R. Fillmore, "Natural language processing algorithm to extract multiple myeloma stage from oncology notes in the veterans affairs healthcare system", *JCO Clin. Cancer Inform.,* vol. 8, no. 8, 2024.e2300197
[http://dx.doi.org/10.1200/CCI.23.00197] [PMID: 39038255]

[34] M.M.A. Cardoso, J. Machado-Rugolo, L. Thabane, N.C. da Rocha, A.M.P. Barbosa, D.S. Komoda, J.T.C. de Almeida, D.S.P. Curado, S.A.T. Weber, and L.G.M. de Andrade, "Application of natural language processing to predict final recommendation of Brazilian health technology assessment reports", *Int. J. Technol. Assess. Health Care,* vol. 40, no. 1, 2024.e19 [http://dx.doi.org/10.1017/S0266462324000163] [PMID: 38605654]

[35] J.I. Park, J.W. Park, K. Zhang, and D. Kim, "Advancing equity in breast cancer care: natural language processing for analysing treatment outcomes in under-represented populations", *BMJ Health Care Inform.,* vol. 31, no. 1, 2024.e100966 [http://dx.doi.org/10.1136/bmjhci-2023-100966] [PMID: 38955389]

[36] O. Aouina, J. Hilbey, and J. Charlet, “SemOntoMap: A hybrid approach for semantic annotation of clinical texts,” in Studies in Health Technology and Informatics, J. Mantas, A. Hasman, G. Demiris, K. Saranto, M. Marschollek, T. N. Arvanitis, I. Ognjanović, A. Benis, P. Gallos, E. Zoulias, and E. Andrikopoulou, Eds. Amsterdam, Netherlands: IOS Press, 2024. [http://dx.doi.org/10.3233/SHTI240789]

SUBJECT INDEX

www.ingramcontent.com/pod-product-compliance
Lightning Source LLC
LaVergne TN
LVHW070945210926
848482LV00002B/104
9798898814946